HEALTHY CHILDREN 2000

*National Health Promotion and
Disease Prevention Objectives
Related to Mothers, Infants,
Children, Adolescents, and Youth*

The Jones and Bartlett Series in Health Sciences

Aquatic Exercise
Sova

Aquatics
Sova

Aquatics Activities Handbook
Sova

Basic Law for the Allied Health Professions
Cowdrey

Basic Nutrition: Self-Instructional Modules, Second Edition
Stanfield

Biological Bases of Human Aging and Disease
Kart/Metress/Metress

The Biology of AIDS, Third Edition
Fan/Conner/Villarreal

The Birth Control Book
Belcastro

Children's Nutrition
Lifshitz

Contemporary Health Issues
Banister/Allen/Fadl/Bhakthan/Howard

Drugs and Society, Third Edition
Witters/Venturelli/Hanson

Essential Medical Terminology
Stanfield

First Aid and CPR
National Safety Council

First Aid and Emergency Care Workbook
Thygerson

Fitness and Health: Life-Style Strategies
Thygerson

Golf: Your Turn for Success
Fisher/Geertsen

Health and Wellness, Fourth Edition
Edlin/Golanty

Healthy People 2000
U.S. Department of Health and Human Services

Healthy People 2000-- Summary Report
U.S. Department of Health and Human Services

Human Anatomy and Physiology Coloring Workbook and Study Guide
Anderson

Interviewing and Helping Skills for Health Professionals
Cormier/Cormier/Weisser

Introduction to Human Disease, Third Edition
Crowley

Introduction to Human Immunology
Huffer/Kanapa/Stevenson

Introduction to the Health Professions
Stanfield

Medical Terminology (with Self-Instructional Modules)
Stanfield/Hui

The Nation's Health, Third Edition
Lee/Estes

Personal Health Choices
Smith/Smith

Principles and Issues in Nutrition
Hui

Sexuality Today
Nass/Fisher

Sports Equipment Management
Walker/Seidler

Step Aerobics
Brown

Teaching Elementary Health Science, Third Edition
Bender/Sorochan

Weight Management the Fitness Way
Dusek

Weight Training for Strength and Fitness
Silvester

Writing a Successful Grant Application
Reif-Lehrer

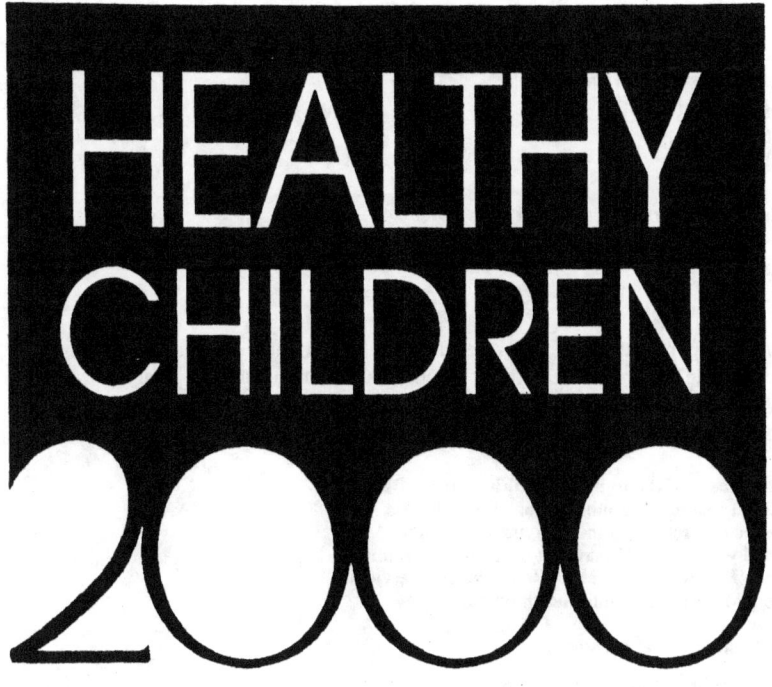

National Health Promotion and Disease Prevention Objectives Related to Mothers, Infants, Children, Adolescents, and Youth

U.S. Department of Health and Human Services
Public Health Service
Health Resources and Service Administration
Maternal and Child Health Bureau

JONES AND BARTLETT PUBLISHERS
BOSTON   LONDON

Editorial, Sales, and Customer Services Offices
Jones and Bartlett Publishers
One Exeter Plaza
Boston, MA 02116

Jones and Bartlett Publishers International
P.O. Box 1498
London W6 7RS
England

All rights reserved. No part of the material protected by this copyright notice may be reproduced or utilized in any form, electronic or mechanical, including photocopying, recording, or by any information storage and retrieval system, without written permission from the copyright owner.

Library of Congress Cataloging-in-Publication Data
Healthy children 2000 : national health promotion and disease
   prevention objectives related to mothers, infants, children,
   adolescents, and youth / U.S. Department of Health and Human
   Services, Public Health Service, Health Resources and Services
   Administration, Maternal and Child Health Bureau.
       p. cm.
     Includes bibliographical references.
     ISBN 978-0-86720-756-9

     1. Children--Health and hygiene--United States. 2. Youth--Health
and hygiene--United States. 3. Mothers--Health and hygiene--United
States. 4. Health promotion--Government policy--United States
5. Health promotion--United States--Planning. 6. Medicine
Preventive--Government policy--United States. 7. Medicine,
Preventive--United States--Planning. I. United States. Public
Health Service. II. United States. Maternal and Child Health
Bureau.
RJ102. H453 1992
362. 1 '9892' 00973--dc20   92-25698
                                                               CIP
Reprinted from the
Department of Health and Human Services.
Publication No. HRSA-M-CH 91-2

Healthy Children 2000 has been adapted from *Healthy People 2000: National Promotion and Disease Prevention Objectives*

Healthy People 2000 *is a statement of national opportunities. Although the Federal Government facilitated its development, it is not intended as a statement of Federal standards or requirements. It is the product of a national effort, involving 22 expert working groups, a consortium that has grown to include almost 300 national organizations and all the State health departments, and the Institute of Medicine of the National Academy of Sciences, which helped the U.S. Public Health Service to manage the consortium, convene regional and national hearings, and receive testimony from more than 750 individuals and organizations. After extensive public review and comment, involving more than 10,000 people, the objectives were revised and refined to produce this report.*

Printed in the United States of America
96 95 94 93 92   10 9 8 7 6 5 4 3 2 1

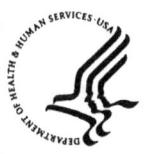

DEPARTMENT OF HEALTH & HUMAN SERVICES   Public Health Service

Office of the Assistant Secretary
for Health
Washington DC 20201

September 10, 1991

Dear Colleague:

Healthy Children 2000 is a special compendium of approximately 170 national health promotion and disease prevention objectives affecting mothers, infants, children, adolescents and youth contained in *Healthy People 2000*, the set of 300 objectives originally published in September, 1990.

That over half of the objectives in *Healthy People 2000* are included in this volume attests to the importance placed on these segments of the population by the consortium of more than 300 public, private and voluntary health agencies and organizations that came together to propose ways and means of improving the health status of Americans over the decade of the 1990s.

A child's health, as well as the health of the adult whom the child subsequently becomes, is profoundly affected by the child's conception, gestation, and birth, and by the nurturing and care the child receives within the family and within the community. The family is the primary unit for the delivery of health services to infants, children, and youth. Our growing recognition of the psychological and social components of health has enhanced our awareness of the family's importance.

The family is not only the principal influence upon a child's development, it is also the intermediary between the child and the outside world, including the health care system. Children benefit from a family-centered approach to care, an approach where the providers and systems are sensitive to this central role of families.

It is essential to provide community supports for the family, including a safe environment within which families and children can develop, and appropriate community-based services organized into a rational system. It is hoped that the strategies suggested in this volume will assist communities to meet their responsibilities.

Healthy Children 2000 is intended for use by policy makers and program managers across the country, by care providers in the public and private sectors, and by all who advocate and have a concern for child health interests. They must collaborate with each other and with the families and children themselves in order to achieve these ambitious health objectives.

Since the future of our Nation is so closely tied to the health of our children, we must make every effort to realize the promise of *Healthy Children 2000*. I commit the Public Health Service to work with you toward achievement of these objectives in the coming decade.

James O. Mason
James O. Mason, M.D., Dr.P.H.
Assistant Secretary for Health

Contents

Introduction	1
1. Physical Activity and Fitness	9
2. Nutrition	17
3. Tobacco	31
4. Alcohol and Other Drugs	47
5. Family Planning	59
6. Mental Health and Mental Disorders	73
7. Violent and Abusive Behavior	81
8. Educational and Community-Based Programs	97
9. Unintentional Injuries	105
10. Occupational Safety and Health	*
11. Environmental Health	121
12. Food and Drug Safety	*
13. Oral Health	129
14. Maternal and Infant Health	137
15. Heart Disease and Stroke	*
16. Cancer	157
17. Diabetes and Chronic Disabling Conditions	165
18. HIV Infection	181
19. Sexually Transmitted Diseases	191
20. Immunization and Infectious Diseases	203
21. Clinical Preventive Services	213
22. Surveillance and Data Systems	*
References	223

* *Priority area chapters marked with an asterisk appear in* Healthy People 2000, *but not in this document. They are listed here only to provide a complete priority area list. Other sections of* Healthy People 2000 *that have been omitted are not listed here.*

Introduction

Introduction*

The year 2000 appears ahead on the calendar of our Nation's history as a turning point. It may well be like any other year in the ongoing lives of people who inhabit this country and the world. But from the perspective of history, the year 2000 will bring to its conclusion a tumultuous century, characterized by astounding scientific achievements, devastating world wars, and explosive population growth. It will inaugurate at once a new century and a new millennium, a future so vast in its human and historic dimensions that it defies prediction while posing momentous questions about social and economic viability and human vitality in the face of a new era.

The year 2000 connotes change. Its arrival contains enough power to shape that change, motivating actions that can improve American lives. The beginning of the twenty-first century beckons both with challenge and opportunity for improved health of Americans.

Healthy People 2000 offers a vision for the new century, characterized by significant reductions in preventable death and disability, enhanced quality of life, and greatly reduced disparities in the health status of populations within our society. It is the product of a national effort, involving professionals and citizens, private organizations and public agencies from every part of the country.

This report does not reflect the policies or opinions of any one organization, including the Federal Government, or any one individual. It is the product of a national process. It is deliberately comprehensive in addressing health promotion and disease prevention opportunities in order to allow local communities and States to choose from among its recommendations in addressing their own highest priority needs.

During the 1980s, there were major declines in death rates for three of the leading causes of death among Americans: heart disease, stroke, and unintentional injuries. Infant mortality also decreased, and some childhood infectious diseases were nearly eliminated. Gains in these areas give hope that the 1990s will see more progress, especially for diseases that have so far not declined.

Unintentional injuries have declined. In the last decade and a half, traffic fatalities dropped by one-third, partly reflecting increased use of seatbelts, lower speed limits, and declines in alcohol abuse.

Progress has been made in the health status of children as well. In 1987, we achieved a record low rate of 10.1 infant deaths per 1,000 live births. Although still higher than rates in many other developed countries, this figure represents a 65-percent decline since 1950. Preventable childhood diseases, such as mumps, measles, and rubella, are now unusual in this country due to widespread use of vaccines. Immunization levels among school children exceed 95 percent for most of these diseases.

Changing trends point to still other areas that require attention. In the past decade, rising rates of syphilis and the emergence of HIV infection point to the need for new strategies to address these public health problems.... Among the 15 priority areas that were the focus of the 1990 objectives, areas in which progress seemed to lag included pregnancy and infant health, nutrition, physical fitness and exercise, family planning, [and] sexually

---

* *The text of this introduction has been excerpted from various sections of* Healthy People 2000: National Health Promotion and Disease Prevention Objectives, *including chapters 1 through 6 of Part I and introductions to pertinent chapters of Part II. Within this document, omissions within paragraphs are marked with ellipses; in the interest of readability in this greatly condensed introduction, omissions of one or more complete paragraphs are not marked. Throughout the rest of this volume, omissions between paragraphs are marked with a line of asterisks. Also, editorial interpolations are contained with brackets.*

transmitted diseases. . . . On the other hand, priority areas related to high blood pressure control, immunization, control of infectious diseases, unintentional injury prevention and control, smoking, and alcohol and drugs showed substantial progress.

The Nation's Health: Age Groups

Responding effectively to the health challenges of the 1990s will require a clear understanding of the health-related threats and opportunities facing all Americans. One way to grasp the dimensions and the realities of the tasks laid out in this report is to consider the special problems of infants, children, adolescents and young adults, adults, and older adults. The health profiles of these age groups can help us remember that the improvements envisioned here are not generalizations about the population, but prescriptions for healthier lives for each of us—newborn babies, boys and girls, teenagers and young people, women and men, and people in their later years.

Maternal and Infant Health

One of the most heartening indicators of our Nation's improvement in health during the 20th century has been the steady decline in the infant mortality rate. Between 1950 and 1987, the infant mortality rate in the United States dropped from 29.2 per 1,000 live births to 10.1. Eight years after *Healthy People* (1979) posed the challenge of a 35-percent reduction in infant mortality by 1990, we had achieved a reduction of 28 percent in that rate.

Yet comparison of even our 1987 rate with that of other industrialized nations demonstrates the continued importance of efforts in this regard. Moreover, the continuing disparities between minority and majority populations represent a major health challenge. In 1987, the mortality rate for black infants was still over twice that of whites, and rates for some American Indian tribes and for Puerto Ricans were also considerably higher than for white infants.

Improving the health of mothers and infants is a national challenge.

Women who receive prenatal care in the first trimester have better health and have better pregnancy outcomes than women who receive little or no prenatal care. Prenatal care should include three basic components: (1) early and continuing risk assessment; (2) health promotion; and (3) medical, nutritional, and psychosocial interventions and followup.

Approximately one-half of pregnancies in the United States are unintended, either mistimed or unwanted; unintended pregnancy is associated with low birth weight and infant death. The United States' high unintended pregnancy rate may be due to lack of knowledge among sexually active people, failure to translate knowledge into behavior, or lack of family planning services and information.

To achieve further reductions in infant mortality and morbidity, health care providers and individuals must focus on modifying the behaviors and lifestyles that affect birth outcomes. Couples who wish to have children need to know more about reproduction, contraception, and the importance of reducing risks before pregnancy. For example, they should receive comprehensive risk assessments that identify health problems or unhealthy behaviors that are best addressed before pregnancy, such as smoking, substance abuse, poor nutrition, family/genetic history, medical problems and chronic illness, psychosocial problems, and short pregnancy interval.

Very low birth weight (less than 1,500 grams) is associated with 40 percent of all infant deaths. Very low birth weight declined slightly from 1970 to 1981 but rose by about 0.9 percent per year from 1981 to 1986. Low-birth-weight babies are nearly twice as likely to have severe developmental delay or congenital anomalies. These babies are also at a significantly greater risk of such long-term disabilities as cerebral palsy, autism, mental retardation, and vision and hearing impairments, and other developmental disabilities.

Increasing rates of HIV infection and cocaine addiction in newborns are also of concern. By January 1990, more than 2,000 babies had been born with HIV infection, and some hospitals from urban communities reported rates of cocaine-addicted babies as high as 20 percent. The long term consequences of these alarming trends are inestimable.

Infant mortality rates provide a summary measure of the effects of major health threats to the developing fetus and newborn baby. But for every 10 babies who die, 990 live. Some of those who live have been harmed, often permanently, by unhealthy beginnings. The quality, not just the quantity, of their lives is a function of health during both the prenatal and infant periods.

Significant reduction of the infant mortality rate and the elimination of racial and ethnic differences in pregnancy outcome will not occur through simple continuation of current effort. A national, State, and local commitment to improving birth outcomes and maintaining healthy infants is imperative. Affecting infant mortality rates requires the removal of financial, educational, social, and logistic barriers to care. Part of the national effort to reduce infant mortality must be assuring that health services are received by those who need them.

Children

Childhood is a critical time for healthy human development. Not only are children dependent on other individuals for their food, clothing and protection, but they are influenced by the behavioral patterns that they witness. The vulnerability of children places them at special risk for preventable problems including unintentional injuries, homicide, child abuse and neglect, and lead poisoning. They are also at risk for developmental problems, which can affect them throughout their lives.

The health profile of American children has shifted markedly in the past 40 years. Once dominated by the threat of major infectious diseases, such as polio, diphtheria, scarlet fever, pneumonia, measles, and whooping cough, today, widespread immunization has virtually eliminated many of these diseases. Others are in steep decline.

Between 1977 and 1987, the rate of childhood deaths declined 21 percent, exceeding the 1990 target set in *Healthy People*. Replacing infectious diseases are injury-related morbidity and mortality. Unintentional injuries are currently the leading cause of death in childhood. Nearly half of all childhood deaths are unintentional injuries, and about half of these are due to motor vehicle accidents. Unintentional injuries are preventable, and the rates of childhood deaths in motor vehicle crashes have decreased substantially as a result of prevention strategies of the last decade. These include an increased use of child safety seats, safer automobile design and reduced speed limits. Other causes of injury-related deaths among children—drowning, falls, poisoning, fires—have also declined as a result of improved protections, with the sole exception of child homicide.

Violence toward children has become of increasing concern as an American health issue, with rapidly rising rates of reported cases of child deaths due to violence. The periodic Study of National Incidence of Child Abuse and Neglect estimated that, in 1986, nearly 2 percent of children—or more than 1,000,000—were demonstrably harmed by abuse or neglect. The most common kind of abuse identified was physical, followed by emotional and sexual; the most common kind of neglect was educational, followed by physical and emotional. Substantial increases in reported physical and sexual abuse cases have occurred since 1980, but the 1986 study concluded that this was due more to improved reporting, reflecting greater public and professional awareness of the problem, than to an actual increase in child abuse. On the other hand, the study also demonstrated that many incidents of child maltreatment still go unreported.

Psychological, emotional, and learning disorders are on the rise among children, as are chronic physical conditions such as hearing and speech impairment. Low-income children are at a significantly higher risk for such problems.

Children in families with incomes below $5,000 per year had an average of 9.1 disability days in 1980 compared to only 4 days for children in families with incomes of $25,000 or more.

An accurate profile of the health of U.S. children, therefore, must go beyond mortality and morbidity data. It must also consider emotional, psychological, and learning problems, the social and environmental risks to which they are related, and the total costs to the Nation.

Improving the health of American children requires a wide range of social and economic interventions. For example, more and better preschool education for disadvantaged children and children with disabilities could help to detect and prevent developmental problems. Educational and support programs for parents in high-risk environments hold promise for reducing child abuse and other health problems, such as lead poisoning. The complex developmental problems besetting children in these environments demand concerted efforts by many different sectors of society. Primary care health providers, social service professionals, health educators, housing officials, community groups, and concerned individuals can each make a difference in the health of American children.

Adolescents and Young Adults

The years from 15 through 24 are a time of changing health hazards. Caught up in change and experimentation, young people also develop behaviors that may become permanent. Attitudes and patterns related to diet, physical activity, tobacco use, safety, and sexual behavior may persist from adolescence into adulthood.

The dominant preventable health problems of adolescents and young adults fall into two major categories: injuries and violence that kill and disable many before they reach age 25 and emerging lifestyles that affect their health many years later.... Thus, particular attention should be given to prevention of motor vehicle crash injuries, assault, homicide, and suicide. To improve chances of a healthy adulthood, emphasis also should be placed on reducing tobacco, alcohol, drug abuse, and improving nutrition.

From 1977 to 1987, the death rate among people aged 15 through 24 declined 14 percent. The leading causes of death among adolescents and young adults include injuries, homicide, suicide, cancer, and heart disease. Deaths due to cancer and heart disease have declined dramatically among adolescents since the 1950s, and although they are still among the leading causes of death in this age group, they are overshadowed by deaths caused by unintentional injuries, homicide, and suicide.

Unintentional injuries account for about half of all deaths among people aged 15 to 24; three-quarters of these deaths involve motor vehicles. More than half of all fatal motor vehicle crashes among people in this age group involve alcohol. Young white men had the highest death rates for motor vehicle crashes in 1987, at 59 per 100,000. The rate for young black men was much lower: 36 per 100,000. The rate was lower yet for women of both races.

Motor vehicle crash deaths decreased in this age group in the early 1980s, possible because of the raised minimum drinking age in many States and decreasing alcohol use. The recent trend, however, is upward. The raised speed limit on rural interstate highways may be a factor in this trend. Further, nearly 60 percent of 8th and 10th graders reported not using seatbelts on their most recent ride.

Homicide is the second leading cause of death among all adolescents and young adults, and it is the number one cause among black youth. The homicide rate for young black men increased by 40 percent between 1984 and 1987 to nearly 86 per 100,000, more than 7 times the rate for young white men. Race, however, appears not to be as important a risk factor for violent death as socioeconomic status. Racial differences in homicide rates are significantly reduced when socioeconomic factors are taken into account. As with motor vehicle accidents, about half of all homicides are associated with alcohol use. Nationwide, 10 percent are drug-related, but in many cities this rate is substantially higher. Over half of all homicide victims are relatives or acquaintances of the perpetrators. Most are killed with firearms.

Suicide is the second leading cause of death among young white men aged 15 to 24, and rates continue to climb. From 1950 to 1987 the death rate from suicide in this group increased from under 7 to about 23 per 100,000 population. The rate of suicides among black adolescents and young adults is half of that among whites. White men between 20 and 24 years of age are more likely to commit suicide than their counterparts aged 15 through 19, but the gap between these two groups is narrowing. In general, suicides have decreased among older youth and increased among the younger cohort.

Both white and black young women have relatively low suicide rates (4.7 and 2.3 respectively in 1987), although young women attempt suicide unsuccessfully approximately three times more often than young men. As is the case with homicides, 60 percent of suicides among adolescents and young adults are committed with firearms.

Many of the most important risk factors for chronic disease in later years also have their roots in youthful behavior. The earlier cigarette smoking begins, for example, the less likely the smoker is to quit.

The use of snuff and chewing tobacco has increased dramatically in recent years among teenage boys. Between 1970 and 1986, snuff use increased fifteen-fold and chewing tobacco use increased fourfold among young men aged 17 through 19. In 1987, the prevalence of smokeless tobacco use among young men aged 18 through 24 was nearly 9 percent. Among younger adolescent boys aged 12 through 17, nearly 7 percent had used some form of smokeless tobacco within the last month.

The use of alcohol and illicit drugs by adolescents and young adults has been declining and awareness of the dangers of drinking and taking drugs has grown among high school seniors. However, among those aged 18 through 24, drinking is more prevalent than in any other age group. Alcohol use and experimentation with illicit drugs starts early.

Although the average age of first use of alcohol and marijuana is 13, pressure to begin use starts at even younger ages.

Sexual activity among teenagers poses special risks including unwanted pregnancy and sexually transmitted diseases, including HIV infection. Unintended pregnancies among teenagers can adversely affect the well-being of teenage girls and their babies. Rates of sexually transmitted diseases, such as gonorrhea and syphilis, are highest among people aged 15 through 29.

Although the 1980s brought some improvements in the health status of adolescents and young adults, many other young people still must face a constellation of problems, including alcohol and other drug abuse, school failure, delinquency, peer group violence, and unwanted pregnancy. While education about risks to health is important, programs for adolescents and young adults must go beyond education to include in-depth counseling and support. Especially for youth in high-risk environments, comprehensive programs are needed to provide positive alternatives to alcohol and other drug abuse, teenage pregnancy, and lifestyles conducive to violence. Also important are programs that can reach school dropouts, who may have the highest risks of all.

Healthy People 2000: The Challenge and Goals

The Nation has within its power the ability to save many lives lost prematurely and needlessly. Implementation of what is already known about promoting health and preventing disease is the central challenge of *Healthy People 2000*.

But *Healthy People 2000* also challenges the Nation to move beyond merely saving lives. The health of a people is measured by more than death rates. Good health comes from reducing unnecessary suffering, illness, and disability. It comes as well from an improved quality of life. Health is thus best measured by citizens' sense of well-being. The health of a Nation is measured by the extent to which the gains are accomplished for all the people.... The purpose of *Healthy People 2000* is to commit the Nation to the attainment of three broad goals that will help bring us to our full potential, [namely to:]

- Increase the span of healthy life for Americans
- Reduce health disparities among Americans
- Achieve access to preventive services for all Americans

The challenge of *Healthy People 2000* is to use the combined strength of scientific knowledge, professional skill, individual commitment, community support, and political will to enable people to achieve their potential to live full, active lives. It means preventing premature death and preventing disability, preserving a physical environment that supports human life, cultivating family and community support, enhancing each individual's inherent abilities to respond and to act, and assuring that all Americans achieve and maintain a maximum level of functioning.

We have a broad array of opportunities to achieve our goals.... *Healthy People 2000* uses the three approaches of health promotion, health protection, and preventive services as organizing categories, but running through the priority areas and the objectives is a common theme of shared responsibility for carrying out this national agenda. Achievement of the agenda depends heavily on changes in individual behaviors. It requires use of legislation, regulation, and social sanctions to make the social and physical environment a healthier place to live. It calls on medical and health professionals to prevent, not just to treat, the diseases and conditions that result in premature death and chronic disability. All are necessary. None is sufficient alone to achieve *Healthy People 2000*'s goals and objectives.

The challenge spelled out in *Healthy People 2000* calls upon communities to translate national objectives into State and local action. [This volume] offers community implementation strategies for putting the objectives of *Healthy People 2000* into practice and encourages communities to establish achievable community health targets.

Physical Activity and Fitness

1

Contents

* * *

1.3	Moderate physical activity
1.4	Vigorous physical activity
1.5	Sedentary lifestyle
1.6	Muscular strength, endurance, and flexibility
1.7	Weight loss practices
1.8	Daily school physical education
1.9	School physical education quality

* * *

[Research Needs]

1. Physical Activity and Fitness

* * *

Risk Reduction Objectives

1.3*   Increase to at least 30 percent the proportion of people aged 6 and older who engage regularly, preferably daily, in light to moderate physical activity for at least 30 minutes per day. (Baseline: 22 percent of people aged 18 and older were active for at least 30 minutes 5 or more times per week and 12 percent were active 7 or more times per week in 1985)

Note: Light to moderate physical activity requires sustained, rhythmic muscular movements, is at least equivalent to sustained walking, and is performed at less than 60 percent of maximum heart rate for age. Maximum heart rate equals roughly 220 beats per minute minus age. Examples may include walking, swimming, cycling, dancing, gardening and yardwork, various domestic and occupational activities, and games and other childhood pursuits.

Baseline data source: Behavioral Risk Factor Surveillance System, CDC.

Physical activity is defined as any bodily movement produced by skeletal muscles that results in caloric expenditure.[1] Caloric expenditure utilizes energy. Energy utilization enhances weight loss or control and is important in preventing and managing obesity, coronary heart disease, and diabetes mellitus. Engaging regularly in light to moderate physical activity for at least 30 minutes per day will help to ensure that calories are expended and confer health benefits.[2,3] For example, daily physical activity equivalent to a sustained walk for 30 minutes per day would result in an energy expenditure of about 1050 Calories per week (1.5 miles X 100 kcal per mile X 7 days per week = 1050 kcal per week). If caloric intake remains constant, this would translate into a weight loss of roughly one-third pound per week. Furthermore, epidemiologic studies suggest that a weekly expenditure of 1000 Calories could have significant individual and public health benefit for coronary heart disease prevention, especially for those who are originally sedentary.[4]

A minimum level of intensity for light to moderate physical activity is set by the example of a sustained walk. This level of activity is feasible for most people. Those willing and able can perform even more vigorous types of physical activity for the purpose of improving and/or maintaining cardiorespiratory fitness (see Objective 1.4). However, light to moderate activities confer considerable health benefit, are more likely to be adopted and maintained than intense activities, and are less likely to result in injury.[5]

Although light to moderate physical activity for a sustained period of at least 30 minutes is preferable, intermittent physical activity also increases caloric expenditure and may be important for those who cannot fit 30 minutes of sustained activity into their schedules. The point is to encourage physical activity as part of a daily routine. People engaging in light to moderate physical activity less often than daily also receive health benefits, but if the frequency falls below three days per week, they may be less likely to maintain a regular pattern of activity over time.[6]

Most Americans engage in less physical activity than is proposed by this objective. Currently only 22 percent of people aged 18 and older engage in at least 30 minutes of activity 5 or more times per week and only 12 percent report that they are this active 7 or more times per week. Similar rates prevail for older adults and low-income individuals.

Increasing public awareness about the many benefits of light to moderate physical activity could help to attain this objective. For example, Americans need to recognize the importance of daily physical activity to weight management, to know that walking is a form of exercise most people can do, and to understand that one needs to remain active throughout life. It is also important for people to realize that starting out slowly, and gradually increasing the frequency and duration of their physical activity over time is the key to successful behavior change.[7] In the case of walking, the message becomes "if you are not used to daily walking, then walk slowly and take short, frequent walks, gradually increasing distance and speed." Educational messages should be appropriately tailored to reach older adults, people with disabilities, and racial and ethnic minorities.

For young children, attaining this objective will require public awareness messages targeted to parents. Parents should be encouraged to exercise with their children (e.g., daily family walks), to advocate for daily school physical education (see Objective 1.8), and to involve their children in the physical activity programs of community organizations.

*This objective also appears as Objective 15.11 in *Heart Disease and Stroke* and as Objective 17.13 in *Diabetes and Chronic Disabling Conditions*.

1.4 **Increase to at least 20 percent the proportion of people aged 18 and older and to at least 75 percent the proportion of children and adolescents aged 6 through 17 who engage in vigorous physical activity that promotes the development and maintenance of cardiorespiratory fitness 3 or more days per week for 20 or more minutes per occasion. (Baseline: 12 percent for people aged 18 and older in 1985; 66 percent for youth aged 10 through 17 in 1984)**

Special Population Target

Vigorous Physical Activity	1985 Baseline	2000 Target
1.4a Lower-income people aged 18 and older (annual family income <$20,000)	7%	12%

Note: Vigorous physical activities are rhythmic, repetitive physical activities that use large muscle groups at 60 percent or more of maximum heart rate for age. An exercise heart rate of 60 percent of maximum heart rate for age is about 50 percent of maximal cardiorespiratory capacity and is sufficient for cardiorespiratory conditioning. Maximum heart rate equals roughly 220 beats per minute minus age.

Baseline data sources: For people aged 18 and older, the National Health Interview Survey, CDC; for youth aged 10 through 17, the National Children and Youth Fitness Study I, ODPHP.

Regular vigorous physical activity helps achieve and maintain higher levels of cardiorespiratory fitness than light to moderate physical activity. Cardiorespiratory fitness or aerobic capacity describes the body's ability to perform high intensity activity for a prolonged period of time without undue stress or fatigue. Having higher levels of cardiorespiratory fitness helps enable people to carry out their daily occupational tasks and leisure pursuits more easily.

The vigorous physical activities that help to achieve and maintain cardiorespiratory fitness can also contribute substantially to caloric expenditure, and probably provide additional protection against coronary heart disease over less vigorous forms of regular physical activity.[8,9] Vigorous physical activities include brisk walking, jogging/running, lap swimming, cycling, dancing, skating, rowing, jumping rope, cross-country skiing, hiking/backpacking, racquet sports, and competitive group sports (soccer, basketball, volleyball). Activities such as stair climbing; strenuous housework, yardwork, and occupational tasks; and children's games (tag, kickball) and other childhood pursuits may also qualify as vigorous activities if they are sustained and elevate the heart rate to at least 60 percent of the maximum heart rate for age.

Higher levels of cardiorespiratory fitness can be achieved by increasing the frequency, duration, or intensity of activity over that suggested in this objective (i.e., more than three times per week or more than 20 minutes per session or at a higher intensity), but the relationship is not linear. Progressively larger increases in frequency, duration, or intensity are needed to induce a steady increase in cardiorespiratory fitness. The frequency of musculoskeletal injury also rises with more frequent, prolonged, and intense activity.[5]

This objective is designed to encourage vigorous physical activity participation for at least three times per week. Unfortunately, those that meet the minimal frequency and duration proposed in this objective may secure a strong cardiorespiratory system, but they may not achieve the weight control or physiologic benefits secured by daily activity (see Objective 1.3). On the other hand, daily vigorous physical activity performed for 30 minutes per day will surely provide daily energy expenditure, but there is also an increased injury risk.[5] Therefore, vigorous physical activity should be incorporated into the daily activity pattern proposed in Objective 1.3 in a manner that will not result in injury.

Monitoring progress toward this objective must take into account the decline in maximal cardiorespiratory capacity with age.[10] A method for this has been developed and used in surveys that obtain information about physical activities performed without measuring pulse rates.[11]

1.5 Reduce to no more than 15 percent the proportion of people aged 6 and older who engage in no leisure-time physical activity. (Baseline: 24 percent for people aged 18 and older in 1985)

Special Population Targets

No Leisure-Time Physical Activity	1985 Baseline	2000 Target
1.5b People with disabilities	35%†	20%
1.5c Lower-income people (annual family income <$20,000)	32%†	17%

†Baseline for people aged 18 and older

Note: *For this objective, people with disabilities are people who report any limitation in activity due to chronic conditions.*

Baseline data source: National Health Interview Survey, CDC.

Although the protective effect of a more active lifestyle is seen for both occupational and leisure-time physical activity, the amount of physical activity at work and in the home has declined steadily. For most people, the greatest opportunity for physical activity is during leisure. Unfortunately, 24 percent of men and women aged 18 and older report no leisure-time physical activity. The prevalence of leisure-time sedentarism increases with advancing age—33 percent of people aged 45 through 64 and 43 percent of those aged 65 and older engage in no leisure-time physical activity.[12] People with disabilities and lower-income individuals are also more likely to be sedentary at leisure.

It is important for those who are sedentary during their leisure-time to take the first step towards developing a pattern of regular physical activity. Public education efforts need to address the specific barriers that inhibit the adoption of physical activity by different population groups. Older adults, for example, need information about safe walking routes, appropriate foot care and footwear for those with foot problems, appropriate levels of activity for those with coronary heart disease and other chronic conditions, and the availability of group activities in the community.

1.6 **Increase to at least 40 percent the proportion of people aged 6 and older who regularly perform physical activities that enhance and maintain muscular strength, muscular endurance, and flexibility. (Baseline data available in 1991)**

Muscular strength, muscular endurance, and joint flexibility are accepted components of health-related fitness although the type, frequency, duration, and intensity of activities necessary for specific age and gender groups remains to be determined. Regular participation in home maintenance, yardwork, gardening, and selected occupational activities may satisfy this objective in adults. Participation in games and other active childhood pursuits may satisfy this objective in children. Satisfying this objective may require combinations of activities as not all activities will both increase muscular strength and endurance and enhance flexibility.

Muscular strength and endurance describe the ability of skeletal muscles to perform hard and/or prolonged work. Strength and endurance greatly affect the ability to perform the tasks of daily living without undue physical stress and fatigue. Regular use of skeletal muscles helps to improve and maintain strength and endurance.[13,14] Engaging in regular physical activity and engaging in a variety of physical activities can help to satisfy this objective. Although weight training (exercising with free weights or weight machines) can increase muscle strength and endurance, weight training is not necessary to meet this objective and may not be appropriate for all age groups and individuals.[15]

Flexibility describes the range of motion in a joint or sequence of joints. Those with greater flexibility may have a lower risk of future back injury.[16]... Joint movement through the full range of motion helps to improve and maintain flexibility. Stretching exercises and engaging regularly in a variety of physical activities may help to satisfy this objective.

Physical activities that improve muscular strength, muscular endurance, and flexibility also improve the ability to perform tasks of daily living.... Increasing the public's awareness of all of these potential benefits may help to encourage the pursuit of activities that will promote muscular strength, muscular endurance, and flexibility.

1.7* **Increase to at least 50 percent the proportion of overweight people aged 12 and older who have adopted sound dietary practices combined with regular physical activity to attain an appropriate body weight. (Baseline: 30 percent of overweight women and 25 percent of overweight men for people aged 18 and older in 1985)**

Baseline data source: National Health Interview Survey, CDC.

Overweight occurs when too few calories are expended and too many consumed for individual metabolic requirements.[17] The results of weight loss programs focused on dietary restrictions alone have not been encouraging. Physical activity burns calories, increases the proportion of lean to fat body mass, and raises the metabolic rate.[18] Therefore, a combination of both caloric control and increased physical activity is important for attaining a healthy body weight.[19]

Neither frequent fluctuations in body weight nor extreme restrictions in food intake are desirable. Overweight people should increase their physical activity and should avoid calorie-dense foods, especially those high in fat. Diets that are lower in fat and higher in vegetables, fruits, and grains can facilitate weight reduction. Extremely low-calorie diets, cyclic weight reduction, and fad weight-loss regimes of unscientific merit should be avoided. Practices should be adopted that are safe and that lead to long-term maintenance of appropriate weight. Extreme behaviors as exhibited in bulimia or anorexia nervosa should be medically treated.

Self-help groups and programs that apply the principles of behavior modification (e.g., goal setting, self-monitoring, stimulus control, reinforcement) may help overweight individuals to sustain the physical activity and dietary practices needed to reach an appropriate body weight.

The target for this objective is very ambitious, but given the potential health benefits of weight loss in the overweight person, this objective deserves special priority. Attaining this objective will help to reduce the prevalence of overweight in the total population (see Objective 1.2). The prevention of overweight among those not yet overweight is also vitally important. Objectives 1.3, 1.4, and 1.5 in this priority area and Objectives 2.5 and 2.6 in *Nutrition* address the primary prevention of obesity.

*This objective also appears as Objective 2.7 in *Nutrition*.

Services and Protection Objectives

1.8   Increase to at least 50 percent the proportion of children and adolescents in 1st through 12th grade who participate in daily school physical education. (Baseline: 36 percent in 1984-86)

Baseline data sources: For students in 5th through 12th grade, the National Children and Youth Fitness Study I, ODPHP; for students in 1st through 4th grade, the National Children and Youth Fitness Study II, ODPHP.

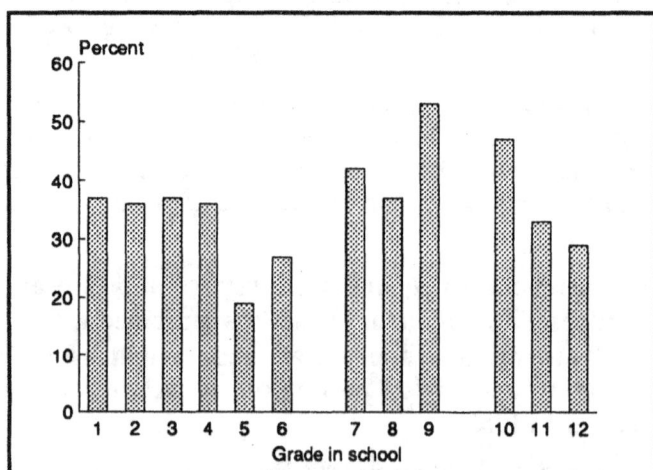

Fig. 1.8

Percentage of students in 1st through 12th grade receiving daily school physical education in 1984-86

Participation in school physical education assures a minimum amount of physical activity for children. Presumably it also encourages extracurricular physical activity by children and continued physical activity into adulthood. Findings from the National Children and Youth Fitness Studies I and II suggest that the quantity, and in particular the quality, of school physical education programs have a significant positive effect on the health-related fitness of children and youth.[20,21] In addition, recent reports suggest that physical education programs in early childhood not only promote health and well-being, but also contribute to academic achievement.[22]

Concern about the amount and quality of youth physical activity and school physical education has been expressed by several groups, including the American Academy of Pediatrics and the American College of Sports Medicine. In 1987, both houses of Congress passed a resolution (H. Con. Res. 97) encouraging State and local educational agencies to provide high quality daily physical education programs for all children in kindergarten through 12th grade. Only one State, Illinois, currently requires daily physical education as part of the curriculum in kindergarten through 12th grade.

Although quantity is not synonymous with quality (see Objective 1.9), the proportion of students receiving daily physical education in school is one measure of the frequency of participation in physical activity and the frequency of exposure to information about how and why to partake in activity. Because time spent engaged in regular, vigorous, and prolonged physical activity outside of school physical education falls off sharply during the fall and winter months, daily school physical education programs can play an important role in helping children and youth maintain a high level of physical activity year-round.

In 1974-75, it was estimated that roughly one-third of students in 5th through 12th grade received physical education daily. As of 1984, the situation had changed little, with only 36 percent of students in 5th through 12th grade receiving physical education daily.[20] In 1986, only 36 percent of students in 1st through 4th grade received daily physical education.[21]

Most children in the lower grades are enrolled in school physical education but many receive it fewer than 5 days per week. In the upper grades, fewer children are enrolled but those who are more often participate in daily physical education classes. Therefore, to achieve this objective, physical education needs to be more frequent for children in the lower grades, whereas enrollment needs to be increased for children in the upper grades.

To achieve this objective equitably for all of America's children, daily adaptive physical education programs should be available for children with special needs. School physical education requirements are also recommended for students in preschool and postsecondary programs.

1.9 **Increase to at least 50 percent the proportion of school physical education class time that students spend being physically active, preferably engaged in lifetime physical activities. (Baseline: Students spent an estimated 27 percent of class time being physically active in 1984)**

Note: Lifetime activities are activities that may be readily carried into adulthood because they generally need only one or two people. Examples include swimming, bicycling, jogging, and racquet sports. Also counted as lifetime activities are vigorous social activities such as dancing. Competitive group sports and activities typically played only by young children such as group games are excluded.

Baseline data source: Siedentop 1983.

Results from the National Children and Youth Fitness Studies I and II revealed that although enrollment in physical education positively affects fitness, the nature of the program is of even greater importance.[20,21] The intent of this objective is to encourage the implementation of high quality physical education programs that will enhance the fitness of children and youth and encourage life-long physical activity.

Although school physical education can help to assure a minimum amount of physical activity for children and youth, studies indicate that only 27 percent of class time is spent in actual physical activity; 26 percent of time is spent in instruction, 22 percent is spent in administrative tasks, and 25 percent is spent waiting.[23] The target of 50 percent is attainable if waiting time is trimmed to less than 5 percent of class time.

Many physical educators stress the importance of dedicating a major portion of the physical education curriculum to lifetime physical activities, especially as the student approaches adulthood. Despite the acknowledged importance of lifetime physical activities, the average student spends more time on lifetime physical activities outside the physical education class (60 percent) than within it.[20] The portion of the physical education curriculum devoted to lifetime fitness in 5th through 12th grade is only 48 percent, 45 percent for boys and 50 percent for girls. The average student is exposed to 5.6 different lifetime activities over a year's time. To a large extent, relays and informal games for younger students and competitive sports for older students are still the mainstay of the physical education program. More class time should be spent engaged in lifetime activities and more emphasis given to developing the knowledge, attitudes, cognitive skills, and physical skills students need to remain physically active throughout life.

* * *

Research Needs

Research is needed, especially for population subgroups, to further define the relationships between physical activity, physical fitness, and:

- the incidence of cardiovascular disease;

* * *

- the incidence of injuries;
- the incidence of obesity and selected types of body fat patterns;
- nutritional patterns;
- the adoption of healthy behavior patterns;
- the prevention and cessation of cigarette smoking;
- the treatment of alcohol and drug abuse;
- the incidence of depressive episodes among depressed people;
- improved mental well-being;
- the cognitive and functional ability of older adults; and
- quality of life.

Research on the determinants of regular physical activity is also needed to identify the knowledge, attitudes, and behavioral and social skills associated with a high probability of adopting and maintaining a regular exercise program.

* * *

Baseline Data Source References

Behavioral Risk Factor Surveillance System, Centers for Disease Control, Public Health Service, U.S. Department of Health and Human Services, Atlanta, GA.

National Health Interview Survey, National Center for Health Statistics, Centers for Disease Control, Public Health Service, U.S. Department of Health and Human Services, Hyattsville, MD.

Siedentop, D. *Developing Teaching Skills in Physical Education.* 2nd edition. Palo Alto, CA: Mayfield, 1983. p. 61.

U.S. Department of Health and Human Services. National children and youth fitness study. *Journal of Physical Education, Recreation, and Dance* 56:44-90, 1985.

U.S. Department of Health and Human Services. National children and youth fitness study II. *Journal of Physical Education, Recreation, and Dance* 58:50-96, 1987.

Nutrition

2

Contents

* * *

2.3 Overweight

2.4 Growth retardation

2.5 Dietary fat intake

* * *

2.7 Weight loss practices

2.8 Calcium intake

* * *

2.10 Iron deficiency

2.11 Breastfeeding

2.12 Baby bottle tooth decay

* * *

2.16 Low-fat, low-calorie restaurant food choices

2.17 Nutritious school and child care food services

* * *

2.19 Nutrition education in schools

* * *

2.21 Nutrition assessment, counseling, and referral by clinicians

[Research Needs]

2. Nutrition

* * *

Health Status Objectives

* * *

2.3* Reduce overweight to a prevalence of no more than 20 percent among people aged 20 and older and no more than 15 percent among adolescents aged 12 through 19. (Baseline: 26 percent for people aged 20 through 74 in 1976-80, 24 percent for men and 27 percent for women; 15 percent for adolescents aged 12 through 19 in 1976-80)

* * *

Note: For people aged 20 and older, overweight is defined as body mass index (BMI) equal to or greater than 27.8 for men and 27.3 for women. For adolescents, overweight is defined as BMI equal to or greater than 23.0 for males aged 12 through 14, 24.3 for males aged 15 through 17, 25.8 for males aged 18 through 19, 23.4 for females aged 12 through 14, 24.8 for females aged 15 through 17, and 25.7 for females aged 18 through 19. The values for adolescents are the age- and gender-specific 85th percentile values of the 1976-80 National Health and Nutrition Examination Survey (NHANES II), corrected for sample variation.[24] BMI is calculated by dividing weight in kilograms by the square of height in meters. The cut points used to define overweight approximate the 120 percent of desirable body weight definition used in the 1990 objectives.

Baseline data sources: National Health and Nutrition Examination Survey (NHANES), CDC; Hispanic Health and Nutrition Examination Survey, CDC; Indian Health Service; for people with disabilities, National Health Interview Survey, CDC.

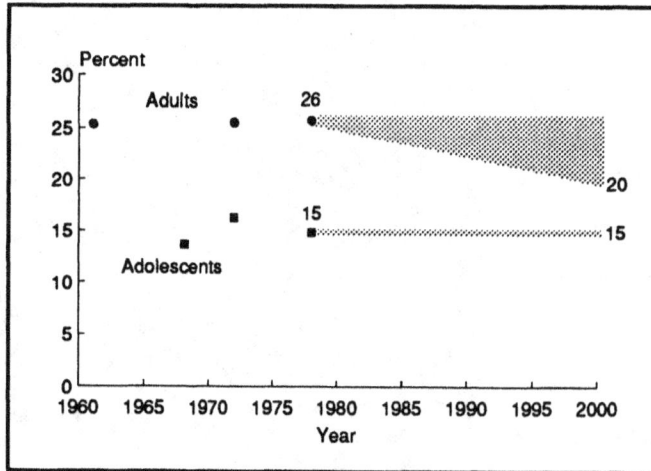

Fig. 2.3

Prevalence of overweight among people aged 20 and older and adolescents aged 12 through 19

Overweight is associated with elevated serum cholesterol levels, elevated blood pressure, and noninsulin-dependent diabetes, and is an independent risk factor for coronary heart disease.[25] Overweight also increases the risk for gallbladder disease and some types of cancer and has been implicated in the development of osteoarthritis of the weight-bearing joints, particularly the knee.

Overweight is multifactorial in origin, reflecting inherited, environmental, cultural, and socioeconomic conditions. The prevalence of overweight increases with advancing age until about age 50 for men and age 70 for women, then declines.[26] Overweight is particularly prevalent in minority populations, especially among minority women. Poverty is related to overweight in women. In 1976-80, 37 percent of women with incomes below the poverty level were overweight compared with 25 percent of those above the poverty level. There is an increased prevalence of overweight among hypertensive and diabetic populations.[25]

Overweight acquired during childhood or adolescence may persist into adulthood and increase the risk for some chronic diseases later in life.[25] Obese children also experience psychological stress. Concern has been expressed that the prevalence of obesity in adolescents may be increasing, but definitive data are lacking. There is also concern that overemphasis on thinness during adolescence may contribute to eating disorders such as anorexia nervosa and bulimia. Therefore, the target for this objective for adolescents is set at no more than 15 percent to prevent an increase in overweight above the 1976-80 baseline. The objective should be achieved through emphasis on physical activity accompanied by properly balanced dietary intake so that growth is not impaired . . . .

* * *

An ideal, health-oriented definition of obesity would be based on the degree of excess body fat at which health risks to individuals begin to increase. No such definition exists.[25] Although several measures of body fat are available, each has limitations. Skinfold thickness measurements reflect the amount of body fat, but are difficult to standardize and require equipment that is not readily available in many settings. Body mass index (BMI) is readily calculated from easily obtainable measurements. Until a better measure of body fat is developed, BMI will be used as a statistically derived proxy for obesity.[27,28]

Additional research is needed to define obesity in children. There is a prepubertal increase in subcutaneous fat that is lost during adolescence in boys, while in girls fat deposition continues. Thus, without measures of sexual maturity, measures of body fat and body weight are equally difficult to interpret in preadolescents and adolescents. Additional research also is needed to define the prevalence and health consequences of obesity in adolescents and older adults.

*This objective also appears as Objective 1.2 in *Physical Activity and Fitness*, as Objective 15.10 in *Heart Disease and Stroke*, and as Objective 17.12 in *Diabetes and Chronic Disabling Conditions*.

2.4 Reduce growth retardation among low-income children aged 5 and younger to less than 10 percent. (Baseline: Up to 16 percent among low-income children in 1988, depending on age and race/ethnicity)

Special Population Targets

	Prevalence of Short Stature	1988 Baseline	2000 Target
2.4a	Low-income black children <age 1	15%	10%
2.4b	Low-income Hispanic children <age 1	13%	10%
2.4c	Low-income Hispanic children aged 1	16%	10%
2.4d	Low-income Asian/Pacific Islander children aged 1	14%	10%
2.4e	Low-income Asian/Pacific Islander children aged 2-4	16%	10%

Note: *Growth retardation is defined as height-for-age below the fifth percentile of children in the National Center for Health Statistics' reference population.*

Baseline data source: Pediatric Nutrition Surveillance System, CDC.

Retardation in linear growth in preschool children serves as an indicator of overall health and development, but may especially reflect the adequacy of a child's diet. Full growth potential may not be reached because of less-than-optimal nutrition, infectious diseases, chronic diseases, or poor health care. Inadequate maternal weight gain during pregnancy and other prenatal factors that influence birth weight also affect the prevalence of growth retardation among infants and young children (see Objectives 14.5 and 14.6 in *Maternal and Infant Health*).

Growth retardation is not a problem for the vast majority of young children in the United States. Given the definition of growth retardation used in this objective, 5 percent of healthy children are expected to be below the fifth percentile of height for age due to normal biologic variation. But a prevalence of more than 5 percent below the fifth percentile for any population subgroup suggests that full growth potential is not being reached by children of that subgroup. This prevalence is exceeded by low-income children in the United States. Among some age and ethnic subgroups of low-income children, up to 16 percent of individuals aged 5 and younger are below the fifth percentile. The prevalence of growth retardation is especially high for Asian and Pacific Islander children aged 12 through 59 months, Hispanic children up to age 24 months, and black infants in the first year of life. The Asian and Pacific Islander children who show the greatest prevalence of low height for age include those of Southeast Asian refugee families. The linear growth status of these children has already shown improvement since the influx of refugee children in the late 1970s, and further improvement is achievable.

Interventions to improve linear growth in populations include better nutrition; improvements in the prevention, diagnosis, and treatment of infectious and chronic diseases; and the provision and use of fully adequate health services. Although the response of a population to interventions for growth retardation may not be as rapid as for iron deficiency or underweight, it should be possible to achieve the objective by the year 2000 in all ethnic, socioeconomic, and age subgroups. Special attention should be given to homeless children, children with disabilities, and other children with special needs.

Risk Reduction Objectives

2.5* Reduce dietary fat intake to an average of 30 percent of calories or less and average saturated fat intake to less than 10 percent of calories among people aged 2 and older. (Baseline: 36 percent of calories from total fat and 13 percent from saturated fat for people aged 20 through 74 in 1976-80; 36 percent and 13 percent for women aged 19 through 50 in 1985)

Baseline data sources: 1976-80 National Health and Nutrition Examination Survey (NHANES II), CDC; 1985 Continuing Survey of Food Intakes by Individuals (CSFII), USDA.

Considerable evidence associates diets high in fat with increased risk of obesity, some types of cancer, and possibly gallbladder disease. There is strong and consistent evidence for the relationship between saturated fat intake, high blood cholesterol, and increased risk for coronary heart disease.[25] Clinical, animal, and epidemiologic studies demonstrate that high intakes of saturated fatty acids increase the levels of serum total and low-density-lipoprotein (LDL) cholesterol. In turn, high blood cholesterol levels increase the risk of coronary heart disease. Saturated fat intake is the major dietary determinant of serum total cholesterol and LDL cholesterol levels in populations. Lowering saturated fat intake can help to reduce total and LDL cholesterol levels, and thus coronary heart disease (see *Heart Disease and Stroke*). The impact of polyunsaturated fatty acids and monounsaturated fatty acids on serum cholesterol is still being studied; both reduce blood cholesterol levels when substituted for saturated fatty acids. Polyunsaturated fatty acids may independently reduce blood cholesterol levels.

Epidemiologic and experimental animal studies suggest that dietary fat can influence the risk of some cancers, particularly cancers of the breast, colon, and prostate. The amount of fat consumed rather than the specific type of fat appears to be responsible for the risk of some types of cancer. Although the precise quantification of the contribution of dietary fat to the overall risk of cancer is not yet possible, there is general consensus that prudent dietary guidelines for fat intake should be encouraged.

Dietary fat contributes more than twice as many calories as equal amounts by weight of either protein or carbohydrate, and some studies indicate that diets high in fat are associated with higher prevalences of overweight. Weight control may be facilitated by decreasing calorie intake, especially by choosing foods relatively low in fat and calories.[25]

This objective is consistent with good nutritional practices for general health and may lower the risk of heart disease, cancer, and other chronic conditions such as obesity. However, certain population groups need particular attention to assure adequate essential nutrient intake while consuming reduced-fat diets. These groups include children, women, and older adults.

This objective recommends that healthy children follow the recommended eating patterns that are lower in fat and saturated fat as they begin to eat with the family, usually at age 2 or older. Because eating habits developed during childhood can influence lifetime eating practices, it is considered prudent to move toward these recommended eating patterns. However, as food intake varies from day to day, these recommendations are meant to represent an average of nutrient intake over several days.[29] Implementation activities should recognize that this objective applies to the diet for a day or more, not to a single meal or a single food.

Infants and children younger than age 2 have dietary requirements different from those of older people. Infants whose diet is primarily mother's milk or formula often appropriately consume 40 percent or more of calories from fat, and this well-established pattern of infant nutrition should be continued. Diets that contain less than 30 percent of calories from dietary fat may not be appropriate for children younger than age 2 and no restriction of dietary fat is proposed. Care must be taken to ensure the caloric and nutrient needs of the growing child.

The targets of 30 percent of calories or less from fat and less than 10 percent of calories from saturated fat are consistent with established recommendations [29,30] and are believed attainable. To attain this objective, health professionals, food industry organizations, government agencies, and other organizations must collaborate and provide consistent information to the public on how to reduce dietary fat intake and eat a nutritionally adequate diet. In 1988, only 64 percent of people aged 18 and older could identify the major sources of saturated fat, although 72 percent were aware of the association between dietary fat and/or cholesterol and heart disease.[31] Unfortunately, knowledge does not always translate into behavior change. To increase the likelihood of behavior change, nutrition education programs should incorporate the principles and techniques of behavior modification.

*This objective also appears as Objective 15.9 in *Heart Disease and Stroke* and as Objective 16.7 in *Cancer*.

* * *

2.7*   Increase to at least 50 percent the proportion of overweight people aged 12 and older who have adopted sound dietary practices combined with regular physical activity to attain an appropriate body weight. (Baseline: 30 percent of overweight women and 25 percent of overweight men for people aged 18 and older in 1985)

Baseline data source: National Health Interview Survey, CDC.

* * *

*This objective also appears as Objective 1.7 in *Physical Activity and Fitness.*

2.8   Increase calcium intake so at least 50 percent of youth aged 12 through 24 and 50 percent of pregnant and lactating women consume 3 or more servings daily of foods rich in calcium, and at least 50 percent of people aged 25 and older consume 2 or more servings daily. (Baseline: 7 percent of women and 14 percent of men aged 19 though 24 and 24 percent of pregnant and lactating women consumed 3 or more servings, and 15 percent of women and 23 percent of men aged 25 through 50 consumed 2 or more servings in 1985-86)

Note: The number of servings of foods rich in calcium is based on milk and milk products. A serving is considered to be 1 cup of skim milk or its equivalent in calcium (302 mg). The number of servings in this objective will generally provide approximately three-fourths of the 1989 Recommended Dietary Allowance (RDA) of calcium. The RDA is 1200 mg for people aged 12 through 24, 800 mg for people aged 25 and older, and 1200 mg for pregnant and lactating women.[32]

Baseline data source: Continuing Survey of Food Intakes by Individuals (CSFII), USDA.

Calcium is essential for the formation and maintenance of bones and teeth.[25] The level of bone mass achieved at skeletal maturity (peak bone mass) is a factor modifying the risk for developing osteoporosis. Peak bone mass appears to be related to intake of calcium during the years of bone mineralization.[30] Opinion is divided as to the age at which peak bone mass is achieved. Most of the accumulation of bone mineral occurs in humans by about 20 years of age. However, after the linear growth phase, there is a period of consolidation of bone density that continues until approximately age 30 to 35. A high peak bone mass is thought to be protective against fractures in later life.

Osteoporosis is a multifactorial, complex disorder, but low calcium intake appears to be one important factor in its development. The ideal level of calcium intake for development of peak bone mass is unknown, and it has not yet been established to what extent increased calcium intake will prevent osteoporosis. However, females, particularly adolescent and young adult females, should increase food sources of calcium.[25] In postmenopausal women, the group at highest risk for osteoporosis, estrogen replacement therapy under medical supervision is the most effective means to reduce the rate of bone loss and the risk for fractures.[25] (See Objective 17.18 in *Diabetes and Chronic Disabling Conditions.*)

Children, pregnant and lactating women, and older adults have special needs for calcium based on, respectively, the extra demands of growth, milk production, and the age-related decrease in absorption of calcium. Research is ongoing to determine the dietary calcium requirements for older adults. People with incomes below the poverty level are also of special concern. These individuals, especially women, have consistently lower mean daily calcium intakes than the rest of the population.

Dairy products, including fluid milks, yogurt, and hard and soft cheeses, provide about 55 percent of calcium in U.S. diets.[32] Other major food sources of dietary calcium include canned fish, certain vegetables (e.g., kale, broccoli), legumes (beans and peas), calcium-precipitated tofu, calcium-enriched grain products, lime-processed tortillas, seeds, and nuts. It is uncertain if there are biologically important differences in the absorption of calcium from different foods or diets. With current food selection practices in the United States, use of dairy products constitutes the difference between inadequate and adequate intakes of calcium.

For people who can readily digest milk and milk products, the lower fat forms of these products are among the preferred sources of calcium for attaining the recommended levels of calcium intake. A steady increase in the variety of lower fat dairy products in the marketplace is anticipated. Per capita availability data and comparison of results from the 1977-78 Nationwide Food Consumption Survey and the 1985-86 Continuing Survey of Food Intakes by Individuals indicate that a trend towards increased use of lower fat milk is already occurring.

Most people with lactose intolerance are able to consume small amounts of lactose without distress, and there are a variety of low-lactose and reduced-lactose dairy products available. For example, the Special Supplemental Food Program for Women, Infants, and Children (WIC) already includes low- and lactose-free dairy products in its packages for pregnant women when needed. People who do not (or cannot) consume and absorb adequate levels of calcium from dairy food sources may consider use of calcium-enriched foods, and those with dietary, biochemical, or clinical evidence of inadequate intake should receive professional advice on the proper type and dosage of calcium supplements. Such supplements may be appropriate for some older adults, but doses exceeding the RDA are not advised.[32]

In 1988, only 43 percent of people aged 18 and older were aware of the association between calcium and osteoporosis.[33] The public should be educated about the importance of calcium to health, recommended intakes (in terms of servings), and good food sources of calcium, particularly lower fat dairy products. Educational efforts for racial and ethnic minority groups should emphasize culturally appropriate food sources of calcium.

* * *

2.10   **Reduce iron deficiency to less than 3 percent among children aged 1 through 4 and among women of childbearing age. (Baseline: 9 percent for children aged 1 through 2, 4 percent for children aged 3 through 4, and 5 percent for women aged 20 through 44 in 1976-80)**

Special Population Targets

	Iron Deficiency Prevalence	1976-80 Baseline	2000 Target
2.10a	Low-income children aged 1-2	21%	10%
2.10b	Low-income children aged 3-4	10%	5%
2.10c	Low-income women of childbearing age	8%†	4%
	Anemia Prevalence	1983-85 Baseline	2000 Target
2.10d	Alaska Native children aged 1-5	22-28%	10%
2.10e	Black, low-income pregnant women (third trimester)	41%‡	20%

†*Baseline for women aged 20-44*
‡*1988 baseline for women aged 15-44*

Note: Iron deficiency is defined as having abnormal results for 2 or more of the following tests: mean corpuscular volume, erythrocyte protoporphyrin, and transferrin saturation.[34] *Anemia is used as an index of iron deficiency. Anemia among Alaska Native children was defined as hemoglobin <11 gm/dL or hematocrit <34 percent. For pregnant women in the third trimester,* *anemia was defined according to CDC criteria.[35] The above prevalences of iron deficiency and anemia may be due to inadequate dietary iron intakes or to inflammatory conditions and infections. For anemia, genetics may also be a factor.*

Baseline data sources: National Health and Nutrition Examination Survey (NHANES), CDC; for Alaska Native children, CDC 1988; for low-income pregnant women, Pregnancy Nutrition Surveillance System, CDC.

Chronic iron deficiency in childhood may have adverse effects on growth and development. The prevalence of iron deficiency is higher in black children compared to white children, and is substantially higher in children from families with incomes below the poverty level. A reduction in the prevalence of iron deficiency among young children can be achieved by increasing the proportion of new mothers who breastfeed (see Objective 2.11), increasing the use of iron-fortified formulas when formulas are used, and delaying the introduction of whole cow milk feedings until 9 to 12 months of age. Trends in the prevalence of anemia, primarily related to iron deficiency, indicate that progress is being made in this area.[36] However, continued efforts are needed to assure that these trends continue, especially among low-income children.

Women of childbearing age are at increased risk for iron deficiency because of iron loss in menstruation and because of the iron requirements of pregnancy. Maternal iron deficiency during pregnancy and lactation increases the likelihood that the infant will be iron deficient in the early years of life. A reduction in iron deficiency among women of childbearing age can be achieved by nutrition education to encourage selection of iron-rich foods and by adequate supplementation with iron during pregnancy.

2.11* Increase to at least 75 percent the proportion of mothers who breastfeed their babies in the early postpartum period and to at least 50 percent the proportion who continue breastfeeding until their babies are 5 to 6 months old. (Baseline: 54 percent at discharge from birth site and 21 percent at 5 to 6 months in 1988)

Special Population Targets

Mothers Breastfeeding Their Babies:	1988 Baseline	2000 Target
During Early Postpartum Period—		
2.11a Low-income mothers	32%	75%
2.11b Black mothers	25%	75%
2.11c Hispanic mothers	51%	75%
2.11d American Indian/Alaska Native mothers	47%	75%
At Age 5-6 Months—		
2.11a Low-income mothers	9%	50%
2.11b Black mothers	8%	50%
2.11c Hispanic mothers	16%	50%
2.11d American Indian/Alaska Native mothers	28%	50%

Baseline data sources: Ross Laboratories Mothers Survey; for American Indians/Alaska Natives, Pediatric Nutrition Surveillance System, CDC.

*For commentary, see Objective 14.9 in *Maternal and Infant Health*.

2.12* Increase to at least 75 percent the proportion of parents and caregivers who use feeding practices that prevent baby bottle tooth decay. (Baseline data available in 1991)

Special Population Targets

Appropriate Feeding Practices	Baseline	2000 Target
2.12a Parents and caregivers with less than high school education	—	65%
2.12b American Indian/Alaska Native parents and caregivers	—	65%

*For commentary, see Objective 13.11 in *Oral Health*.

* * *

Services and Protection Objectives

* * *

2.16 Increase to at least 90 percent the proportion of restaurants and institutional food service operations that offer identifiable low-fat, low-calorie food choices, consistent with the *Dietary Guidelines for Americans*. (Baseline: About 70 percent of fast food and family restaurant chains with 350 or more units had at least one low-fat, low-calorie item on their menu in 1989)

Baseline data source: Survey of Chain Operators, National Restaurant Association.

Restaurants, including fast food restaurants, and institutional food service operations at worksites, hospitals, nursing homes, postsecondary institutions, correctional facilities, and military installations play a critical role in the dietary intake of the U.S. population. In 1985, 40 percent of all meals were consumed outside the home. On a typical day, 45.8 million people, a fifth of the U.S. population, are served at fast food establishments. Because so many individuals eat food outside the home, it is important to encourage food service personnel to offer healthful food choices. If people are to choose a diet that promotes health and reduces the risk of some diseases, then food choices based on the *Dietary Guidelines for Americans*[37] should be offered in these settings. Therefore, the concepts of these guidelines and the principles for healthful menu planning and food preparation need to be promoted and reinforced to restaurant owners and managers and to culinary training and food service management and personnel.

Baseline data for this objective are limited. However, a national survey of worksites found that approximately 10 percent of worksites with 50 or more employees offered nutrition education activities for employees that included healthy food service selections.[62] Limited data are also available from a survey of 35 fast food and family restaurants with 350 or more units.[551] A substantial proportion of the respondents offered an entree salad or salad bar (71 percent), reduced or low calorie dressings (71 percent), fruit juice (71 percent), and low fat milk (76 percent). Fifty-two percent served a grilled chicken sandwich, 29 percent featured fresh fruit, 29 percent offered low fat frozen yogurt, and 24 percent offered skim milk. In addition, 62 percent used either vegetable oil and/or vegetable shortening exclusively for frying operations.

2.17 Increase to at least 90 percent the proportion of school lunch and breakfast services and child care food services with menus that are consistent with the nutrition principles in the *Dietary Guidelines for Americans*. (Baseline data available in 1993)

The *Dietary Guidelines for Americans*[37] is the primary expression of Federal nutrition policy. As such, it represents the best principles of healthy dietary practices and offers appropriate guidance for meal planning in schools and other food service programs for children. For many children, school meals make a significant contribution to their total day's nutrient intake. Child care settings for preschoolers and before and after school programs for older children also contribute substantially to the nutrient intake of America's children. Thus, these meals must be well balanced and in keeping with all of the principles of sound nutrition.

School food service personnel, and particularly cafeteria managers, are to a large extent the gatekeepers to schoolchildren's food supply. Although meal planning in many schools already incorporates the principles of the *Dietary Guidelines*, such planning should be universal. It is especially important that school meals provide choices that include low fat foods, vegetables, fruits, and whole-grain products. New foods may need to be introduced gradually to increase their acceptance by students.

School fundraising activities that involve food sales, onsite vending machine offerings, and food offerings at concession stands during recreational and other events should also reflect the principles of the *Dietary Guidelines*. In addition, schools should provide students with preschool through 12th grade nutrition education (see Objective 2.19) and point-of-choice nutrition information in the school cafeteria.

* * *

2.19 Increase to at least 75 percent the proportion of the Nation's schools that provide nutrition education from preschool through 12th grade, preferably as part of quality school health education. (Baseline data available in 1991)

Most food preferences and many dietary habits are established during childhood. Educating school age children about nutrition is important to establishing healthy eating habits early in life. Providing nutrition education from preschool through 12th grade will reach children during the years when they are beginning to make their own decisions and to eat more food away from home.

Currently, many students understand that there is a connection between good nutrition and good health, but a large number do not understand that a diet high in fat, sugars, or salt may increase the risk for certain chronic diseases.[38] Furthermore, although the majority know that a nutritious diet leads to good health, this knowledge is not reflected in their food-buying and meal patterns. One survey found that only 21 percent of students say they think a lot about whether the food they choose is good for them.[38] When they shop for snacks or food for themselves, 65 percent say they buy candy. Another survey of a nationally representative sample of eighth and tenth graders found that 48 percent of the girls and 32 percent of the boys had not eaten breakfast on 5 or more days during the preceding week.[39] On average, students reported eating three snacks per day. More than half of these snacks were foods high in fat and/or sugars. Nearly 4 out of every 10 students ate fried foods four or more times a week.

Although few studies have examined the impact of school nutrition education on behavior, nutrition education can increase students' knowledge about nutrition and can help shape appropriate attitudes. A well-designed curriculum can help students develop the behavioral skills they need to plan, prepare, and select healthful meals and snacks. Optimally, school nutrition education should include educational cafeteria experiences as well as classroom work. The required nutrition education can be provided in a variety of classroom units. While it is advantageous to include nutrition education as a component of quality health education, integration into science and related curricula can serve to reinforce principles and messages learned in health units. To further enhance the likelihood that students adopt healthy dietary practices, students must have access to healthful food choices (see Objective 2.17) and the support of those around them.

To attain this objective, all States and school districts should require nutrition education. Only 12 States required nutrition education in 1985. Achieving this objective also requires that teachers be knowledgeable about nutrition and how to teach nutrition. Thus, nutrition coursework should be included in the core curriculum for the professional preparation of teachers of all grades and emphasized in continuing education activities for teachers.

For a definition of quality school health education, see *Educational and Community-Based Programs*.

* * *

2.21 **Increase to at least 75 percent the proportion of primary care providers who provide nutrition assessment and counseling and/or referral to qualified nutritionists or dietitians. (Baseline: Physicians provided diet counseling for an estimated 40 to 50 percent of patients in 1988)**

Baseline data source: Lewis 1988.

Primary care providers are optimally positioned in the health care system to provide preventive services, including nutrition assessment and counseling. Primary care providers include general practitioners, family physicians, internists, pediatricians, geriatricians, obstetrician/gynecologists, physician assistants, nurse practitioners, and nurses. The public views physicians in particular as credible sources of health information. In 1987, Americans visited physicians an average of 5.3 times per year, and 76 percent visited a physician within the preceding year.[40] Nutrition advice from other health professionals (e.g., pharmacists, dentists) reaches even more people and reinforces important nutrition messages. Nutrition counseling by qualified nutritionists and dietitians, who are trained to help people make dietary changes, is important for many patients.

Dietary modifications can be achieved through primary care interventions. Dietary assessment, advice, counseling, and followup by physicians and/or dietitians/nutritionists have been found to be effective in reducing patient dietary fat intake and serum cholesterol.[41] Yet only 26 percent of adults report that "eating proper foods" was often or sometimes discussed during visits to a doctor or other health professional for routine care.[42] A recent national survey of internists found that 66 percent routinely obtained and recorded information about diet for patients new to their practice.[43] A meta-analysis of 9 physician surveys, 2 chart audit studies, and 1 consumer survey estimated that physicians provide diet counseling for only 40 to 50 percent of patients.[44] Physicians also fail to refer many of their patients to qualified nutritionists or dietitians for counseling.

The U.S. Preventive Services Task Force recommended that physicians and other clinical service providers include nutrition counseling and referral as a standard part of their practice.[45] The Task Force recommended:

> "Clinicians should provide periodic counseling regarding dietary intake of calories, fat (especially saturated fat), cholesterol, complex carbohydrates

and fiber, and sodium. Specifically, patients should receive a diet and exercise prescription designed to achieve and maintain a desirable weight by keeping caloric intake balanced with energy expenditures. Adolescents and adults, in particular, should be given dietary guidance on how to reduce total fat intake to less than 30 percent of total calories and dietary cholesterol to less than 300 mg/day. Saturated fat consumption should be reduced to less than 10 percent of total calories. To achieve these goals, patients should emphasize consumption of fish, poultry prepared without skin, lean meats, and low-fat dairy products. . . . Patients should be encouraged to eat a variety of foods that emphasize consumption of whole grain products and cereals, vegetables and fruits. Those who are at risk for dental caries, especially children, should limit their consumption of foods high in refined sugars. It is also reasonable to recommend eating foods low in sodium and limiting the amount of salt added in food preparation and at the table. Adolescent girls and women should receive counseling on methods to ensure adequate calcium and iron intake; parents should be encouraged to include iron-enriched foods in the diets of infants and young children; and pregnant women should receive specific nutritional guidelines to enhance fetal and maternal health. . . . Clinicians who lack the time or skills to perform a complete dietary history, to address potential barriers to changes in eating habits, and to offer specific guidance on food selection and preparation, should either have patients seen by other trained providers in the office or clinic or should refer patients to a registered dietitian or qualified nutritionist for further counseling."

Although many physicians consider diet modification important for their patients, they often feel ill-prepared to counsel patients about dietary behaviors. When asked about their confidence in dealing with dietary change, 35 percent of Massachusetts primary care physicians reported being "very prepared" to counsel patients and only 7 percent reported feeling "very successful" in this regard.[99] Thus for many physicians, referring patients for nutrition assessment and counseling represents appropriate clinical practice. To ensure high rates of referral, office systems should be established to prompt and facilitate referral.

* * *

Research Needs

Nutrition research is needed to determine the following:

- The role of specific dietary factors in the etiology and prevention of chronic diseases, including cancer, osteoporosis, and stroke.

- The childhood dietary patterns that will best provide adequate intake of calories and nutrients essential for growth and development, and also prevent later development of chronic diseases.

- The effects of maternal nutrition on the health of the developing fetus.

* * *

- The effects of nutrition on age-related impairment of organ system functions (e.g., cardiovascular, gastrointestinal/oral cavity, immune, musculoskeletal, and nervous systems).

* * *

- Healthful dietary patterns translated from nutrient requirements.

- Biochemical markers of dietary intake to improve ability to monitor the effects of dietary intervention.

- Effective educational methods to translate dietary recommendations into appropriate food choices and sustained behavioral changes for various subpopulations.

- Food labels that are more informative and useful to the public.

- The relationship of total body fat and body fat distribution to health outcomes (i.e., a health-related definition of obesity).

- The epidemiology of weight gain and successful weight loss, the health effects of weight loss and regain (weight cycling), and the healthy nutritional practices that best promote weight loss.

- The etiology, epidemiology, prevention, and treatment of eating disorders such as anorexia nervosa and bulimia.

- Medication and nutrition interactions.

- The definition and measurement of hunger.

Baseline Data Source References

Centers for Disease Control (CDC). Centers for Disease Control Pregnancy Nutrition Surveillance System. *Morbidity and Mortality Weekly Report* 37(13):200, 1988.

Continuing Survey of Food Intakes by Individuals (CSFII), Human Nutrition Information Service (HNIS), U.S. Department of Agriculture (USDA), Washington, DC.

Hispanic Health and Nutrition Examination Survey, National Center for Health Statistics (NCHS), CDC, PHS, DHHS, Hyattsville, MD.

Indian Health Service (IHS), PHS, DHHS, Rockville, MD.

Lewis, C.E. Disease prevention and health promotion practices of primary care physicians in the United States. *American Journal of Preventive Medicine* 4(suppl.):9-16, 1988.

National Health Interview Survey (NHIS), NCHS, CDC, PHS, DHHS, Hyattsville, MD.

National Health and Nutrition Examination Survey (NHANES) II, NCHS, CDC, PHS, DHHS, Hyattsville, MD.

Pediatric Nutrition Surveillance System, CDC, PHS, DHHS, Atlanta, GA.

Pregnancy Nutrition Surveillance System, CDC, PHS, DHHS, Atlanta, GA.

Survey of Chain Operators, National Restaurant Association, Washington, DC.

Tobacco

3

Contents

* * *

3.4 Cigarette smoking

3.5 Smoking initiation by youth

* * *

3.7 Smoking cessation during pregnancy

3.8 Children's exposure to smoke at home

3.9 Smokeless tobacco use

3.10 Tobacco-use prevention education and tobacco-free schools

* * *

3.13 Tobacco product sale and distribution to youth

3.14 State plans to reduce tobacco use

3.15 Tobacco product advertising and promotion to youth

3.16 Cessation counseling and followup by clinicians

[Research Needs]

3. Tobacco

***

Risk Reduction Objectives

3.4* Reduce cigarette smoking to a prevalence of no more than 15 percent among people aged 20 and older. (Baseline: 29 percent in 1987, 32 percent for men and 27 percent for women)

Special Population Targets

Cigarette Smoking Prevalence	1987 Baseline	2000 Target

***

3.4h	Women of reproductive age	29%[††]	12%
3.4i	Pregnant women	25%[‡‡]	10%
3.4j	Women who use oral contraceptives	36%[§§]	10%

***

[††]*Baseline for women aged 18-44*
[‡‡]*1985 baseline*
[§§]*1983 baseline*

Note: *A cigarette smoker is a person who has smoked at least 100 cigarettes and currently smokes cigarettes.*

Baseline data sources: National Health Interview Survey, CDC; Worldwide Survey of Substance Abuse and Health Behavior Among Military Personnel, U.S. Department of Defense; Hispanic Health and Nutrition Examination Survey, CDC; for American Indians and Alaska Natives, CDC 1987; for Southeast Asian men, local surveys, CDC[46,47,48]; for women who use contraceptives, Behavioral Risk Factor Surveillance System, CDC.[49]

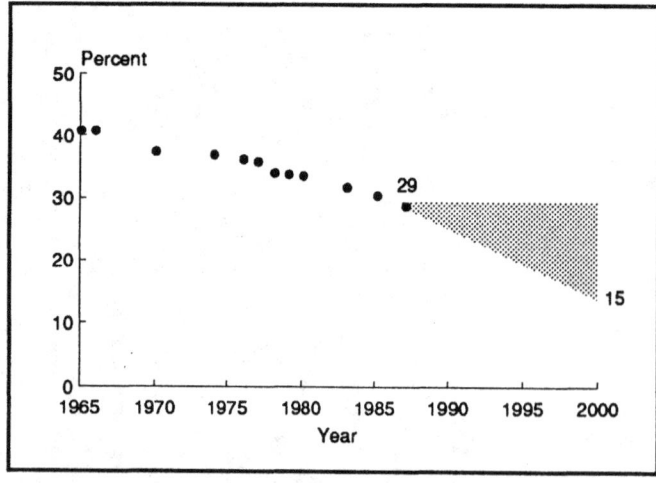

Fig. 3.4

Prevalence of cigarette smoking among people aged 20 and older

Among people aged 20 and older, cigarette smoking prevalence has been declining steadily at a rate of 0.5 percentage points per year since 1965. The decline has been substantially slower among women.[50] By the late 1990s, smoking rates for women will probably exceed the rates for men. In 1987, smoking prevalence for the entire population aged 20 and older was 29 percent. Projection of the 1974 through 1985 trend suggests that smoking prevalence will be 22 percent in the year 2000.[51] The target of 15 percent, although challenging, is believed attainable with intensified effort, given the changing social attitudes regarding tobacco use.

* * *

Women of reproductive age are targeted as a primary prevention strategy to reduce the prevalence of smoking during pregnancy. Approximately 29 percent of women aged 18 through 44 smoked cigarettes in 1987.[52]

National data on smoking during pregnancy are scarce and estimates vary. The 1980 National Natality Survey reported that 29 percent of all married women smoked during pregnancy.[53] In 1982, the National Survey of Family Growth found that 32 percent of women aged 15 through 44 smoked during their most recent pregnancy. In the 1985 National Health Interview Survey, 25 percent of women aged 18 through 44 who had given birth within the past 5 years smoked throughout their pregnancy.[42] Limited data suggest that the prevalence of smoking during pregnancy has been decreasing for some but not all groups. Between 1967 and 1980, smoking rates during pregnancy among teenagers remained fairly constant at 38 percent for whites and 27 percent for blacks.[54] Among women over age 20, smoking during pregnancy declined from 34 to 11 percent among black women and declined from 40 to 25 percent among white women. Among white smokers with less than 12 years of education, the prevalence of smoking during pregnancy declined from 48 percent to 43 percent, compared to a decline from 34 to 11 percent for women with 16 or more years of education. In general, women in the lowest age and socioeconomic categories have the highest likelihood of smoking during pregnancy. The National Maternal and Infant Health Survey, begun in 1988, will provide reliable estimates of smoking during pregnancy for the late 1980s. In addition, maternal smoking data from birth certificates will be available for analyses of the effect of smoking on certain pediatric conditions.[55] (See also Objective 14.10 in *Maternal and Infant Health*.)

Women who use oral contraceptives and smoke cigarettes have an increased risk of heart attack and stroke. In 1976-80, 44 percent of women using oral contraceptives smoked cigarettes.[54] In 1983, the Behavioral Risk Factor Surveillance System found that 36 percent of oral contraceptive users aged 18 through 44 smoked cigarettes.[49] The year 2000 target of 10 percent is believed attainable given the apparent downward trend.

*This objective also appears as Objective 15.12 in *Heart Disease and Stroke* and as Objective 16.6 in *Cancer*.

3.5   **Reduce the initiation of cigarette smoking by children and youth so that no more than 15 percent have become regular cigarette smokers by age 20. (Baseline: 30 percent of youth had become regular cigarette smokers by ages 20 through 24 in 1987)**

Special Population Target

Initiation of Smoking	1987 Baseline	2000 Target
3.5a Lower socioeconomic status youth†	40%	18%

†As measured by people aged 20-24 with a high school education or less

Baseline data source: National Health Interview Survey, CDC.

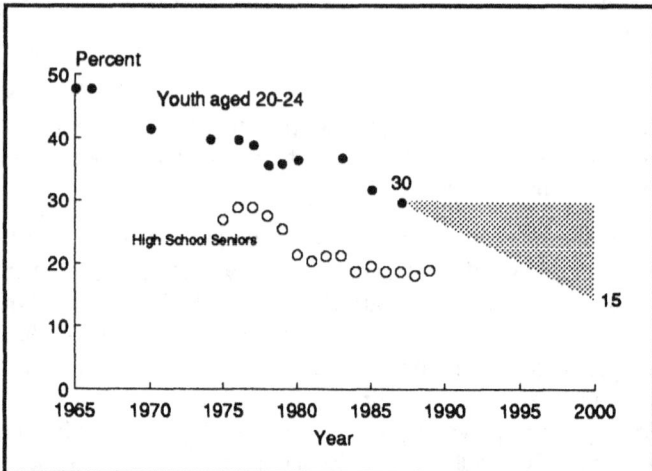

Fig. 3.5

Cigarette smoking prevalence among people aged 20 through 24 and high school seniors

Reducing the initiation of cigarette smoking by youth is an important national priority. If 29 percent of the 70 million children now living in the United States start smoking and continue to smoke cigarettes as adults, then at least 5 million of them will die of smoking-related diseases. Birth cohort studies of ever-smoking rates indicate that initiation is more sensitive to intervention than is quitting behavior. Preventing the initiation of smoking by youth should be a major focus of efforts to reduce the prevalence of cigarette smoking.

Experimentation with smoking is occurring at younger and younger ages and initiation now occurs almost entirely during adolescence. In 1986 and 1987, two surveys of high school students found that for those who had ever smoked, about one-quarter had smoked their first cigarette by the 6th grade, one-half by the 8th grade, three-fourths by the 9th grade, and 94 percent by the 11th grade.[39,58]

In 1988, the National Household Survey on Drug Abuse found that 23 percent of adolescents aged 12 through 17 had smoked at least one cigarette during the preceding year and 12 percent had smoked within the preceding month.[73] In 1987, the National Adolescent Student Health Survey found that 51 percent of 8th graders (aged 13 and 14) and 63 percent of 10th graders (aged 15 and 16) reported having tried cigarettes.[39] Sixteen percent of 8th graders and 26 percent of 10th graders reported having smoked a cigarette during the preceding month, and 8 percent of 8th graders and 18 percent of 10th graders had smoked a pack or more within the preceding month. Annual data from the High School Seniors Survey reveal that reported daily smoking among high school seniors decreased from a peak prevalence of 29 percent in 1976 to 19 percent in 1989.[56,57,58] However, most of the decline occurred between 1977 and 1981, and smoking prevalence among high school seniors has hovered at 18 to 19 percent since 1984.

Differentiating between experimentation and initiation is difficult, and youth surveys all have limitations. The Household Survey on Drug Abuse includes only about 2,000 to 3,000 youth aged 12 through 18, too few for precise estimates. High school surveys do not gather information from young people who have dropped out of school. In 1986-87, 15 percent of whites, 21 percent of blacks, and 37 percent of Hispanics aged 20 through 24 had not finished high school.[59] This nonsurveyed group is known to have a higher smoking rate.[60]

Most adult smokers started to smoke regularly before age 20 and almost all had started by age 24. Accordingly, the proportion of regular smokers in the 20 through 24 age group is considered the most valid and reliable measure of smoking initiation by youth and is used as a proxy measure in this objective. The primary limitation of this measure is the delay of at least 5 years required to reflect actual change in youth behavior.

In 1987, smoking prevalence among people aged 20 through 24 was 30 percent, having decreased an average of 0.69 percentage points per year since 1965.[50] At this rate of decline, smoking prevalence among people aged 20 through 24 is expected to be 20 percent in the year 2000. Because there should be a major emphasis on preventing initiation and because 1987 data suggest that a decline in initiation may have already begun among previously resistant groups, a target of 15 percent has been set for the year 2000. This represents a halving of the 1987 prevalence and will be a major achievement if accomplished.

In 1987, blacks aged 20 through 24 had a smoking prevalence of 26 percent. The rate of decline was 0.79 percentage points per year since 1965, with a substantial drop of 13 percentage points occurring since 1983. This decline exceeds that reported for any other group; hence no special target for black youth has been established.

The 1987 prevalence of cigarette smoking was 40 percent among people aged 20 through 24 whose education had not continued beyond high school. Between 1965 and 1985, initiation among young men in this group declined by 1 percentage point per year but remained constant for young women. However, 1987 data showed the first major decline in smoking prevalence among young women in this age and education category, and the drop was a substantial 5 percentage points from the 1985 estimate. Consequently, the current trend is assumed to be the same for young men and women, at a rate of decrease of 1 percentage point per year. This trend would yield a prevalence of 27 percent in the year 2000 for low socioeconomic status youth. The target for this special population is set at 18 percent and, although challenging, should be attainable given the emphasis placed on prevention of smoking and the increase in school programs in recent years.

* * *

3.7 Increase smoking cessation during pregnancy so that at least 60 percent of women who are cigarette smokers at the time they become pregnant quit smoking early in pregnancy and maintain abstinence for the remainder of their pregnancy. (Baseline: 39 percent of white women aged 20 through 44 quit at any time during pregnancy in 1985)

Special Population Target

	Cessation and Abstinence During Pregnancy	*1985 Baseline*	*2000 Target*
3.7a	Women with less than a high school education	28%[†]	45%

[†]*Baseline for white women aged 20-44*

Baseline data source: Fingerhut, Kleinman, and Kendrick 1990.

Maternal cigarette smoking during pregnancy retards fetal growth and is associated with an increased incidence of low birth weight, prematurity, miscarriage, stillbirth, sudden infant death syndrome, and infant mortality.[50] In the United States, 20 to 30 percent of the incidence of low birth weight[61] and up to 14 percent of preterm deliveries are attributable to maternal cigarette smoking.[50]

Smoking cessation prior to or early during pregnancy can reverse the reduction in infant birth weight associated with maternal smoking. If all pregnant women refrained from smoking, the number of fetal and infant deaths would be reduced by an estimated 10 percent, saving about 4,000 infants each year.[63]

The 1980 National Natality Survey, conducted among a national sample of married mothers of live born infants, found that among women who smoked, 18 percent of white women quit smoking during pregnancy compared with 13 percent of black women. Between 1967 and 1980, there was an increase in the proportion of white women quitting smoking during pregnancy (11 percent to 16 percent), while among blacks the proportion that quit actually declined (17 percent to 11 percent).[54] Among white smokers with less than 12 years of education, there was relatively little change in the proportion that quit during pregnancy (11 percent to 9 percent), but among smokers with 16 years or more of education, the proportion more than doubled (12 percent to 27 percent).

Intervention studies indicate that up to 27 percent of pregnant women who smoke at the time of enrollment into prenatal care may quit smoking for the duration of their pregnancy with intensive smoking cessation counseling and followup.[64] Use of a serialized self-help program for pregnant women recently yielded a quit rate of 26 percent.[65]

Analysis of a followback of the women who reported a recent pregnancy in the 1985 National Health Interview Survey demonstrated that 39 percent of white women who were smokers at the start of their pregnancy quit.[66] This objective seeks to increase quitting during pregnancy by 50 percent. While challenging, this objective has been the basis of several recent smoking and health initiatives, and its high profile in the health community makes it attainable. (See also Objective 3.4i and Objective 14.10 in *Maternal and Infant Health*.)

Smoking cessation programs for pregnant women should also address the issue of postpartum relapse. The National Health Interview Survey Followback Study found that only one-third of the women who quit smoking during pregnancy were still abstinent 1 year postpartum, with the majority relapsing in the first 3 months after delivery.

3.8 **Reduce to no more than 20 percent the proportion of children aged 6 and younger who are regularly exposed to tobacco smoke at home. (Baseline: More than 39 percent in 1986, as 39 percent of households with one or more children aged 6 or younger had a cigarette smoker in the household)**

Note: Regular exposure to tobacco smoke at home is defined as the occurrence of tobacco smoking anywhere in the home on more than three days each week.
Baseline data source: Adult Use of Tobacco Survey, CDC.

Environmental tobacco smoke is a cause of disease, including lung cancer, in healthy nonsmokers, and is a significant health risk for children.[67,68] The children of parents who smoke are more likely to develop lower respiratory tract infections, to be hospitalized or see a doctor for these conditions during the first year of life, and to develop middle ear infections than children of parents who do not smoke. Parental smoking may compromise lung function in young children and the developing lungs of the growing child. It may also contribute to the rise of chronic airflow obstruction later in life.[67,68]

The major source of smoke exposure for young children is their home. Both passive smoking and being nursed by a smoking mother contribute to the amount of tobacco constituents absorbed by infants.[69,70] In the most recent and comprehensive study of passive smoke exposure of infants, the amount smoked in the same room or vehicle or even the same house as the infant was the major predictor of infants' urinary cotinine levels.[69] Smoking around the infant and putting the infant in a room where smoking occurred recently increased the infant's absorption of environmental tobacco smoke. The authors concluded that "simply blowing smoke away from the infant, going into another room to smoke, or increasing the ventilation in a room will probably not prevent the infant from eventually absorbing tobacco smoke." If people who have contact with children must smoke, they should smoke outdoors or in areas that do not contribute air to places where the child might be.[69,71]

Although a baseline estimate for this objective is not yet available, 39 percent of households with one or more children aged 6 or younger had a cigarette smoker in the household in 1986.[72] The proportion of children aged 6 and younger exposed to tobacco smoke at home is almost certainly higher.

3.9   **Reduce smokeless tobacco use by males aged 12 through 24 to a prevalence of no more than 4 percent. (Baseline: 6.6 percent among males aged 12 through 17 in 1988; 8.9 percent among males aged 18 through 24 in 1987)**

Special Population Target

Smokeless Tobacco Use	1986-87 Baseline	2000 Target
3.9a American Indian/Alaska Native youth	18-64%	10%

Note: For males aged 12 through 17, a smokeless tobacco user is someone who has used snuff or chewing tobacco in the preceding month. For males aged 18 through 24, a smokeless tobacco user is someone who has used either snuff or chewing tobacco at least 20 times and who currently uses snuff or chewing tobacco.

Baseline data sources: For males aged 12 through 17, National Household Survey on Drug Abuse, ADAMHA; for males aged 18 through 24, National Health Interview Survey, CDC; for American Indian and Alaska Native youth, CDC 1988.

Smokeless tobacco includes primarily moist or dry snuff and chewing tobacco. Oral cancer has been shown to occur several times more frequently among smokeless tobacco users than among nonusers and may be 50 times as frequent among long-term snuff users.[68] All smokeless tobacco products contain substantial amounts of nicotine; their use can support nicotine dependence and may lead to cigarette use.

The consumption of smokeless tobacco in the United States increased 40 percent between 1970 and 1986. Most new users of smokeless tobacco products are adolescent males. In 1988, 6.6 percent of males aged 12 through 17 had used some form of smokeless tobacco in the preceding month.[73] The prevalence of smokeless tobacco use among males aged 18 through 24 was 8.9 percent in 1987.[52]

Between 1970 and 1986, the prevalence of snuff use increased fifteenfold and chewing tobacco use increased more than fourfold among men aged 17 through 19.[50] In contrast, the prevalence of use among men aged 50 and older declined by almost half for each type of product. Attaining the target of 4 percent set for this objective will be a challenge as it requires reversing an upward trend.

Smokeless tobacco use among women was less than 1 percent in 1987.[52] Use of smokeless tobacco by minority groups varies. Black and Hispanic adolescent populations report lower usage rates than whites. In contrast, Native American schoolchildren have reported prevalences of regular smokeless tobacco use ranging from 18 to 64 percent.[74]

Services and Protection Objectives

3.10 Establish tobacco-free environments and include tobacco use prevention in the curricula of all elementary, middle, and secondary schools, preferably as part of quality school health education. (Baseline: 17 percent of school districts totally banned smoking on school premises or at school functions in 1988; antismoking education was provided by 78 percent of school districts at the high school level, 81 percent at the middle school level, and 75 percent at the elementary school level in 1988)

Baseline data source: National School Boards Association 1989.

Tobacco-free environments in schools reinforce student knowledge of the health hazards of tobacco use and exposure to environmental tobacco smoke, promote a tobacco-free environment as the norm, and discourage students from starting to use tobacco. In 1988, a survey of 2,000 school districts found that 95 percent had a written policy or regulation on tobacco smoking in schools, and 17 percent totally banned smoking (i.e., no smoking allowed by anyone on school premises or at school functions).[75,76]

School-based health education programs have demonstrated that they can at least delay the onset of tobacco use among adolescents.[50,77] Tobacco use prevention can be included in the curriculum as a stand-alone program, as part of a substance abuse prevention program, or as part of a school health education curriculum.[50,77] However it is presented, a minimum of two 5-session blocks of classes on tobacco prevention, delivered in separate school years between 6th and 9th grade is recommended.[77]

Effective programs emphasize the short-term consequences of tobacco use (e.g., decreased stamina, stained teeth, foul-smelling breath and clothes, and the potential for addiction).[50,77] Social factors influencing use (e.g., parents, peers, and media) and the social consequences of use (e.g., most adolescents disapprove of peers who use tobacco) should be emphasized.[50,77] Effective programs also include an experiential component. Students can be taught to resist pressure exerted by peers or adults to use tobacco through modeling, role play, and guided rehearsal of appropriate refusal skills.[77]

Adequate teacher training is vital to the success of prevention programs. Peer involvement can also contribute to optimal results. A peer leader to assist the trained teacher with the curriculum is ideal. Parental support for tobacco prevention education is also important, and parental involvement may contribute to program success among younger students (5th grade and below).[77]

Additional emphasis needs to be placed on the cessation of smoking and smokeless tobacco use among youth. One particularly important goal is preventing the transition from experimental to regular use. As with prevention, emphasis on the short-term physiological consequences of tobacco use and the social factors influencing behavior may be more effective than information on the long-term health consequences of tobacco use in helping adolescents stop.[50]

In 1988, antismoking education was provided by 78 percent of school districts at the high school level, 81 percent at the middle/junior high school level, and 75 percent at the elementary school level.[76] The nature of the antismoking education provided is unknown. A second 1988 survey of randomly selected school districts in a small sample of States found that whereas 98 percent of the districts reported that their health curriculum included a review of the health hazards of cigarette smoking, only 83 percent included a review of the health hazards of smokeless tobacco use.[78] Furthermore, although about 70 percent of the districts addressed these topics in 7th through 9th grade, these topics were most often addressed in 10th grade (74 percent) and were covered in 5th and 6th grade in only half of the districts.

Optimally, tobacco use prevention education should be included as part of quality school health education. For a definition of quality school health education, see *Educational and Community-Based Programs*.

* * *

3.13 Enact and enforce in 50 States laws prohibiting the sale and distribution of tobacco products to youth younger than age 19. (Baseline: 44 States and the District of Columbia had, but rarely enforced, laws regulating the sale and/or distribution of cigarettes or tobacco products to minors in 1990; only 3 set the age of majority at 19 and only 6 prohibited cigarette vending machines accessible to minors)

Note: Model legislation proposed by DHHS recommends licensure of tobacco vendors, civil money penalties and license suspension or revocation for violations, and a ban on cigarette vending machines.[79]

Baseline data source: CDC 1990.

Current data indicate that four out of five smokers begin smoking before the age of 21. Two-thirds of men who have ever used smokeless tobacco started before age 21. Moreover, preadolescents are known to experiment with both cigarettes and smokeless tobacco. Given the high percentage of tobacco users who begin before adulthood, prevention efforts must focus on children and young adolescents. Individuals who start smoking early have more difficulty quitting, are more likely to become heavy smokers, and are more likely to develop a smoking-related disease. Many adolescents who smoke do not understand the nature of tobacco addiction and are unaware of, or underestimate, the important health consequences of smoking.[50]

To protect children and adolescents, appropriate public health policies must be established for the advertisement, sale, and distribution of tobacco products. These policies should reduce children's and adolescents' opportunities to experiment with tobacco products and develop a pattern of regular use by making these products less available.[50]

Strict observance of prohibitions against the sale of tobacco to minors may be the most powerful means for reducing the initiation of smoking by children.[50,80] Purchases from retailers or vending machines appear to be the main source of cigarettes for children. Restrictions on child tobacco use are fewer now than at any time in many past decades, despite what is known about the dangers of tobacco use, its addictive nature, and the early age of initiation. This situation is in sharp contrast to virtually all other tobacco-related public policy measures, which have been strengthened since the release of the 1964 Surgeon General's Report.[50]

All States should have in place, and enforce, State laws requiring at least age 19 as the minimum age for purchase of tobacco products. An age cut-off of 19 (as opposed to younger cut-offs) facilitates the elimination of tobacco from high schools. Selling or otherwise providing tobacco products to children and adolescents where age verification is difficult or impossible, such as through vending machines, should not be allowed. As Indian Nations are sovereign and are exempted from many State laws, Tribal Councils should similarly enforce prohibition of tobacco sales to Indian youth living on reservations.

3.14 **Increase to 50 the number of States with plans to reduce tobacco use, especially among youth. (Baseline: 12 States in 1989)**

Baseline data source: Association of State and Territorial Health Officials.

The health effects of tobacco use are well-documented. Tobacco use also has an impact on the community at large. Tobacco use affects the overall quality of community life by posing health threats to large numbers of people, by increasing disability, by reducing years of productivity, and by diverting resources that could be used for other pressing medical and social problems.

Effective tobacco use prevention and cessation efforts require community action, just as other public health issues usually are addressed at the State and local level. Because social factors strongly influence decisions to quit and the ability to remain tobacco free, the community can—and should—provide an environment that discourages tobacco use. Preventing tobacco addiction among youth emphasizes even more clearly the need for State and local planning.

The purpose of a State plan for prevention and cessation of tobacco use is to identify, and eventually put in place, a system of antitobacco use measures that is responsive to local conditions, and that is effective and ongoing. A wide range of strategies are needed, including educational, behavioral, social, and regulatory measures, all oriented to reducing, and eventually eliminating, tobacco use and its consequences. As outlined in the *Guide to Public Health Practice: State Health Agency Tobacco Prevention and Control Plans*, elements essential to State plans to reduce tobacco use include comprehensive planning, evaluation, funding, and community involvement.

Achieving the goal of a tobacco-free society requires increasing the priority of tobacco use as a public health issue, and improving the community's ability to promote healthier behavior. Through a State plan, tobacco prevention needs can be identified and addressed, resources can be used more efficiently and effectively, and the combined commitment of diverse groups and agencies can generate a high level of awareness of tobacco control as a community issue.

Development of a strong community norm for not using tobacco requires visible and diverse activities which continue over time. For example, a statewide approach to the prevention of tobacco use among youth might include school-based educational efforts, policies that restrict the sale of tobacco products to minors and that limit the enticements for youth to start using tobacco, and economic disincentives to purchase tobacco, such as State and local excise taxes.

Other objectives in this chapter describe school-based educational efforts (see Objective 3.10), policies that restrict the sale of tobacco products to minors (see Objective 3.13), and policies that limit the enticements for youth to start using tobacco (see Objective 3.15). Pricing policies that discourage the initiation of tobacco use by youth are another important element of many State plans.

Excise (sales) taxes raise the purchase price of tobacco products and can serve as an economic disincentive for tobacco product consumption. Cigarette price increases primarily affect smoking prevalence; the effect on the number of cigarettes per smoker appears minimal. Adolescents are especially sensitive to price changes in tobacco products. Thus, excise tax increases are an important tool for delaying and preventing the initiation of tobacco use by youth.

Although the short-term effects of an increase in tobacco product excise taxes may be modest, the long-term impact can be substantial. Furthermore, if tax increases are maintained in terms of real dollars, they can continue to discourage generations of youth from initiating tobacco use. In 1985, an analysis of the potential impact of increasing the

Federal excise tax on cigarettes from 16 to 32 cents per pack estimated that almost 3.5 million Americans would forego smoking, including more than 800,000 teenagers and almost 2 million people aged 20 through 35.[81] If a 16-cent increase were maintained in real value over time, more than 480,000 premature smoking-induced deaths would be averted for Americans aged 12 and older today.

Excise tax increases offer the added benefit of generating public revenue with relatively low administrative costs. A portion of the funds can be earmarked for tobacco use prevention programs to further deter tobacco use by youth. The capacity to simultaneously raise revenue and enhance public health has made the tobacco excise tax a particularly attractive public policy tool at both Federal and State levels.

The Federal Government has taxed cigarettes since 1864. The Federal excise tax on cigarettes is currently 16 cents per pack, having been raised from 8 cents to 16 cents in 1983, the first increase since 1951. In 1985, Federal excise taxes were imposed on snuff (24 cents per pound) and chewing tobacco (8 cents per pound). These are equivalent to a 1.8-cent tax on a 1.2-ounce can of snuff and a 1.0-cent tax on a 2-ounce pack of chewing tobacco. In addition to the Federal tax, all States, the District of Columbia, 369 towns, and 20 counties currently impose excise taxes on cigarettes.[50] As of July 30, 1990, State excise tax rates ranged from 2 cents per pack in North Carolina to 41 cents in Texas and averaged 22 cents per pack. Increasingly, States also tax the sale of smokeless tobacco. In 1964, only 14 States taxed smokeless tobacco. By 1990, this number had increased to 34.

In real terms, the Federal excise tax on cigarettes decreased by 68 percent from 1964 to 1982, and the average State tax on cigarettes declined by more than 40 percent over the past 15 years. To serve as an effective deterrent over time, excise taxes on tobacco products should be structured to increase or at least not to decrease in real terms. Replacing unit taxes on cigarettes and other tobacco products with equivalent-yield ad valorem taxes would allow revenues to keep pace with inflation-induced increases in product prices.

3.15 **Eliminate or severely restrict all forms of tobacco product advertising and promotion to which youth younger than age 18 are likely to be exposed. (Baseline: Radio and television advertising of tobacco products were prohibited, but other restrictions on advertising and promotion to which youth may be exposed were minimal in 1990)**

Baseline data source: Federal Trade Commission, reported by the Office on Smoking and Health, CDC.

Public health concern about tobacco advertising is based on the premise that such advertising perpetuates and increases cigarette consumption. Cigarette advertising may increase cigarette consumption by recruiting new smokers, inducing former smokers to relapse, making it more difficult for smokers to quit, and increasing the level of smokers' consumption by acting as an external cue to smoke.[82,83] While the tobacco industry denies that its advertising is targeted to children and adolescents, cigarette advertising is heavy in many magazines with large adolescent readerships.[83,84] Furthermore, tobacco advertisers typically employ image-based ads, which are most effective with young people and have the greatest impact on children whose poor performance in school increases the distance between their ideal and current self-image.[85]

Cigarettes are one of the most heavily advertised and promoted products in the United States.[79] In constant dollars, expenditures for cigarette advertising and promotion have increased threefold since 1975 and continue to grow. The total expenditure for cigarette advertising and promotion in 1988 was $3.3 billion, a 27-percent increase over 1987 expenditures.[79] Many experts consider promotional activities as effective or even more effective than traditional advertising in influencing smoking behavior.[86] The proportion of total expenditures spent on promotional activities (e.g., free samples, sponsorship of events) increased from 26 percent in 1975 to 68 percent in 1988.

Free samples or coupons place tobacco products directly into the hands of the consumer. Although the tobacco industry's voluntary codes prohibit the distribution of cigarette samples to individuals under 21 years of age and the distribution of smokeless tobacco to people younger than 18, widespread violation of these codes is evident.[87]

Tobacco companies also sponsor sporting, cultural, and other special events. Rock concerts, rodeos, skiing competitions, and golf and tennis tournaments help to deliver the youth market to sponsoring tobacco companies, which reinforce their presence by putting brand names on promotional products such as T-shirts and hats. Television coverage of these events broadcasts product names and logos to millions of adolescents for hours at a time.

Tobacco advertising and promotion also adversely affect media coverage of tobacco-related health issues. Studies have shown a significant inverse relationship between magazine and newspaper dependence on tobacco advertising revenue and coverage of smoking and health topics.[50,88] Tobacco sponsorship of organizations and events also appears to discourage organizations from speaking out and educating their constituents about smoking and health.

Preventing the exposure of youth to tobacco advertising and promotion could be accomplished by advertising limitations (e.g., prohibiting tobacco advertising in publications with a substantial teenage readership, prohibiting tobacco sponsorship of sporting events with a substantial teenage and preteenage audience, prohibiting billboards within a certain distance of schools) or by a total ban on tobacco advertising and promotion. Also, prohibiting the use of imagery in ads and allowing only words and a picture of the product itself (i.e., tombstone advertising) would protect minors from the pictorial themes now used to glamorize tobacco use.[50,83,84]

3.16 **Increase to at least 75 percent the proportion of primary care and oral health care providers who routinely advise cessation and provide assistance and followup for all of their tobacco-using patients. (Baseline: About 52 percent of internists reported counseling more than 75 percent of their smoking patients about smoking cessation in 1986; about 35 percent of dentists reported counseling at least 75 percent of their smoking patients about smoking in 1986)**

Baseline data sources: For internists, Wells et al. 1986; for dentists, Secker-Walker et al. 1989.

This objective capitalizes on the unique position of the primary care provider. About 70 percent of adult smokers visit a physician every year. Primary care providers see both motivated and unmotivated users of tobacco, are considered credible sources of health information and advice, and often see patients during a "teachable moment." Furthermore, 71 percent of all heavy smokers surveyed stated that they would stop if their doctor so urged them.[89]

Brief smoking cessation counseling by primary care physicians has been shown to be effective.[90,91] Such counseling may include information about the dangers of tobacco use and the benefits of stopping, personalized cessation advice, selection of a target date, written self-help materials, appropriate referral, and, when indicated, a pharmacologic aid to quitting. Followup visits or telephone calls, especially during the first 4 to 8 weeks, make cessation attempts more likely to succeed.[45,92] Use of office reminder systems can increase both the provision of cessation advice by providers and the rate of quitting among their patients.[93]

The U.S. Preventive Services Task Force recommended that smoking cessation counseling be included as part of the periodic health examination.[45] If every primary care provider offered the brief intervention outlined above to all of their tobacco using patients, then approximately 1 million Americans, over and above the 1.3 million that quit annually, would stop using tobacco in a year.[91,94,95] Advice from all types of primary care providers (e.g., physicians, physician assistants, nurse practitioners, and nurse midwives) and oral health care providers (e.g., dentists, dental hygienists) would reach even more people and serve to repeat the message for many patients.

Although the health benefits of smoking cessation are well-established, physicians frequently fail to advise smokers to quit. In seven studies that relied on physician self-report (including two national surveys of family practitioners), the proportion of smokers counseled to stop smoking ranged from 52 percent to 97 percent.[44] A recent national survey of internists found that 98 percent of internists routinely obtained and recorded the smoking histories of patients new to their practice and 70 percent discussed reducing or stopping tobacco use at every visit with tobacco-using patients.[43] Even lower percentages of smokers counseled were found in three chart audit studies (63 percent) and three consumer surveys (about 40 percent of smokers said they received counseling from a physician).[44] Furthermore, although physicians accurately acknowledge abstinence from smoking as a primary means of preventing disease,[96] many patients do not receive such advice until serious health problems exist. Results from a national survey of internists, for example, indicate that while 82 percent of the internists report that they counsel more than 75 percent of smokers with heart disease, only 52 percent of the internists counsel more than 75 percent of all their patients who smoke.[97] These providers appear to be oriented more toward tertiary rather than primary prevention.

Several reports suggest doctors may lack the preparation to adequately facilitate patient cessation.[98,99,100,101] The National Cancer Institute has developed a program to educate medical and dental clinicians about tobacco-use intervention. Such a program can be applied to all health care situations. A wide variety of materials are available from the National Cancer Institute and other organizations for use by health care providers in counseling patients to quit.[102] Training on cessation should be available in all health care undergraduate, graduate, and continuing education programs.[103,104]

* * *

Research Needs

Research on the initiation of tobacco use

- Develop/refine risk-based classifications for children and adolescents that describe the full continuum of initiation risk (e.g., pre-contemplators, contemplators, experimenters, regular users).

- Identify the determinants of experimentation and initiation (i.e., the determinants of progression along the risk continuum described above).

- Evaluate the effectiveness of combined interventions (e.g., school-based programs and mass media) on smoking initiation, and determine which intervention elements are effective in delaying onset, maintaining delayed onset, and preventing initiation.

Research on regular smokers trying to quit

- Identify quit attempt determinants.
- Identify barriers to making a quit attempt (e.g., lifetime quitting history, perceived self-efficacy).
- Evaluate the effectiveness of different interventions (particularly advice from primary care providers, mass media campaigns, and telephone counseling) in motivating smokers to make a quit attempt.

Research on preventing relapse

- Assess the magnitude of the relapse problem.
- Develop classifications for recent quitters and former smokers based on length of time abstinent that describe and predict relapse risk.
- Identify the determinants of relapse for former smokers at all levels of relapse risk.
- Develop and evaluate innovative programs to prevent relapse by former smokers at all levels of relapse risk.
- Establish valid criteria for when to label a former smoker a "confirmed ex-smoker."

Research on tobacco policies

Evaluate the effectiveness of public policies in reducing the initiation of tobacco use and/or increasing tobacco use cessation. In particular, evaluate:

- Policies that affect children's access to tobacco products.
- Policies that affect children's exposure to advertising and promotion of tobacco products.
- Policies that restrict smoking in the workplace.

* * *

Baseline Data Source References

Adult Use of Tobacco Survey, Office on Smoking and Health, Centers for Disease Control, Public Health Service, U.S. Department of Health and Human Services.

Association of State and Territorial Health Officials, McLean, Virginia.

Behavioral Risk Factor Surveillance System, Centers for Disease Control, Public Health Service, Department of Health and Human Services.

Centers for Disease Control. Indian Health Service facilities become smoke-free. *Morbidity and Mortality Weekly Report* 36:348-350, 1987.

Centers for Disease Control. Prevalence of oral lesions and smokeless tobacco use in Northern Plains Indians. *Morbidity and Mortality Weekly Report* 37:608-611, 1988.

Centers for Disease Control. State laws restricting minors' access to tobacco. *Morbidity and Mortality Weekly Report* 39:349-353, 1990.

Federal Trade Commission, Washington, DC.

Fingerhut, L.A.; Kleinman, J.C.; and Kendrick, J.S. Smoking before, during, and after pregnancy. *American Journal of Public Health*, 80(1990):541-544.

Hispanic Health and Nutrition Examination Survey, National Center for Health Statistics, Centers for Disease Control, Public Health Service, Department of Health and Human Services.

National Health Interview Survey, National Center for Health Statistics, Centers for Disease Control, Public Health Service, Department of Health and Human Services.

National Household Survey on Drug Abuse, National Institute on Drug Abuse, Alcohol, Drug Abuse, and Mental Health Administration, Public Health Service, Department of Health and Human Services.

National School Boards Association. *Smoke-Free Schools: A Progress Report*. Alexandria, VA: the Association, 1989.

Secker-Walker, R.H.; Solomon, L.J.; and Hill, H.C. A statewide survey of dentists' smoking cessation advice. *Journal of the American Dental Association* 118:37-40, 1989.

U.S. Department of Defense. *Worldwide Survey of Substance Abuse and Health Behavior Among Military Personnel. Report of the Research Triangle, Institute to the Office of the Assistant Secretary of Defense (Public Affairs)*. Washington DC: the Department, 1988.

Wells, K.B.; Lewis, C.E.; Leake, B.; Schleiter, M.K.; Brook, R.H. The practices of general and subspecialty internists in counseling about smoking and exercise. *American Journal of Public Health* 76:1009-1013, 1986.

Alcohol and Other Drugs

Contents

4.1	Alcohol-related motor vehicle crash deaths

* * *

4.5	Average age of first use
4.6	Use by young people
4.7	Heavy drinking by high school seniors and college students
4.8	Alcohol consumption
4.9	Perception of social disapproval by high school seniors
4.10	Perception of harm by high school seniors
4.11	Anabolic steroid use
4.12	Access to treatment programs
4.13	Alcohol and drug education in schools

* * *

4.16	Policies to reduce minors' access to alcohol
4.17	Restrictions on promotion of alcohol to youth
4.18	Alcohol concentration tolerance levels
4.19	Screening, counseling, and referral by clinicians for alcohol/drug problems
	[Research Needs]

4

4. Alcohol and Other Drugs

* * *

Health Status Objectives

4.1   Reduce deaths caused by alcohol-related motor vehicle crashes to no more than 8.5 per 100,000 people. (Age-adjusted baseline: 9.8 per 100,000 in 1987)

Special Population Targets

Alcohol-Related Motor Vehicle Crash Deaths (per 100,000)	1987 Baseline	2000 Target
* * *		
4.1b People aged 15-24	21.5	18

Baseline data source: Fatal Accident Reporting System, U.S. Department of Transportation.

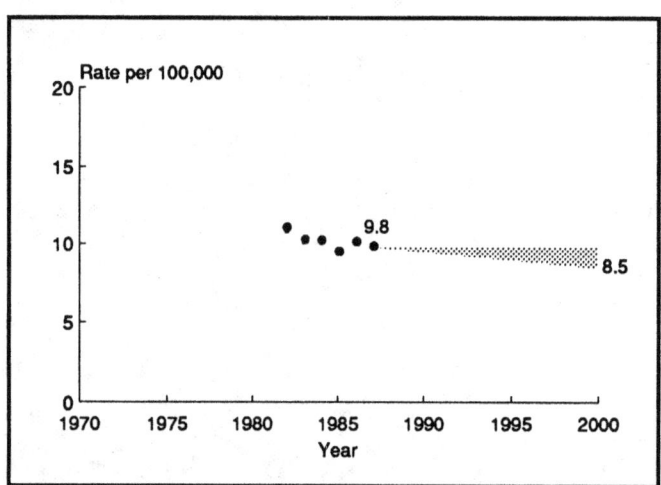

Fig. 4.1

Age-adjusted alcohol-related motor vehicle crash death rate

This objective is stated in terms of fatalities because of the availability of reliable and precise data regarding deaths caused by motor vehicle crashes. Injuries are also a serious problem. Although decreases in deaths may indicate parallel reductions in injuries, improvements in occupant protection and emergency medical services may prevent deaths while the incidence of crash-related injuries is actually increasing. In general, there is a need to improve surveillance of injuries caused by motor vehicle crashes, including those involving alcohol.

In 1987, motor vehicle crashes were the fifth leading cause of death in the United States, and approximately half of these were alcohol-related.[105] Many more people were seriously injured and permanently disabled. Alcohol-related traffic crashes are the leading cause of death and spinal cord injury for young Americans.

The alcohol-related proportion of crash deaths dropped by 10 to 15 percent between 1982 and 1986 because of the emergence of highly visible citizen activist groups, the media attention that such groups generated, and resulting increases in deterrence activities involving legislation, increased enforcement of alcohol-impaired driving laws (including roadside sobriety checkpoints), and more frequent use of sanctions such as license suspensions and revocations. For instance, State laws that uniformly establish age 21 as the minimum alcohol purchase age were associated with an overall reduction of nearly 13 percent in the fatal accident involvement rate for youth under 21.[106] In 1988, the Surgeon General of the U.S. Public Health Service explicitly recognized the contribution of alcohol advertising to the problem of drinking and driving and called for increased regulation of alcohol advertising.[107]

The levels of citizen activism, enforcement, and sanctioning activity have declined to some extent in recent years. As a result, progress in further reducing alcohol-related crashes has slowed since 1985.[106] These shifts in alcohol-related crash deaths show how united citizen, private business, and government concern and action can bring attention to a problem and develop strategies to address it.

Much more remains to be done. Other needed measures include increased media attention to alcohol-impaired driving laws and their enforcement, enforcement of alcohol beverage control laws regarding access to alcohol by minors, and increased testing of drivers involved in fatal and serious injury cases.

* * *

Risk Reduction Objectives

4.5   **Increase by at least 1 year the average age of first use of cigarettes, alcohol, and marijuana by adolescents aged 12 through 17. (Baseline: Age 11.6 for cigarettes, age 13.1 for alcohol, and age 13.4 for marijuana in 1988)**

Baseline data source: National Household Survey of Drug Abuse, ADAMHA.

Drug use among young people appears to develop in predictable stages, consistent with the "gateway" concept.[108] This concept suggests that experimentation with drugs usually begins with cigarettes, alcohol, or marijuana, and then progresses to other drugs. Young people engage in relatively little experimentation with most illicit drugs before the final 3 years of high school. Less than 11 percent of the class of 1986 had tried any illicit drug except marijuana before they entered the 10th grade. However, 50 percent of the high school seniors who had ever used marijuana already had used it before entering high school, while an even greater percentage of pre-high school students had already used alcohol.[109]

This objective is particularly important because the use of drugs at preteen ages, especially use of these gateway drugs, appears to predict both greater involvement with alcohol and with other drugs and less likelihood of recovery. The use of cigarettes, alcohol, and marijuana is correlated with other health problems including adolescent suicide, homicide, school dropout, motor vehicle crashes, delinquency, early sexual activity, sexually transmitted diseases, and problem pregnancy.[110] People who begin smoking in childhood are more inclined toward heavy smoking or drinking at an earlier age than those who start later. They also are more likely to abuse other drugs. Young adults are unlikely to develop alcohol and drug problems if age of first use is delayed beyond childhood and adolescence.[111]

Marijuana use exemplifies the age-at-first-use phenomenon. Use of marijuana prior to age 15 has been associated with both heavier use after 15 and the use of other drugs.[111,112]

4.6 **Reduce the proportion of young people who have used alcohol, marijuana, and cocaine in the past month, as follows:**

Substance/Age	1988 Baseline	2000 Target
Alcohol/aged 12-17	25.2%	12.6%
Alcohol/aged 18-20	57.9%	29%
Marijuana/aged 12-17	6.4%	3.2%
Marijuana/aged 18-25	15.5%	7.8%
Cocaine/aged 12-17	1.1%	0.6%
Cocaine/aged 18-25	4.5%	2.3%

Note: The targets of this objective are consistent with the goals established by the Office of National Drug Control Policy, Executive Office of the President.

Baseline data source: National Household Survey of Drug Abuse, ADAMHA.

Mind-altering and addictive substances have been shown to jeopardize physical, mental, and social development during the formative years and to endanger the successful transition from school to the workplace. Moreover, use of these substances, including alcohol, is illegal for young people and thus may have long-term implications for such things as employment and schooling.[113]

Of particular concern is drug use among school dropouts, lower income, inner-city youth whose rates of use do not appear to have declined as much as rates among general population youth. Also of particular concern is the increasing rate of use among pregnant teenagers whose pregnancies must be considered at high risk even without drug involvement.[114,115]

4.7 **Reduce the proportion of high school seniors and college students engaging in recent occasions of heavy drinking of alcoholic beverages to no more than 28 percent of high school seniors and 32 percent of college students. (Baseline: 33 percent of high school seniors and 41.7 percent of college students in 1989)**

Note: Recent heavy drinking is defined as having 5 or more drinks on 1 occasion in the previous 2-week period as monitored by self-reports.

Baseline data source: Monitoring the Future (High School Senior Survey), ADAMHA.

Heavy drinking among youth has been conclusively linked to such problems as motor vehicle crashes and deaths, physical fights, destroyed property, academic troubles, job troubles, and troubles with law enforcement authorities.[109] In recent years, binge drinking among high school seniors has only declined in modest increments. About one-third of high school seniors reported having 5 or more drinks in a row on at least one occasion in the past 2 weeks.[109]

The declining pattern of alcohol use among high school seniors is an indication of the feasibility of a 25-percent reduction target for the young adult population. The development of school-based and community-based prevention programs and the increase in awareness through media and other communication channels may account for the gradual decline. The possibility of serious medical and economic consequences for individuals, families, and society make prevention and early intervention essential.

4.8   Reduce alcohol consumption by people aged 14 and older to an annual average of no more than 2 gallons of ethanol per person. (Baseline: 2.54 gallons of ethanol in 1987)

Baseline data source: National Institute on Alcohol Abuse and Alcoholism, ADAMHA.

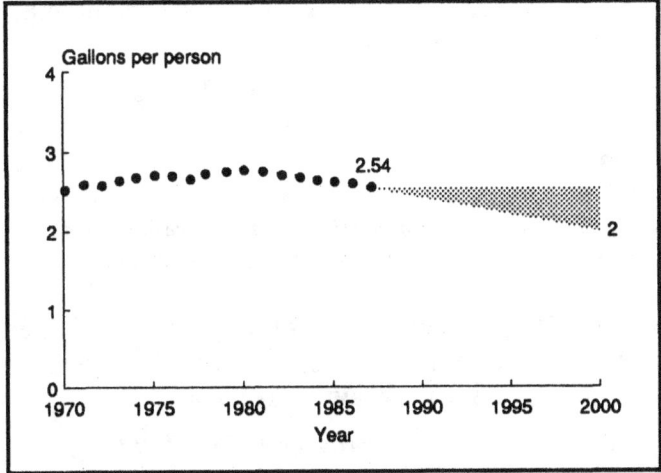

Fig. 4.8

Average consumption of ethanol per person per year

While any drinking by people under 21 years of age is illegal and undesirable, existing statistics provide estimates of per capita consumption for the population over age 14. These estimates are based on population figures as they relate to information on beverage sales, tax receipt data, or both, which come primarily from States, with some data from beverage industry sources.

The overall downward trend, after a peak in 1981 at 2.76 gallons per person over age 14, masks substantial differences in consumption trends for types of alcoholic beverages. For example, wine has shown an increase in the past 10 years with no evidence of any decline, partly due to soaring wine cooler sales since their introduction in 1983. Beer consumption increased from 1977 to 1981 but declined slightly in following years. Spirits consumption declined 20.5 percent between 1978, the peak year, and 1986.[4] The decreasing trend in alcohol consumption can be attributed to a variety of factors, including changing lifestyles and heightened awareness of the health and safety risks of alcohol consumption.

Consumption of alcohol can be influenced by laws and regulations, particularly those that have an impact on alcoholic beverage prices and minimum drinking age laws. Studies on the effects of the price of alcohol on consumption and alcohol-related problems among people aged 16 to 21 concluded that "higher real prices for beer, the most popular alcoholic beverage among youth, would reduce not only the number of young people who drink but also the incidence of heavy drinking and of frequent drinking."[117] The price of alcoholic beverages can most effectively be increased by increased taxation. Studies on the effects of minimum legal drinking ages on alcohol consumption by young people aged 16 to 21 reported that "frequency of consumption of beer is inversely related to the minimum legal age for its purchase."[117]

Now that the legal drinking age has been raised to 21 in all States, progress on the objective can be achieved through stricter enforcement of the minimum age laws. For example, tracking procedures can be implemented that maintain a statistical record of establishments reported to have made illegal sales of alcoholic beverages to youths.

Alcohol advertising can also influence youths as well as adults in their decisions about drinking. Sponsorships and promotions on college campuses by alcohol producers and the use of celebrities and youth-oriented musical groups in advertising create a prodrinking environment.[107]

4.9 Increase the proportion of high school seniors who perceive social disapproval associated with the heavy use of alcohol, occasional use of marijuana, and experimentation with cocaine, as follows:

Behavior	1989 Baseline	2000 Target
Heavy use of alcohol	56.4%	70%
Occasional use of marijuana	71.1%	85%
Trying cocaine once or twice	88.9%	95%

Note: Heavy drinking is defined as having 5 or more drinks once or twice each weekend.
Baseline data source: Monitoring the Future Study (High School Senior Survey), ADAMHA.

4.10 Increase the proportion of high school seniors who associate risk of physical or psychological harm with the heavy use of alcohol, regular use of marijuana, and experimentation with cocaine, as follows:

Behavior	1989 Baseline	2000 Target
Heavy use of alcohol	44%	70%
Regular use of marijuana	77.5%	90%
Trying cocaine once or twice	54.9%	80%

Note: Heavy drinking is defined as having 5 or more drinks once or twice each weekend.
Baseline data source: Monitoring the Future Study (High School Senior Survey), ADAMHA.

Recently, investigators reported that the 10-year decline (from 1978 to 1987) in marijuana use by high school seniors can be directly attributed to the dramatic increase in the perceived risk of psychological and physical harm and the increased perception of social disapproval associated with regular use of marijuana.[118] A similar relationship seemed to occur between increased perceived risk of use and decreased reported use of cocaine from 1986 to 1987. In a comparable fashion, these two prevention factors, if emphasized at the national level, may also be instrumental in the future prevention of tobacco and alcohol use, particularly by adolescents.

Although lifestyle factors such as truancy, religious values, or political beliefs are linked to individual differences in the use of marijuana, these factors do not explain the general downward trend in marijuana use since 1978. Rather, "if perceived risks and disapproval associated with regular marijuana use had not risen substantially in recent years, the decline in actual use would not have occurred."[118]

It is important to note that current users uniformly deny the risks of using marijuana. Thus, whereas the trend in increased perceptions of risk is encouraging, additional efforts must be made to alter the behavior of users.

4.11 Reduce to no more than 3 percent the proportion of male high school seniors who use anabolic steroids. (Baseline: 4.7 percent in 1989)

Baseline data source: Monitoring the Future Study (High School Senior Survey), ADAMHA.
Anabolic steroids have legitimate therapeutic uses and therefore can be prescribed appropriately. Their inappropriate use as a part of regimens for body-building and strength-enhancing pose new problems, especially among young men engaged in athletic pursuits. To date, they appear not to have become a part of the illicit drug culture and are not procured principally through illegal channels. Control of the risks they pose as a result

of inappropriate use is a matter of proper regulation, as well as professional and consumer awareness, to ensure drug safety.

It is estimated that there are over one million current or previous users of anabolic-androgenic steroids in the United States, with approximately one-half this group comprised of adolescents. The role of anabolic steroid use in the etiology of various diseases is unclear, but studies have associated it with changes in the physiology of organs and body systems with potential for subsequent health problems. The best documented effects include those on the liver, serum lipids, and the reproductive system. Other suspected areas of concern include cerebrovascular accidents and prostatic changes. A recent population-based study demonstrated that a significant proportion of adolescent users report behaviors, perceptions, and opinions which are consistent with psychological dependence on this drug.[119]

Services and Protection Objectives

4.12 **Establish and monitor in 50 States comprehensive plans to ensure access to alcohol and drug treatment programs for traditionally underserved people. (Baseline data available in 1991)**

While many alcohol and other drug abuse treatment programs exist, access to these programs is limited by structural, economic, linguistic, and cultural barriers. These barriers preclude provision of adequate services and thus limit the potential for controlling and reducing alcohol and drug abuse in the Nation. The following populations have the most trouble getting appropriate treatment:

- People with low incomes. Coverage for alcohol and drug abuse services under private and public financing programs is consistently less in amount and scope of benefits than coverage for general health care services. Thus, treatment is greatly dependent upon the individuals' or families' ability to pay. For the uninsured working population and the Nation's homeless population, financing of treatment poses an intractable barrier.

- Women. Women have limited access to drug and alcohol services because of their unique needs, especially pregnant women and mothers with young children. Because of the specific risks to the fetus of alcohol and drug use during pregnancy, programs are needed that specifically address the needs of pregnant women.

- Youth. Adolescent drug and alcohol users have unique needs and problems that cannot be adequately addressed in programs designed for adults. Treatment models specifically designed to serve the needs of youthful users have only recently begun to be developed but can be expected to expand during the 1990s. Special attention to the treatment needs of homeless, runaway, and school-dropout youth is needed.

- Minorities. Nonwhite and non-English-speaking minority populations require treatment programs that take into account specific cultural influences on alcohol and other drug use and that impose no language barriers. Concerted attention should be given to the development of multilingual, multicultural treatment programs.

- Inmates in correctional facilities. A large proportion of incarcerated offenders have varying degrees of alcohol and drug abuse problems. The majority of treatment programs available in prisons, however, are underfunded and understaffed.

When offenders are released, the probability is great that their untreated alcohol and drug problems will reemerge along with criminal behavior.

Data are scarce for determining the number of people in these populations who are not currently being treated because of a lack of appropriate, accessible services. New data systems to measure the prevalence of alcohol and drug problems may help to improve this situation, though these systems will need to be designed specifically to capture information about the needs of these special populations who are at highest risk. The State Substance Abuse Services Plans, analyzed by the Office for Treatment Improvement of the Alcohol, Drug Abuse, and Mental Health Administration will be analyzed to establish a baseline and track this objective.

4.13 **Provide to children in all school districts and private schools primary and secondary school educational programs on alcohol and other drugs, preferably as part of quality school health education. (Baseline: 63 percent provided some instruction, 39 percent provided counseling, and 23 percent referred students for clinical assessments in 1987)**

Baseline data source: *Report to Congress and the White House on the Nature and Effectiveness of Federal, State, and Local Drug Prevention/Education Programs*, U.S. Department of Education, 1987.

Legislation passed by Congress and signed by the President declares alcohol and other drug education and prevention to be essential components of a comprehensive strategy to reduce demand for and use of drugs in the United States. This commitment to prevention and education is underscored by funding provided for these programs; a total of $355 million was appropriated by Congress in fiscal year 1989 for prevention programs supported by the Department of Education alone.

A quality school health education program should provide factual information about the harmful effects of drugs, support and strengthen students' resistance to using drugs, carry out collaborative drug-abuse prevention efforts with parents and other community members, and be supported by strong school policies as well as services for confidential identification, assessment, referral to treatment, and support groups (often provided through a student assistance program) for drug users. For a definition of quality school health education, see *Educational and Community-Based Programs*.

Traditionally, alcohol and other drug education programs have focused on junior and senior high school students. However, as indicated by statistics for the average age of first use of the gateway drugs, prevention must also be directed to elementary school students. It is particularly crucial to prevent or at least delay the use of alcohol and other drugs by children and teenagers because rapid growth can amplify the physiological and psychological effects.

State boards of education, governing boards of State university systems, and State legislatures can play a crucial role by mandating school drug and alcohol policies and alcohol and other drug education and prevention programs. About three-quarters of the States have already taken action to require such education. States can also set minimum curriculum standards for drug and alcohol education and require teaching certification in the subject. States can disseminate data on effective prevention practices and assist local educational agencies and communities in surveying drug use and evaluating prevention programs.

* * *

4. Alcohol and Other Drugs

4.16 Increase to 50 the number of States that have enacted and enforce policies, beyond those in existence in 1989, to reduce access to alcoholic beverages by minors.

Note: Policies to reduce access to alcoholic beverages by minors may include those that address restriction of the sale of alcoholic beverages at recreational and entertainment events at which youth make up a majority of participants/consumers, product pricing, penalties and license-revocation for sale of alcoholic beverages to minors, and other approaches designed to discourage and restrict purchase of alcoholic beverages by minors.

Although changes in laws regulating minimum drinking age in all States have had some effect on consumption of alcoholic beverages by adolescents and young adults, they have not eliminated access to alcohol nor deterred many adolescents from drinking.[120] Other interventions are needed as well to restrict access to and discourage use of alcoholic beverages by young people under age 21. Localities and States can enact restrictions on sale of alcoholic beverages at entertainment recreational events where teenagers compose the majority of participants and observers.

An understanding of characteristics of environments that promote or reduce alcohol consumption and alcohol use problems is relevant to the development of effective prevention policies and programs. For adolescents, clearly some influences are beyond direct control of State policies, such as family attitudes toward drinking, peer value systems, and individual risk characteristics. However, policies can be designed to shape environmental factors that either facilitate or help to control use of alcoholic beverages by teenagers.

Many young people are able to make their own direct purchases, despite laws and ordinances making sale to minors illegal. More effective enforcement procedures, with effective sanctions imposed on those establishments that fail to obey these laws, can be imposed to curtail access. Policies that hold parents responsible for their children's possession and use of alcoholic beverages can also become the basis for local programs to reduce the prevalence of drinking behavior among youth.

Among the other policy-related changes that States can consider are regulations of the types of establishments that may sell alcoholic beverages. Such means as use of zoning ordinances, restriction of hours of sale, and determinations of whether alcoholic beverages may be sold for on-site or off-site consumption can be used to address the patterns of adolescent purchasing and drinking behaviors. In addition, changes in price—including Federal, State and local taxes—may affect both alcohol consumption patterns and alcohol-involved automobile crashes. Evidence about the association between price and alcohol consumption comes from the results of natural experiments (e.g., comparisons of alcohol consumption in States with differing taxes on alcohol), as well as from econometric research, which uses available data to make projections about the possible impact of price changes on consumption and alcohol use problems through statistical modeling.

Econometric studies examined the effects of price on alcohol consumption and alcohol-involved automobile crashes. These studies used the existing prices of alcoholic beverages in the young people's places of residence as a base and derived estimates from available data on alcohol use among youth aged 16 to 21 in the United States between 1975 and 1981.[121,122] Controlling for other variables that may be related to alcohol use and fatal motor vehicle crashes, such as age, sex, and family income, these studies have projected that higher real prices for beer would reduce the incidence of heavy drinking and frequent drinking among young people, as well as the number of young people who drink.[122,123]

Stable Federal excise taxes combined with only modest increases in State and local excise taxes have contributed to a decline in the real price of alcoholic beverages.[121] The Federal tax on alcohol in beer and wine has remained constant since 1951, and the tax on alcohol in distilled spirits was increased in 1985 after remaining unchanged for nearly 35 years.[121] Further, the Federal excise tax on alcohol in beer, the most popular beverage among youths who use alcohol, is less than one-third the tax on alcohol in distilled spirits.[121] Between 1960 and 1980, the real price of beer fell by 27 percent; the real price of wine, by 20 percent; and the real price of spirits, by 48 percent.[124] To serve as an effective deterrent over time, excise tax on alcohol products should be structured to increase or at least not to decrease in real terms. Indexing alcohol taxes would allow the price of alcohol to keep pace with inflation.

In terms of fatal automobile crashes, it is estimated that a 100-percent increase in the real beer tax (approximately $1.50 per 24-unit case of 12-ounce cans) would reduce highway mortality among 15- to 17-year-old drivers by about 18 percent; among 18- to 21-year-old drivers, by about 27 percent; and among 21- to 24-year-old drivers, by about 19 percent.[125] A tax amounting to approximately 35 percent of the retail price of beer is projected to halve the number of alcohol-related fatalities among 16- to 21-year-old drivers, a 50-percent tax would eliminate approximately 75 percent of these deaths.[126]

Higher prices for alcohol were also found to be related to lower rates of heavy drinking. Cirrhosis mortality, an indicator of 10 to 20 years of heavy drinking by individuals, is found to be lower in 30 States that raised distilled spirits taxes, compared to States that did not raise taxes.[124] It is projected that an increase of $1 in State distilled spirits tax rates from 1962 to 1977, would have reduced cirrhosis mortality by nearly 2 percent in a State, and that doubling the Federal distilled spirits tax would have reduced cirrhosis mortality by 20 percent in the Nation.

Taxes on alcohol are estimated to cover only about half the lifetime discounted costs that drinkers impose on others through collectively financed health insurance, pensions, disability, group life insurance, fines, motor vehicle accidents, and criminal justice costs.[127] Specifically, these "external costs" total $0.48 per ounce of alcohol consumed, approximately twice the current average (State plus Federal) excise and sales taxes on alcoholic beverages. These external costs are dominated by costs associated with alcohol-related traffic crashes.

Equalizing the taxes for wine and beer to those for spirits, adjusting the level for inflation since 1970, and adding the average current State alcohol tax level, would total 70 cents per ounce of ethanol, a level consistent with the recommendations of the Surgeon General's Workshop on Drunk Driving.[107]

4.17 Increase to at least 20 the number of States that have enacted statutes to restrict promotion of alcoholic beverages that is focused principally on young audiences. (Baseline data available in 1992)

Experts have directed specific attention to public policy approaches to reduce illicit use of alcohol by young people.[107] In addition to taxation measures to increase the price of alcohol, these include measures to restrict or control the serving of alcoholic beverages in settings where young people comprise the majority of possible consumers, and limitations on promotion focusing principally on young audiences. Establishing a baseline and tracking of this objective will be carried out by the Office of Alcohol and State Programs, National Highway Traffic Safety Administration, U.S. Department of Transportation.

Advertisements and promotion have been found to stimulate alcohol consumption of adults and adolescents to at least a modest degree.[128] Although advertising appears to have a more limited effect on excessive, hazardous, and problematic drinking, it may be a significant contributing factor in creating or reinforcing these adverse alcohol use patterns.

Although single young males are more likely to report frequent heavy drinking and drinking-related problems,[129] and drivers under the age of 21 have the highest rates of alcohol-involved fatal traffic crashes,[130] little research has examined alcohol advertisements targeted specifically at college students.[131] The average number of inches of national alcohol advertising per college newspaper issue was lower in 1984-85 than in 1977-78, but during both periods the amount of space devoted to alcohol advertising greatly exceeded advertising for books and soft drinks. In the 1977-78 period, 34.6 column inches per issue were devoted to alcohol advertising, compared to 1.4 for books and 1.2 for soft drinks.[132] During 1984-85, 23.8 inches were devoted to alcohol, 1.3 to books, and 0.5 to soft drinks.[131]

At the time of the 1984-85 study, not all States had raised their minimum drinking age for alcoholic beverages to 21. However, extensive alcohol advertising was found even at colleges in States where the minimum drinking age was 21. There were no significant differences in total column inches devoted to alcohol advertising between the States with a drinking age of 21 and those with a lower minimum.[131] Furthermore, in 1984-85, where space devoted to national alcohol advertising was compared with all national advertising, a greater proportion of national advertising was given to alcohol advertising in schools with lower male enrollments.

4.18 **Extend to 50 States legal blood alcohol concentration tolerance levels of .04 percent for motor vehicle drivers aged 21 and older and .00 percent for those younger than age 21. (Baseline: 0 States in 1990)**

Baseline data source: National Institute on Alcohol Abuse and Alcoholism, ADAMHA.

A blood alcohol concentration of 0.10 percent significantly affects the ability to drive by impairing vision, perception, judgment, reaction time, and the ability to brake and control speed. The Surgeon General's Workshop on Drunk Driving recommended changes in State laws relating to acceptable blood alcohol concentration tolerance levels in drivers.[107] Those States that have adopted lower legal levels for drivers under age 21 have already experienced decreases in fatalities among this age group.

4.19 **Increase to at least 75 percent the proportion of primary care providers who screen for alcohol and other drug use problems and provide counseling and referral as needed. (Baseline data available in 1992)**

Recommendations from a number of professional associations and the U.S. Preventive Services Task Force concur that primary health care providers have an important responsibility regarding counseling to prevent alcohol and other drug abuse problems, case finding, and referral to self-help resources and treatment services.[45] Particular concern is directed toward adolescent patients and pregnant women. Though baseline data are unavailable, several local studies of physician practice report that as many as about 34 percent of physicians provide counseling to those patients whom they believed to be drinking alcohol excessively.[133] Patient records confirm this counseling for about 18 percent.[134] This objective supports increasing the proportion who regularly provide such counseling related to alcohol as well as other drug use. The Office of Disease Prevention and Health Promotion will initiate a survey of primary care providers to establish baseline data and track this objective in 1992.

* * *

Research Needs

If progress is to continue toward reducing disability and death related to alcohol and other drug use, the following areas must be addressed to achieve a sound research base:

- The interaction of biological, family (parental and other modeling), environmental, and psychological processes that are associated with the risk of, or resistance to, using alcohol and other drugs and the transition from use to abuse of drugs.

- The relationship between community/environmental factors and the support of or barriers to alcohol abuse and other drug-using behaviors.

- Etiology of the use of cocaine and cocaine derivatives as well as new drugs that are increasingly used, including steroids.

- Evaluation of interventions to understand more fully the extent to which new skills (e.g., coping skills, parental skills) produce resistance to alcohol abuse and drug use and maintenance of this resistance over time.

- Evaluation of the effectiveness of state-of-the-art model prevention intervention strategies.

- The physical, social, economic and psychological consequences of illicit drug use.

In addition, renewed commitment is needed to assure diffusion of the results of etiologic and intervention research to service practitioners and educators.

Baseline Data Source References

Fatal Accident Reporting System, National Highway Traffic Safety Administration, U.S. Department of Transportation, Washington, DC.

Monitoring the Future Study (High School Senior Survey), Alcohol, Drug Abuse, and Mental Health Administration, Public Health Service, U.S. Department of Health and Human Services, Rockville, MD.

National Household Survey of Drug Abuse, National Institute on Drug abuse, Alcohol, Drug Abuse, and Mental Health Administration, Public Health Service, U.S. Department of Health and Human Services, Rockville, MD.

National Institute on Alcohol Abuse and Alcoholism, Alcohol, Drug Abuse, and Mental Health Administration, Public Health Service, U.S. Department of Health and Human Services, Rockville, MD.

Report to Congress and the White House on the Nature and Effectiveness of Federal, State, and Local Drug Prevention/Education Program. Washington, DC: U.S. Department of Education, 1987.

Family Planning

5

Contents

5.1	Adolescent pregnancy
5.2	Unintended pregnancy
5.3	Infertility
5.4	Adolescent postponent of sexual intercourse
5.5	Adolescent abstinence from sexual intercourse
5.6	Contraception use by sexually active adolescents
5.7	Effective family planning
5.8	Family discussion of human sexuality
5.9	Counseling about adoption
5.10	Age-appropriate preconception counseling by clinicians
5.11	Clinic services for HIV and other sexually transmitted diseases
	[Research Needs]

5. Family Planning

* * *

Health Status Objectives

5.1 Reduce pregnancies among girls aged 17 and younger to no more than 50 per 1,000 adolescents. (Baseline: 71.1 pregnancies per 1,000 girls aged 15 through 17 in 1985)

Special Population Targets

Pregnancies (per 1,000)	*1985 Baseline*	*2000 Target*
5.1a Black adolescent girls aged 15-19	186†	120
5.1b Hispanic adolescent girls aged 15-19	158	105

†*Non-white adolescents*

Note: For black and Hispanic adolescent girls, baseline data are unavailable for those aged 15 through 17. The targets for these two populations are based on data for women aged 15 through 19. If more complete data become available, a 35-percent reduction from baseline figures should be used as the target.

Baseline data source: The Alan Guttmacher Institute, calculated using birth data from the National Vital Statistics System, characteristics of abortion patients compiled by the Centers for Disease Control, and abortion data collected by the Alan Guttmacher Institute.

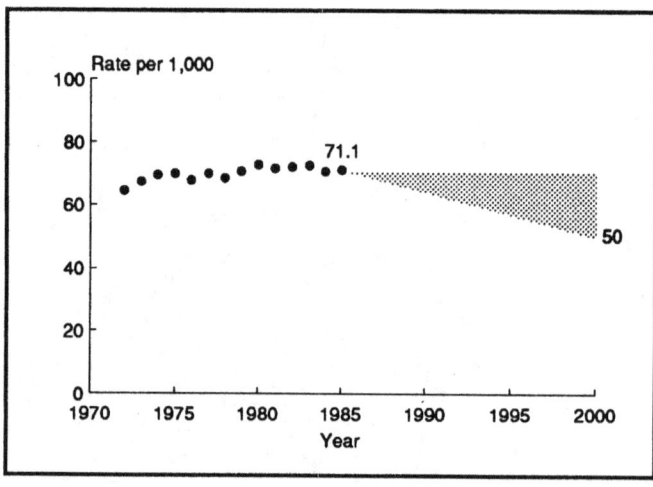

Fig. 5.1

Pregnancy rate among adolescent girls aged 15 through 17

Few situations are as life-changing for a young women and her family as an unintended, out-of-wedlock pregnancy. The manner in which she, her family, and her partner resolve the crisis may have life-long consequences for the people involved and for the broader community.

This objective targets reductions in pregnancies among all adolescents under age 18, with the assumption that most of such pregnancies are unintended pregnancies among unmarried teens. Although the baseline data for this objective do not exclude pregnancies among those who are married, married adolescents constitute only 1.9 percent of the entire population of adolescent girls aged 15 through 17.[135] In 1981, an estimated 84 percent of pregnancies among young women under age 20 were unintended.[136] Further, 96 percent of abortions among women aged 19 and younger are to unmarried women.[137]

When pregnancy rates for all teenagers aged 15 through 19 (110 per 1,000 women in 1985) are compared to rates among Hispanic women (158 per 1,000 women in 1985), Hispanic rates appear to be higher than the total population. Thus, a special population target for Hispanic teenagers has been included in this objective. However, teenage Hispanic women are more likely to have married than either black or white teenage women. Approximately 4 percent of Hispanic women aged 15 through 17 have married, compared to approximately 2 percent of white women and 1 percent of black women aged 15 through 17. Twenty-one percent of Hispanic women aged 18 and 19 have married, while 15 percent of white women and 3 percent of black women aged 18 and 19 have done so.[135]

Nearly 70 percent of births to Hispanic women aged 17 are to unmarried women.[138] Thus, it is assumed that this objective can be achieved without reducing intended pregnancies among married women.

When the pregnancy rate for black teenagers is compared to that of all teenagers, pregnancy rate differences are even more profound. The Alan Guttmacher Institute estimates that there were 186 pregnancies per 1,000 nonwhite women aged 15 through 19 in 1985. Approximately 80 percent of these nonwhite women are black.[137] Further evidence of disparity is available by examining the proportions of women who have ever been pregnant. By age 20, nearly 40 percent of all women have ever been pregnant;[137] approximately 60 percent of black women have ever been pregnant by age 20.[139] However, not all of these pregnancies are among unmarried women. The targets for both black and Hispanic teenagers can be met by reducing unintended pregnancies. Intended pregnancies are not targeted for reduction.

Recent research suggests that the higher frequency of poor health outcomes among adolescents who give birth do not stem from intrinsic medical risk, but from socioeconomic and behavioral factors, such as low income, low levels of education, and poor nutritional patterns.[139,140] Thus, while it may be possible to control these factors and demonstrate that healthy teens can have healthy pregnancies, some of the factors that may predispose a young woman to become pregnant also place her and her baby at risk for poor health outcomes. The negative effects of unintended adolescent pregnancy include induced abortion (43 percent of pregnancies among young women aged 15 through 17 end in abortion),[137] emotional and psychological disruption, social and economic effects on the adolescent and her child, and economic consequences for society at large.

The social and economic consequences of adolescent pregnancy have been extensively studied in recent years. Well planned studies consistently show that adolescent pregnancy and child-rearing generally retard an adolescent's achievement of social and economic independence.[141] Interruption of an adolescent's progress toward social and economic independence is usually caused by interruption of formal schooling. In addition to the personal costs to teen parents and their babies, societal costs of teen childbearing are immense. In 1985, an estimated $16.6 billion in public funds were spent to support families begun by teenage mothers, with virtually all of these costs associated with public assistance programs including Aid to Families with Dependent Children, Medicaid, and Food Stamps.[142]

This objective and its special population targets are particularly challenging. Pregnancy rates among young women aged 15 through 17 showed virtually no change between 1979 and 1985, hovering around 70 per 1,000 women (70.1 in 1979 and 71.1 in 1985). The effectiveness of various efforts to reduce rates of adolescent pregnancy will vary depending on the type of community involved. Programs should be tailored to local standards and values. No simple, one-dimensional approach is likely to succeed, given the complexity of the issue and the number of factors influencing an individual's decision to become sexually active. A successful approach is one that promotes development of mature, responsible individuals who understand the consequences of their actions, and who are goal-oriented and self-disciplined. Mature teens understand that their actions today have consequences for tomorrow and that the choices they make today will be with them for the rest of their lives.

5.2 **Reduce to no more than 30 percent the proportion of all pregnancies that are unintended. (Baseline: 56 percent of pregnancies in the previous 5 years were unintended, either unwanted or earlier than desired, in 1988)**

Special Population Target

Unintended Pregnancies	1988 Baseline	2000 Target
5.2a Black women	78%	40%

Baseline data source: National Survey of Family Growth, CDC, adjusted for underreporting of abortion using an adjustment factor from the Alan Guttmacher Institute.

Measuring whether or not pregnancies are intended is an uncertain process. Unintended pregnancies include those pregnancies that women report they did not want at all (unwanted pregnancies) and those that they report were earlier than they wanted (mistimed). Assessing unintended pregnancy is important as an indication of the extent to which couples are able to control the timing and spacing of their pregnancies.

Abstinence is the most effective means of avoiding unintended pregnancy and sexually transmitted diseases. Without effective contraception, 89 percent of couples who engage in sexual intercourse regularly will conceive within one year.[143,144] To use contraception effectively, couples must understand the effectiveness of alternate methods and the correct way to use their chosen method. Even "perfect use" (correct and consistent) can result in unintended pregnancy. In 1987, approximately 43 percent of unintended pregnancies occurred among couples who were using a contraceptive method the month the pregnancy began.[145]

Teenagers account for about one third of unintended pregnancies with three quarters of teenage pregnancies occurring among teens who are not practicing contraception. Women aged 20 through 24 account for the largest proportion of unintended pregnancies (36 percent); women aged 25 through 34 account for about 27 percent. Women aged 35 through 44 account for only four percent of all unintended pregnancies.[146] In 1988, approximately 39 percent of unintended pregnancies during the previous 5 years were to married women.[147]

Effective family planning and the avoidance of unintended pregnancy can improve infant health. The Institute of Medicine's 1985 report *Preventing Low Birthweight* found "that the reduction in infant mortality in the United States over the past 20 years is due in part to effective family planning."[150] For example, data from the United States 1960 Live Birth Cohort Study showed that 27 percent of the reduction in infant mortality between 1965 and 1967 was due to changes in women's age and parity (number of children born to each woman), which was attributed to individual contraceptive practice. For many women, contraception increases the interval between births. Having a short interval between births is a well established risk factor for low birth weight. In so far as contraception lengthens birth intervals, it can contribute to a reduction in low birth weight. A study of national data found low birth weight in 19 percent of births that occurred within one year of a previous birth, a proportion 3 to 4.5 times higher than the proportion found for longer interval births.[149]

Women who plan their pregnancies tend to seek prenatal care earlier than women who become pregnant unintentionally. Data from the 1980 Natality Survey indicate that married women who wanted a child at the time they became pregnant were more likely to receive early prenatal care than women who would have preferred to become pregnant at a later time. Women who had not planned to have any more children showed the longest delays in seeking prenatal care. The study attributed about one-third of the black-white difference in the reported number of prenatal visits to higher levels of unintended pregnancy among black women.[150]

Approaches to reducing rates of unintended pregnancy include reducing rates of sexual activity, approaching sexual activity with a greater sense of responsibility, and increased effective use of family planning methods. For unmarried people, for whom the consequences of unintended pregnancy are generally the most serious (particularly adolescents), postponement of sexual activity is the most effective means of preventing unintended pregnancy. For married couples and other sexually active people, better understanding of fertility and improved use of family planning methods are needed.

5.3 Reduce the prevalence of infertility to no more than 6.5 percent. (Baseline: 7.9 percent of married couples with wives aged 15 through 44 in 1988)

Special Population Targets

	Prevalence of Infertility	1988 Baseline	2000 Target
5.3a	Black couples	12.1%	9%
5.3b	Hispanic couples	12.4%	9%

Note: Infertility is the failure of couples to conceive after 12 months of intercourse without contraception.

Baseline data source: National Survey of Family Growth, CDC.

Infertility affects an estimated 2.4 million married couples and an unknown number of potential parents among unmarried couples and singles. When infertility estimates include couples who are surgically sterile, approximately 14 percent of couples with wives aged 15 through 44 are infertile. Diagnosis and treatment of infertility is costly: in 1987, Americans spent about $1 billion to combat infertility.[151] The overall incidence of infertility remained relatively constant between 1965 and 1982, with only one group, married couples with wives aged 20 through 24, experiencing an increase in infertility (from 3.6 percent in 1965 to 10.6 percent in 1982). The reason for this increase is not clear. Possible explanations include a link to the increase in the gonorrhea rate (which tripled between 1960 and 1977), the use of intrauterine devises (IUDs) which may increase the risk of pelvic inflammatory disease, complications or infections following childbirth or abortion, and environmental factors such as radiation, toxic chemicals, and pollution.[152]

An analysis of cycle III of the National Survey of Family Growth revealed that the proportion of women with fecundity impairments who want to have more children is higher among Hispanic women than non-Hispanic women (6.4 percent versus 4.3 percent) and higher among nonblack women than black women (4.6 percent versus 3.8 percent). The proportion who want more children is higher among those women at or above 150 percent of the poverty level than among poorer women (5.1 percent versus 2.7 percent). Black women in need of infertility services are less likely to have obtained services than nonblack women (30 percent versus 51 percent) and Hispanic women are less likely than non-Hispanic women (39 versus 50 percent) to receive needed services.[153]

Three factors most often contribute to infertility among women: problems in ovulation, blocked or scarred fallopian tubes, and endometriosis (presence in lower abdomen of tissue from the uterine lining). In men, the most frequent causes are abnormal or too few sperm. For as many as one in five infertile couples, a cause is never found. Infertility arising from sexually transmitted diseases—an estimated 20 percent of the cases in the United States—is the most preventable.[154] The reduction in infertility targeted by this objective roughly parallels reductions in sexually transmitted diseases targeted in the sexually transmitted disease priority area. The sexually transmitted disease objectives target 30 percent and 20 percent reductions, respectively, in the incidence of gonorrhea and chlamydia. Such reductions could reduce the infertility rate by approximately 5 percent. Additional, nonquantified reductions in infertility are possible through improved preconception counseling, especially counseling related to prevention of sexually transmitted diseases.

Despite recent advances in the medical treatment of infertility, outcomes for individual couples entering treatment are still uncertain. Among treatments for infertility are fertility awareness and fertility monitoring, medical induction of ovulation, surgical procedures to correct blockage of the fallopian tubes, artificial insemination, and *in vitro* fertilization and other assisted reproductive techniques. These alternatives vary in cost, potential risks, invasiveness, effectiveness, and acceptability to people on moral and religious grounds.

Given the high cost of infertility services and their generally low success rates, more attention should be given to improving adoption opportunities. Adoption is frequently not considered by couples due to a lack of information or to misinformation about the adoption process. At present, 25 percent of children in foster care are under age six and three percent are under age one. Black children are over-represented in the foster care population, comprising 33 percent of all children.[155] Greater efforts should be made to reach black couples who want children with information about adoption. Improving adoption outreach services could help solve two important problems: assuring that couples who want children will have them and reducing the number of children placed in foster care without permanent homes. Since children in foster care are at higher risk for physical and emotional problems, families would be more motivated to assume the responsibility of adoption if post-adoption services and reimbursement for health care expenses were made available.

Risk Reduction Objectives

5.4* Reduce the proportion of adolescents who have engaged in sexual intercourse to no more than 15 percent by age 15 and no more than 40 percent by age 17. (Baseline: 27 percent of girls and 33 percent of boys by age 15; 50 percent of girls and 66 percent of boys by age 17; reported in 1988)

Baseline data sources: National Survey of Family Growth, CDC; National Survey of Adolescent Males.

One in ten young women aged 19 and younger become pregnant each year, and approximately 40 percent will experience at least one pregnancy before age 20. Initiation of sexual activity at a young age is a primary risk factor for unintended pregnancy. By age 21, approximately one in five young people have acquired a sexually transmitted disease. Because only some teenagers are sexually active, this amounts to a rate of at least 25 percent among those who are (see *Sexually Transmitted Diseases*). Sexually transmitted diseases can have profound long term consequences, including infertility and cancer. HIV infection, also one of the sexually transmitted diseases, is incurable and deadly.

Sexual relationships among teenagers are often characterized by extreme impermanence. As a result, 58 percent of sexually active young women aged 15 through 19 have had two or more sexual partners and seven percent have had 10 or more partners.[152] According to the most recent data from the National Survey of Family Growth, three quarters of young women have had sexual intercourse by their twentieth birthday. Teenagers report that social pressure is the chief reason why their peers do not wait until they are older to have sexual intercourse.[156] Sexual activity at young ages is more common among young people from low socioeconomic status families, and among adolescents who smoke, use alcohol or other drugs, or have evidence of delinquency.[157,158,159,160,161]

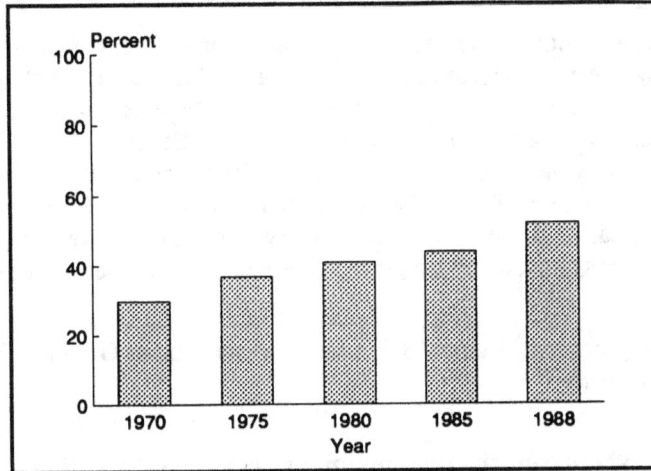

Fig. 5.4
Percentage of adolescent girls aged 15 through 19 who have had sexual intercourse

There are some indications that early sexual intercourse by adolescents can have negative effects on social and psychological development. One study found that early sexual intercourse among adolescent white males was associated inversely with self-reported grades in school.[162] An inverse association was also found between white females' college aspirations and sexual experience. Initiation of sexual intercourse by teenagers is associated with a number of factors, including academic achievement, religiousness, relationships between parents and their children, puberty, and other developmental characteristics, race, and socioeconomic status. For example, teenagers who score high on intelligence tests, are academically motivated, and are doing well in school are less likely to initiate sexual activity at a young age.[141,158,163,164,165,166,167,168] Young people are more likely to be sexually experienced if they perceive themselves to be in poor communication with their parents.[164,169]

Adolescents who report their discipline received at home as "not strict at all" are more than twice as likely to participate in nonmarital intercourse than adolescents who report a moderate amount of strictness and rules. Also, teenagers who report their parents as "extremely strict" are slightly more likely to be involved in nonmarital sex than those reporting moderate discipline. Women aged 15 through 19 are more likely to be sexually active if they are not regular church attenders and if they report that religion is not very important to them.[169] Sexual activity at the youngest ages may be the result of sexual abuse or incest. The issue of coercion has important implications for how sexual abstinence is promoted among teenagers. In the case of coercive relationships, teenagers must be taught not only to say "no," but also to say no effectively and, whenever possible, to translate it into action. Victims of coercive/abusive relationships may need help in bringing these relationships to the attention of people who can help them. Parents, family members, physicians, school nurses, social workers, teachers, and others who are in contact with young adolescents they know to be sexually active should be aware of the possibility of abuse. All States have statutes that require physicians, other professionals, and citizens to report suspected abuse.

Research supports widely held beliefs that adolescents can respond positively to directive counseling from adults about sexuality. For example, one study found that when staff of contraceptive clinics employed authoritative guidance in helping clients to select contraceptive methods, clients' contraceptive use was substantially improved.[170] Other research supports the creation of environments within communities that support teen decisions to postpone sexual activity. Some successful programs have taken a community approach involving parents, the media, the schools, and the clergy in preventing teen pregnancy. One study found that such an approach was successful in reducing teen sexual activity and improving contraceptive use among teens who were sexually active.[171]

Although the theoretical effectiveness rates of some contraceptives are quite high, adolescents are not generally effective users of contraception. In addition, the most effective method of contraception and the method most commonly used by young women, the oral contraceptive pill, does not protect against sexually transmitted diseases. Conversely, barrier methods, particularly the condom, provide substantial protection against sexually transmitted diseases, but are most likely to be used ineffectively or sporadically by adolescents. Thus, decreasing the level of sexual activity should significantly improve adolescent health by decreasing unintended pregnancies and sexually transmitted diseases.

*This objective also appears as Objective 18.3 in *HIV Infection* and as Objective 19.9 in *Sexually Transmitted Diseases*.

5.5   **Increase to at least 40 percent the proportion of ever sexually active adolescents aged 17 and younger who have abstained from sexual activity for the previous 3 months. (Baseline: 26 percent of sexually active girls aged 15 through 17 in 1988)**

Baseline data source: National Survey of Family Growth, CDC.

Many factors are strongly associated with sexual activity before marriage, including characteristics such as puberty, age, race, and socioeconomic status, religiousness, intelligence and academic achievement, and dating behavior; family characteristics such as family background and parental support and control; and the influence of peers.[139] When young adolescent girls begin having sexual intercourse, it is generally infrequent and unpredictable.[139] Some adolescents who have had recent intercourse view the event as atypical behavior which they are unlikely to repeat.[172]

Negative consequences of nonmarital sexual intercourse can include elevated risk of acquiring a sexually transmitted disease and suffering impaired fertility as a result of sexually transmitted infections. Therefore, abstaining from further nonmarital sexual intercourse protects adolescents from a variety of risks to health.

Peers of the same gender are a major influence on adolescent attitudes about sexual activity. The proportion of their same-sex peers that teenagers believe are sexually active and how sexually active they believe them to be are powerful predictors of sexual experience among adolescent boys and girls.[139] However, individual behavior and attitudes are more closely related to what adolescents think their friends are doing than what they are actually doing.

Recent studies[173] of sexual victimization as a factor in adolescent pregnancy suggest that coercive sexual relationships are more common than previously believed.[173] Even in noncoercive sexual relationships among adolescents, there may be strong feelings of ambivalence or opposition to continuing sexual activity. According to a recent study of adolescents in Utah, half of the adolescents who reported that they were sexually active stated that they desired not to be.[172]

Programs that address these feelings of ambivalence about sexual activity, present these feelings as normal, and encourage teens to postpone further sexual activity can help teens avoid further risks to their health.

5.6 **Increase to at least 90 percent the proportion of sexually active, unmarried people aged 19 and younger who use contraception, especially combined method contraception that both effectively prevents pregnancy and provides barrier protection against disease. (Baseline: 78 percent at most recent intercourse and 63 percent at first intercourse; 2 percent used oral contraceptives and the condom at most recent intercourse; among young women aged 15 through 19 reporting in 1988)**

Note: Strategies to achieve this objective must be undertaken sensitively to avoid indirectly encouraging or condoning sexual activity among teens who are not yet sexually active.
Baseline data source: National Survey of Family Growth, CDC.

The only certain way to prevent teenage pregnancy is through abstinence from sexual intercourse. Abstinence also provides absolute protection from sexually transmitted diseases, including AIDS. Mutually faithful monogamy with an uninfected partner will also protect people from sexually transmitted diseases. However, for sexually active teenagers who will not postpone sexual activity and who do not wish to become pregnant or infected with a sexually transmitted disease, consistent use of dual methods of contraception is the most effective means of reducing rates of pregnancy and sexually transmitted diseases.

Eighty four percent of teenage pregnancies in 1981 were unintended[136] and less than 5 percent of abortions to women aged 19 and younger occur among married women.[137] Only one third of teenagers who have had sexual intercourse say they use contraceptives all the time. Low-income teenagers are the least likely to use contraceptives consistently. Sexually active teenagers who have talked about sex, pregnancy, and contraception with their parents appear to be more likely than other teenagers to use birth control all the time.[174] Adolescents with a stronger appreciation of the consequences if they or their partner becomes pregnant are also more likely to use contraceptives consistently.[166]

Approximately half of all first nonmarital pregnancies occur in the first six months following initial sexual intercourse; more than one fifth of these pregnancies occur in the first month.[175] Approximately 60 percent of sexually active adolescents who have never used contraceptives become pregnant within 1 year of initiating sexual intercourse, whereas 30 percent of those using a method inconsistently, 14 percent of those always using some method (including withdrawal), and only 7 percent using a medically prescribed method become pregnant.[176,177]

Different methods of contraception have different characteristics in terms of ease of use and effectiveness in preventing pregnancy and sexually transmitted diseases. Due to these differences among contraceptives and contraceptive uses, it is not sufficient merely to recommend a general increase in the use of contraception.

In terms of preventing pregnancy, hormonal contraceptives, such as the oral contraceptive, are the most effective of the commonly available means of reversible contraception. Oral contraceptives, if used correctly and consistently, provide a very high degree of protection from pregnancy. However, oral contraceptives are not effective in reducing transmission of sexually transmitted diseases, including AIDS. Barrier methods, such as the diaphragm, the cervical cap, and the condom are, in general, less effective than hormonal contraceptives in preventing pregnancy. Nevertheless, barrier methods, especially the condom used with a spermicide, can provide substantial protection from sexually transmitted diseases if used correctly. Therefore, for protection against sexually transmitted diseases and unintended pregnancy, sexually active nonmonogamous people should use dual methods of contraception. In this objective, use of condoms in combination with oral contraceptives is a proxy measure for the use of any combination of a barrier method with another method that is effective in preventing pregnancy. For those who do not use oral contraceptives, a combination of two barrier methods such as a condom and a diaphragm can provide a high degree of protection from both pregnancy and sexually transmitted diseases.

The Surgeon General has emphasized that abstinence and mutually faithful monogamy are the only certain ways to prevent AIDS and other sexually transmitted diseases and has also recommended that sexually active people use condoms with a spermicide (such as nonoxynol 9) even if they are also using a highly effective method to prevent pregnancy.

5.7 **Increase the effectiveness with which family planning methods are used, as measured by a decrease to no more than 5 percent in the proportion of couples experiencing pregnancy despite use of a contraceptive method. (Baseline: Approximately 10 percent of women using reversible contraceptive methods experienced an unintended pregnancy in 1982)**

Baseline data source: "Public Sector Savings Resulting from Expenditures for Contraceptive Services."

Even couples who use contraceptive techniques are at risk for unintended pregnancy, especially if they do not use those techniques correctly and consistently. This may be particularly true for young people. A survey of sexually active black high school males found that only 60 percent had used a contraceptive at their last sexual encounter, and most lacked accurate knowledge about the relative effectiveness and availability of various birth control methods.[178] Inconsistent or incorrect use of contraceptives is reported by at least half of women receiving abortion counseling.[179] Although those who do not use contraception comprise only 12 percent of women of childbearing age who are at risk of unintended pregnancy, in 1985, more than half (57 percent) of all unintended pregnancies were to women who were not using a contraceptive method. The remaining 43 percent of unintended pregnancies were to women who experienced contraceptive failure—e.g., they were using a method to prevent pregnancy during the month they conceived.[180]

It has been estimated that as many as one-third of all unintended pregnancies and 500,000 abortions could be prevented each year if the proportion of women at risk for unintended pregnancy and not using contraception were reduced by half.[181] Because unintended pregnancy rates among couples who are not using contraception are so high, even a small increase in the proportion of people at risk for unintended pregnancy who use a contraceptive method could result in relatively large reductions in unintended pregnancies.

Additional reductions in unintended pregnancy are possible through improved use of contraceptive methods. Approximately 10 percent of couples who are using a method to avoid pregnancy fail to prevent conception each year. A comparison of annual contraceptive failure rates is instructive. When used correctly and consistently, the failure rate of oral contraceptives is as low as 0.1 percent; under typical usage conditions, the failure rate (proportion of women who conceive during 1 year of use) is about 3 percent. When used correctly, condoms have a 2 percent failure rate in preventing pregnancy, but the rate may be as high as 12 percent under conditions of typical usage. The diaphragm, in combination with spermicide, has a failure rate of about 3 percent when used correctly and consistently, but the average failure rate is approximately 18 percent. Natural family planning (periodic abstinence) when used correctly and consistently has an expected failure rate of 2 to 10 percent, but an average failure rate of about 20 percent.[144] One study that corrected for underreporting of abortions reports generally higher contraceptive failure rates: 5.8 percent for oral contraceptives; 15.7 percent for condom use; 18.3 percent for the diaphragm; 19.1 percent for natural family planning (including scientifically accepted methods, as well as methods such as calendar rhythm, that are scientifically outmoded); 30 percent for spermicides; and 19.3 percent for other methods (standardized for age, race, and marital status).[180]

In almost all stratifications by race, age, and marital status, contraceptive failure rates are highest among unmarried, nonwhite women. For example, only two percent of married white pill users aged 35 through 44 failed to prevent conception in their first year of pill use compared to 18 percent of unmarried, nonwhite pill users aged 20 and younger.[180] Women with family incomes that are less than twice the Federal poverty level experience contraceptive failure about two-thirds more often than do women with higher incomes, regardless of the method they use. These high failure rates have been associated with such factors as lower education and greater difficulty in obtaining family planning supplies and services.[180] This objective can be accomplished through improved counseling and instruction by primary care providers, including improved counseling services at family planning, sexually transmitted disease, and maternal and infant health clinics. Manufacturers of contraceptives can contribute by assuring that instructions included with their products are clear and explicit. Additional research should be conducted to explain variations in compliance so that products and instructions can be modified to improve successful use.

Services and Protection Objectives

5.8 Increase to at least 85 percent the proportion of people aged 10 through 18 who have discussed human sexuality, including values surrounding sexuality, with their parents and/or have received information through another parentally endorsed source, such as youth, school, or religious programs. (Baseline: 66 percent of people aged 13 through 18 have discussed sexuality with their parents; reported in 1986)

Note: This objective, which supports family communication on a range of vital personal health issues, will be tracked using the National Health Interview Survey, a continuing, voluntary, national sample survey of adults who report on household characteristics including such items as illnesses, injuries, use of health services, and demographic characteristics.

Baseline data source: "American Teens Speak."

Parents are the first and most important educators of their children in matters related to sexual behavior. From them, children receive their first lessons in sexual morality and appropriate sexual conduct, including lessons about the meaning of mutual respect, love, and marital fidelity.

Children also learn about sexuality from other sources, their schools, their peers, and the mass media. Most young people consider their parents their most important source of information about sexuality. Friends are the second most important, school courses rank third, with television considered the fourth most important source.[182]

Parental interest or involvement with their teenager is related to postponement of sexual activity. Students who report parents as very interested in their grades or in their personal achievements (sports, music, dance, etc.) are about twice as likely to report sexual abstinence as those students who say that parents do not feel grades or achievements are important.[183] Many national youth-serving organizations have developed programs of sexuality education that they consider effective.[184]

School-based sex education has been shown to increase knowledge about issues surrounding sexuality, but has not been shown to result in lower rates of sexual intercourse or pregnancy.[185,186,187,188,189] Research consistently shows that family support, family guidance, and family structure have a significant effect on sexual activity. One of the strongest predictors of adolescent sexual attitudes and behavior is the marital status of the parents. Adolescents living with both parents have the least permissive attitudes toward nonmarital sex, followed by those living with a parent who has remarried.[190]

Parents should be given encouragement and all reasonable assistance with fulfilling their responsibility for teaching their children about sexuality. The rising popularity of parent skills classes, along with increased interest in parental involvement in educational programs for their children may present an opportunity for giving parents practical advice about ways of communicating with their children about sex.

5.9 **Increase to at least 90 percent the proportion of pregnancy counselors who offer positive, accurate information about adoption to their unmarried patients with unintended pregnancies. (Baseline: 60 percent of pregnancy counselors in 1984)**

Note: Pregnancy counselors are any providers of health or social services who discuss the management or outcome of pregnancy with a woman after she has received a diagnosis of pregnancy.
Baseline data source: "Orientation of Pregnancy Counselors Toward Adoption."

Adoption provides families for children born to couples who are unprepared to raise a child and seek a loving, stable home for their child and is an important method of family planning for infertile couples. Although many prospective parents are waiting to adopt children, there are relatively few infants available for adoption due to the small number (about 25,000) of infants placed for adoption each year. Of the approximately one million adolescent pregnancies annually, fewer than four percent of the children born are placed for adoption.[152] Forty-three percent of adolescent pregnancies end in abortion.

While a number of factors influence whether or not a woman faced with an unintended pregnancy places the child for adoption, it is clear that despite positive attitudes toward adoption, pregnancy counselors are often poorly informed about adoption. Many pregnancy counselors do not routinely discuss the adoption option with their clients who are faced with unintended pregnancies. This failure to discuss adoption may stem from the counselor's assumption that clients will react unfavorably to the idea of adoption.

Adoption is a practice with a very long tradition in western society. It should be recognized among providers of prenatal care and pregnancy counselors that adoption can work to the benefit of biological parents, the adoptive parents, and most importantly, the child.

5.10* **Increase to at least 60 percent the proportion of primary care providers who provide age-appropriate preconception care and counseling. (Baseline data available in 1992)**

* * *

*This objective also appears as Objective 14.12 in *Maternal and Infant Health*.

5.11* **Increase to at least 50 percent the proportion of family planning clinics, maternal and child health clinics, sexually transmitted disease clinics, tuberculosis clinics, drug treatment centers, and primary care clinics that screen, diagnose, treat, counsel, and provide (or refer for) partner notification services for HIV infection and bacterial sexually transmitted diseases (gonorrhea, syphilis, and chlamydia). (Baseline: 40 percent of family planning clinics for bacterial sexually transmitted diseases in 1989)**

Baseline data source: State Family Planning Directors.

*For commentary, see Objective 19.11 in *Sexually Transmitted Diseases*. This objective also appears as Objective 18.13 in *HIV Infection*.

* * *

Research Needs

* * *

- American women have a comparatively low level of effective contraceptive use and are more likely than their counterparts in other developed countries not to use any method at all. Additional basic research should be conducted to assess nonuse, incorrect use, and effective methods for increasing correct contraceptive use.

- The determinants and consequences of early sexual intercourse are poorly understood. Additional research is needed to better understand early initiation, its consequences, and how it might be prevented.

- Existing contraceptive methods are often unacceptable to men and women because of difficulty or discomfort in use, expense, or undesirable side-effects. Improved contraceptive methods are needed for men and women. Research should focus on developing methods that are easier to use, that have fewer side effects, and that are less expensive.

* * *

Baseline Data Source References

The Alan Guttmacher Institute. Henshaw, S.K.; Kenney, A.M.; Somberg, D.; and Van Vort, J. *Teenage Pregnancy in the United States: The Scope of the Problem and State Responses.* New York: the Institute, 1989.

"American Teens Speak." Harris L. and Associates for Planned Parenthood. American Teens Speak: Sex, Myth, T.V., and Birth Control, New York, 1986. As Cited in *First Things First*. New York: Planned Parenthood Federation of America, Inc., 1989.

National Survey of Family Growth. National Center for Health Statistics, Centers for Disease Control, Public Health Service, U.S. Department of Health and Human Services, Hyattsville, MD.

National Survey of Adolescent Males. In: Sonnenstein, F.L.; Pleck, J.H.; Ku, L.C.; Sexual activity, condom use, and AIDS awareness among adolescent males. *Family Planning Perspectives* 21(4):152-158, 1989.

"Orientation of Pregnancy Counselors Toward Adoption." Mech, E.B. Unpublished study for the Office of Adolescent Pregnancy, Public Health Service, U.S. Department of Health and Human Services, 1984.

Public Sector Savings Resulting from Expenditures for Contraceptive Services. Forrest, J.D., and Singh, S. *Family Planning Perspectives* 22(1):6-15, 1990.

Mental Health and Mental Disorders

6

Contents

6.1	Suicide
6.2	Suicide attempts among adolescents
6.3	Mental disorders among children and adolescents
	* * *
6.7	Depression
	* * *
6.12	Mutual help clearinghouses
6.13	Clinician review of patients' mental functioning
6.14	Clinician review of childrens' mental functioning
	[Research Needs]

6. Mental Health and Mental Disorders

* * *

Health Status Objectives

6.1* Reduce suicides to no more than 10.5 per 100,000 people. (Age-adjusted baseline: 11.7 per 100,000 in 1987)

Special Population Targets

Suicides (per 100,000)		1987 Baseline	2000 Target
6.1a	Youth aged 15-19	10.3	8.2

* * *

Baseline data sources: National Vital Statistics System, CDC; Indian Health Service Administrative Statistics, IHS.

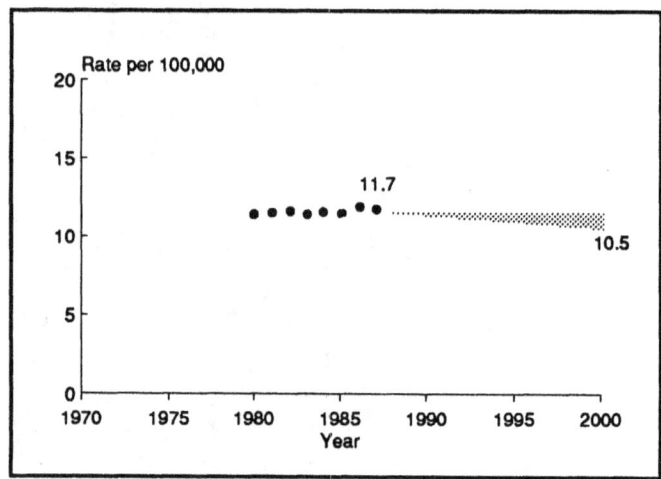

Fig. 6.1

Age-adjusted suicide rate

Suicide is the eighth leading cause of death in the United States and a serious potential outcome of mental illness and mental disorders. In 1987, 30,783 people died of suicide.[40] Mental disorders such as various forms of depression, schizophrenia, panic disorder, and adjustment and stress reactions as well as alcohol and other drug abuse have been implicated in both attempted and completed suicides. For young males, in particular, antisocial personality disorder is also frequently associated with suicidal behavior.

Data from "psychologic autopsies" of completed suicides highlight previous suicide attempts, inadequate treatment, medical illness, precipitous life events, family history of suicide or psychiatric disorders, exposure to suicidal behavior, family violence, and availability of firearms in the home as contributing factors. Stressful life circumstances such as separation or divorce, unemployment, or limited socioeconomic resources can also contribute to suicidal behavior.[191] The most promising current approach to suicide prevention appears to be the early identification and treatment of individuals suffering from mental disorders. Continued research is needed to determine the efficacy of specific treatments as they are applied to specific disorders.

Injuries resulting from gunshots cause a majority of suicidal deaths, and much of the increase in suicide rates since the 1950s can be accounted for by firearm-related deaths.[192,193] Attempted suicides are different, with a predominance of poisoning by pill ingestion and minor lacerations. To determine whether interventions designed to prevent mental illness and promote mental health actually reduce intentional suicide deaths, however, requires consideration of the confounding effects of differential availability, accessibility, and acceptability of lethal weapons as well as community variations in the ownership of guns.[194,195,196]

Other confounding conditions include changes in rates associated with the period in which the suicide takes place or when the individual was born. For example, periods of high unemployment are characterized by high suicide rates; when a high proportion of the population are adolescents, adolescent suicide rates are higher. Cohorts of American males entering adolescence between 1950 and 1980 differed in that each successive cohort went through late adolescence with a higher suicide rate than the preceding cohort, a disparity that continued to age 35.[197]

The overall suicide rate has changed relatively little since 1950. However, the rates vary substantially by gender, age, and race/ethnicity. Men are more likely to commit suicide, with rates generally higher for whites and Reservation Indians. Elderly white men (65 years of age and older) and young, male Reservation Indians are particularly susceptible.[197] Although the rate for male adolescents is comparatively low, there has been a steady increase in suicide among all youth aged 15 to 19 since the 1950s. By 1986, suicide was the second leading cause of death in the 15- to 19-year-old group. Suicide rates among men (but not women) aged 20 through 34 increased dramatically in the last three decades and remained relatively high in the 1980s.[193,197] Special goals have been set for these populations at unusual risk.

* This objective also appears as Objective 7.2 in *Violent and Abusive Behavior*.

6.2* **Reduce by 15 percent the incidence of injurious suicide attempts among adolescents aged 14 through 17. (Baseline data available in 1991)**

Attempted suicide is at once a morbid, potentially lethal, health event, a risk factor for future completed suicide, and a potential indicator of other health problems such as substance abuse, depression, or adjustment and stress reactions.[198] Although much has been written about the increasing rates of youth suicide in the United States, little is known about patterns and trends in the occurrence of suicide attempts among the young. In several surveys of adolescents in the general populations, as many as 10 percent of the respondents report having attempted suicide at least once.[194,552] However, only a small proportion of those who report having attempted suicide also report having actually required medical attention for their injuries. As a group, suicide attempters with serious medical injuries are at higher risk of repeated suicide attempts and completed suicide than are suicide attempters with minor injuries.[199,200] This objective focuses on that part of the spectrum of suicidal behavior among high school students which results in injuries to the victim. The Centers for Disease Control will initiate a system of youth risk behaviors that will establish baseline data and begin tracking this objective beginning in 1991.

* This objective also appears as Objective 7.8 in *Violent and Abusive Behavior*.

6.3 **Reduce to less than 10 percent the prevalence of mental disorders among children and adolescents. (Baseline: An estimated 12 percent among youth younger than age 18 in 1989)**

Baseline data sources: Institute of Medicine; Office of Technology Assessment.

Although an estimated 7.5 million or 12 percent of the Nation's children and adolescents suffer from mental disorders severe enough to warrant treatment, less than one out of eight receives this needed treatment.[201] Included among these disorders are autism, attention deficit and hyperactivity, severe conduct disorders, depression, and alcohol and other drug abuse. More treatment services are needed to reduce the prevalence of these disorders, and more health, education, social, and prevention services are needed to reduce their incidence.

Early diagnosis and effective treatment of those afflicted with these childhood disorders can reduce their duration and recurrence, thus reducing prevalence rates. In addition, as the children's functioning improves, they can be expected to improve their educational, emotional, and psychosocial status, thus decreasing the risk of further deterioration.

A growing segment of children and youth are at exceptionally high risk for psychopathology.[202] More than 20 percent of American children live in poverty, and more than half of these children live in single-parent homes; increasing numbers of children have no home at all. More that 1.5 million children are reported abused and neglected each year. Almost 300,000 children are in foster care, many in up to 30 homes during their childhood years, and approximately 7 million children live with an alcoholic parent. Numerous other risk factors exist. Inadequate prenatal care increases the risk of low birthweight. Low birthweight, combined with poverty and family disorganization, increases the risk of neurologic and psychologic disorders. Babies born to mothers infected with the human immunodeficiency virus or abusing alcohol and other drugs are at vastly increased risk. While a child with only one of these risk factors may develop without problems, each additional factor increases the likelihood of a mental disorder that interferes with the normal developmental process and functioning. Therefore, to achieve a major reduction in the prevalence of mental disorders in children, it is necessary to reduce the factors that put them at risk, to enhance protective factors such as social competency, and to increase the availability of treatment services for those who already have a disorder.

Several programs are effective in preventing social, emotional, and academic difficulties,[203,204,205] including family support programs, parent-infant education programs, early childhood education, school-based social competence promotion, and other social learning programs. Current research is examining whether such intervention programs do, in fact, reduce the incidence of clinically defined mental disorders among the children served.

The lack of knowledge about some childhood disorders such as autism results in few specific preventive efforts. Such, however, is not the case with conduct disorders. About half of all children and adolescents with mental disorders are classified as having severe and persistent conduct disorders. Typically these disorders involve a persistent pattern of behavior in which social rules and the rights of others are violated at a high rate. They include aggression and cruelty in the younger years and delinquent and criminal behavior in adolescence. About half of all children so identified in clinical populations become antisocial adults.[206]

Conduct disorders occur twice as often among males and among children in families where there is marital discord and/or poor parental supervision. The risk is nearly three times as high among children with chronic illness, those with learning disorders, and those who have poor peer relations. Rates are higher among blacks than whites and lower among Asian children than white children; these differences are probably due primarily to socioeconomic factors. Those with more than three of these risk factors are at extraordinary risk for conduct disordered behavior.

A reduction in the rate of conduct disorders (or other mental disorders) will not be achieved by programs designed to alter a single risk factor.[207,208,209] Preventive interventions must address a number of risk factors over an extended period of time, and they must be ongoing and intensive. Several such efforts are underway, and it is likely that such programs can be implemented on a wider scale in the coming decade.

To reduce the incidence and prevalence of childhood mental disorders, including conduct disorders, it will be necessary to achieve many of the other Year 2000 Health Objectives, specifically:

- A reduction in the number of low birthweight and other infants born with neurologic or other physical disorders (see *Maternal and Infant Health*).

- A reduction in the number of children with chronic untreated medical illnesses (see *Maternal and Infant Health, Diabetes and Chronic Disabling Conditions*, and *HIV Infection*).

- An increase in the number of such children who receive special health, education, and social services (see *Diabetes and Chronic Disabling Conditions*).

- A reduction in motor vehicle crashes and other injuries that result in head trauma (see *Unintentional Injuries* and *Violent and Abusive Behavior*).

- An increase in the quality and quantity of educational programs aimed at reducing rates of educational retardation (see *Educational and Community-Based Programs*).

- Interventions that provide economic, educational and social support and guidance for children in high-risk groups, which includes homeless children; those who have lost a parent through death, divorce, or incarceration; and those with older siblings with delinquency records (see *Educational and Community-Based Programs* and *Diabetes and Chronic Disabling Conditions*).

- Reductions in rates of alcohol and other drug abuse among parents and older siblings of all children (see *Alcohol and Other Drugs*).

Secondary prevention of these childhood disorders will be achieved through improvements in diagnosis and treatment. Early treatment and the resulting improvement can alter the trajectory of young children before maladaptive behaviors put them on a course that results in adult psychopathology.

* * *

Risk Reduction Objectives

* * *

6.7 **Increase to at least 45 percent the proportion of people with major depressive disorders who obtain treatment. (Baseline: 31 percent in 1982)**

Baseline data source: Epidemiologic Catchment Area Study, ADAMHA.

Of the total population suffering from a major depressive disorder in any 6-month period, only 31 percent actually receive treatment of any kind, and too often that treatment is inappropriate. Yet, properly implemented psychologic and pharmacologic treatments have been found effective more than 8 times out of 10. A variety of beliefs and concerns hamper help-seeking behaviors. Failure to recognize depressive disorders both by the person suffering depressive symptoms and by the physicians poses significant barriers. Economic access to treatment providers and appropriateness of treatment, whether by a medical care provider or by a mental health provider, can also be problematic. Achievement of this objective will depend on the successful transfer of available knowledge to those who suffer from major depressive disorders as well as to primary health care providers, mental health professionals, and others in the helping professions.[210]

* * *

Services and Protection Objectives

* * *

6.12   **Establish mutual help clearinghouses in at least 25 States. (Baseline: 9 States in 1989)**

Baseline data source: National Council on Self-Help and Public Health.

During the past decade, autonomous mutual help groups have gained increasing recognition as complementary to clinical practice. Often referred to as self-help organizations, their members include people who share or have shared specific physical, mental, or emotional problems. These groups make significant contributions to positive outcomes for persons affected by mental and behavioral disorders, including the family members and formal and informal caregivers of individuals with chronic conditions. An estimated 10 million to 15 million people are members of mutual help groups in the United States, with some 1.9 million adults turning to nonprofessional mutual help resources for personal or emotional problems in the course of a year.[211]

One of the priority recommendations of the Surgeon General's Workshop on Self-Help and Public Health was to establish and strengthen mutual help clearinghouses as a means of expanding this effort. Existing mutual help clearinghouses cover geographic areas that include about 53 percent of the population. They provide information about and referral to thousands of groups and help thousands of people find supportive groups. In addition, they serve an important liaison function between mutual help groups and the mental health and health communities.

6.13   **Increase to at least 50 percent the proportion of primary care providers who routinely review with patients their patients' cognitive, emotional, and behavioral functioning and the resources available to deal with any problems that are identified. (Baseline data available in 1992)**

Between one-half and two-thirds of people who commit suicide visit a physician less than one month before the incident.[200,212] Depression is one of the most common problems seen by primary care physicians, occurring in up to 30 percent of patients.[213] Symptoms of depression, anxiety, and other mental disorders often are not recognized in primary care settings and may go untreated or inappropriately treated. Many people are treated for physical symptoms, such as sleep and appetite problems, headaches, fatigue, and a variety of other unexplained somatic complaints that are often due to undiagnosed depression. Many of those whose depressive disorder is recognized do not receive proper treatment. These situations occur for many reasons including inadequate knowledge about the symptoms of depressive disorders and the availability of effective and appropriate pharmacologic and psychologic treatments, insufficient time spent with patients, lack of medical coverage for mental illness, and the stigma attached to mental illness that keeps physicians from recognizing the illness, or, if recognized, from telling the patient the true diagnosis.

Primary health care providers are urged to be alert to signs of mental and emotional disorders in their patients, giving particular attention to those going through major life transitions such as a recent divorce, separation, bereavement, unemployment, or serious medical illness. Comorbidity of emotional disorders and alcohol and other drug use should also be considered.[212]

Accomplishing this objective will require stronger emphasis on cognitive, emotional, and behavioral disorders as well as on stress pathogenesis as part of health provider education. Despite the fact that stress has been associated with a variety of medical, psychologic, and occupational health complaints, only one American medical school currently requires a stress course as a part of its curriculum.[214] The Office of Disease Prevention and Health Promotion will initiate a survey to establish baseline data and track this objective in 1992.

6.14 **Increase to at least 75 percent the proportion of providers of primary care for children who include assessment of cognitive, emotional, and parent-child functioning, with appropriate counseling, referral, and followup, in their clinical practices. (Baseline data available in 1992)**

Developmental and behavioral assessment is recommended by the American Academy of Pediatrics as a component of well-child care. Although the long-term effectiveness of such screening as currently practiced has not been demonstrated, programs offering early intervention have had encouraging results and small positive effects have been reported for augmented behavioral counseling.[215] Screening without followup is not likely to be effective; therefore this objective addresses not just assessment but referral and followup services as well. The Office of Disease Prevention and Health Promotion will initiate a survey to establish baseline data and track this objective in 1992.

* * *

Research Needs

Research is needed in the field of mental health to determine the following:

- The genetic, neurobiologic, biochemical, and physiologic/molecular contributors to mental health and mental disorders. Social and environmental contributors to mental health and mental disorders.

- Appropriate biomedical and psychosocial interventions that are effective in the diagnosis, treatment, and management of mental disorders.

- The specific biologic mechanisms by which stressful environmental conditions affect mental and physical health, together with pharmacologic, somatic, and physical interventions to prevent or lessen mental and physical effects.

- The barriers to prevention and early identification of cognitive, emotional, and behavioral disorders, including social stigma associated with use of mental health services and care.

* * *

Data Source References

Epidemiologic Catchment Area Survey, National Institute of Mental Health, Alcohol, Drug Abuse, and Mental Health Administration, Public Health Service, U.S. Department of Health and Human Services, Rockville, MD, 1984.

Institute of Medicine, Committee of the Division of Mental and Behavioral Medicine. *Research on Children and Adolescents with Mental, Behavioral, and Developmental Disorders: Mobilizing a National Initiative.* Washington, DC: National Academy Press, 1989.

National Council on Self-Help and Public Health, Washington, DC.

National Vital Statistics System, National Center for Health Statistics, Centers for Disease Control, Public Health Service, U.S. Department of Health and Human Services, Hyattsville, MD

Office of Technology Assessment, U.S. Congress. *Children's Mental Health: Problems and Services—A Background Paper.* Washington, DC: U.S. Government Printing Office, 1986.

Violent and Abusive Behavior

7

Contents

7.1	Homicide
7.2	Suicide
7.3	Weapon-related deaths
7.4	Child abuse and neglect
7.5	Partner abuse
7.6	Assault injuries
7.7	Rape and attempted rape
7.8	Suicide attempts by adolescents
7.9	Physical fighting among youth
7.10	Weapon-carrying by youth
7.11	Inappropriate storage of weapons
7.12	Emergency room protocols
7.13	Child death review systems
7.14	Evaluation and followup of abused children
7.15	Shelter space for battered women
7.16	Conflict resolution education in schools
7.17	Comprehensive violence prevention programs

* * *

[Research Needs]

7. Violent and Abusive Behavior

* * *

Health Status Objectives

7.1 Reduce homicides to no more than 7.2 per 100,000 people. (Age-adjusted baseline: 8.5 per 100,000 in 1987)

Special Population Targets

Homicide Rate (per 100,000)		1987 Baseline	2000 Target
7.1a	Children aged 3 and younger	3.9	3.1
7.1b	Spouses aged 15-34	1.7	1.4
7.1c	Black men aged 15-34	90.5	72.4
7.1d	Hispanic men aged 15-34	53.1	42.5
7.1e	Black women aged 15-34	20.0	16.0

* * *

Baseline data source: National Vital Statistics System, CDC.

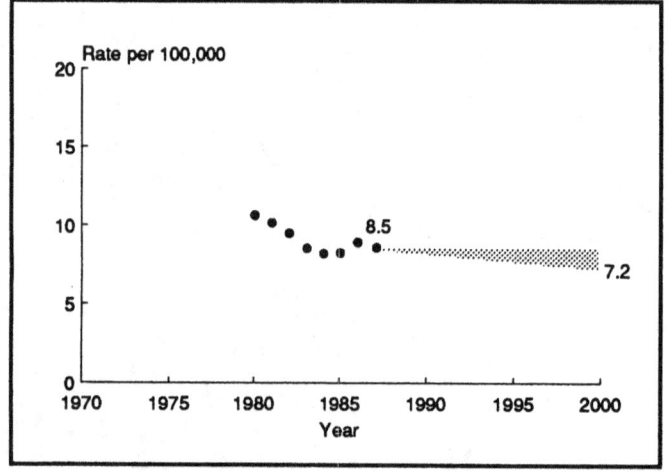

Fig. 7.1

Age-adjusted homicide rate

Homicide is defined here as death due to injuries purposely inflicted by another person, not including deaths caused by law enforcement officers or legal execution. Homicide is the 11th leading cause of death in the United States, accounting for 20,812 deaths in 1987. Men, teenagers, young adults, and minority group members, particularly blacks and Hispanics, are most likely to be murder victims. Most homicides are committed with a firearm, occur during an argument, and occur among people who are acquainted with one another.[216]

Intrafamilial homicide accounts for approximately one out of six homicides, primarily among young adults and blacks. Approximately half of family homicides are committed by spouses. The risk of being killed by one's spouse is 1.3 times higher for wives than for husbands. From 1976 through 1985, spouse homicides declined by more than 45 percent for blacks but remained relatively constant for whites.[217]

Homicides between intimates, regardless of whether the victim is male or female, are often preceded by a history of physical and emotional abuse directed at the woman.[218] When a wife kills a husband it is usually in self-defense. The prevention of homicides among spouses and intimates is directly linked, therefore, to the prevention of abuse of women. Focusing on abuse solely within legally sanctioned marriages, however, will miss abuse that occurs during dating, in nontraditional relationships, and in relationships that have been terminated through separation and divorce.

Among homicide victims under age 4, where the victim and offender relationship is identified, the large majority are killed by a family member or caretaker, whereas older child victims are murdered primarily by acquaintances or strangers.[219]

Child abuse caused an estimated 1,100 deaths in 1986.[229] Half of these resulted from physical abuse and half from neglect. The reported number of child abuse fatalities increased by 23 percent in 1986, an increase that cannot be explained simply as a function of improved reporting systems.[264] More reliable data collection is needed to monitor child abuse deaths among children under age 4.

No cause of death so greatly differentiates black Americans from other Americans as homicide.[220] In 1983, blacks constituted 11.5 percent of the U.S. population but comprised 43 percent of all homicide victims. Death rates from homicide among black men, women, and children far exceed the rates for other citizens of the same age and gender, and homicide is the leading cause of death for blacks aged 15 through 34.[216]

Homicide rates for blacks have declined dramatically since 1970, while white homicide rates have increased.[216] Therefore, while the central focus of public health efforts to prevent homicide should be on facilitating the further decline of black homicide rates, efforts to stem the increasing homicide rate among whites should also be undertaken.

National estimates of the magnitude of Hispanic homicides are currently inadequate. Only the Federal Bureau of Investigation's (FBI) Supplemental Homicide Report System contains Hispanic identifiers; however, information on this identifier is missing for a substantial percentage of the homicide victims reported to the FBI through this system. In 5 Southwestern States (Arizona, California, Colorado, New Mexico, and Texas) between 1977 and 1982 the Hispanic homicide rate was 47 percent of the rate among blacks but almost 3 times the rate of non-Hispanic whites. Hispanic men account for all of the elevated risk faced by Hispanics relative to whites in the Southwest.[221]

Poverty has been identified as an extremely important factor in homicide. This is a critical variable to consider, because if the high incidence of homicide among blacks and other minority groups simply reflects greater poverty, then preventive interventions should be targeted toward all persons living in poverty. Unfortunately, national data sources for homicide do not include socioeconomic information on decedents, making it difficult to monitor progress toward reducing homicide rates in impoverished groups.

Another important factor associated with homicide is the use, manufacture, and distribution of drugs. Violence may occur as a consequence of the pharmacological effects of drugs, of economically motivated crimes to support drug use, or of interactions related to the manufacture, buying, and selling of drugs.[222] No national data sets allow for a determination of the proportion of homicides associated with drug use in these 3 ways. Studies conducted in Miami and New York City, however, indicate that at least 25 percent of the homicides occurring in these cities may be associated with drug use.[223,224]

Healthy Children 2000

7.2* Reduce suicides to no more than 10.5 per 100,000 people. (Age-adjusted baseline: 11.7 per 100,000 in 1987)

Special Population Targets

Suicides (per 100,000)		1987 Baseline	2000 Target
7.2a	Youth aged 15-19	10.3	8.2

* * *

Baseline data sources: National Vital Statistics System, CDC; Indian Health Service Administrative Statistics, IHS.

* * *

* This objective also appears in the *Mental Health and Mental Disorders* priority area as Objective 6.1.

7.3 Reduce weapon-related violent deaths to no more than 12.6 per 100,000 people from major causes. (Age-adjusted baseline: 12.9 per 100,000 by firearms, 1.9 per 100,000 by knives, in 1987)

Baseline data source: National Vital Statistics System, CDC.

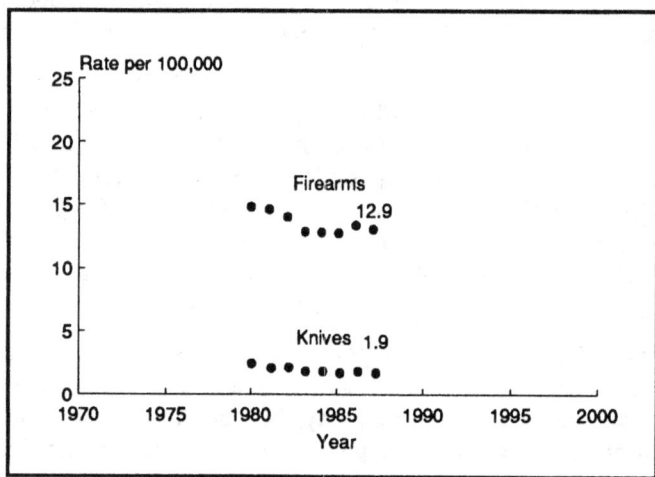

Fig. 7.3

Age-adjusted firearm and knife injury death rates

Violent death can occur as a result of gunshot wounds, knife wounds, poisoning by solids or liquids, deliberate motor vehicle crashes, carbon monoxide poisoning in motor vehicles, arson, drowning, falls, and suffocation or hanging. Among the instruments of violent death, firearms and knives rank far ahead of other means for homicides. Knives are used infrequently in suicidal deaths.[225] Violent and unintentional use of firearms is the second most important contributor, after motor vehicles, to injury deaths.[226] Suicides and homicides account for more than 90 percent of all firearm-related deaths and more than 95 percent of all knife-related deaths. Of the approximately 21,000 homicides that occur in the United States each year, over 60 percent involve firearms and about 20 percent involve knives.[225] In 1985, firearms were the weapons used in 31,566 deaths: 55 percent from suicide, 37 percent from homicide, and 5 percent from unintentionally inflicted injuries; the remainder were due either to legal intervention or the medicolegal cause of death was undetermined.[227] For knives and other cuttings, the total was nearly 5,000 deaths, with only 8 percent from suicide, over 88 percent from homicide, and about 2 percent from unintentional injury.[225] Death rates involving the violent use of firearms with women, teenage boys, and young men as the victims were highest during the

1980s;[228] men between the ages of 15 and 34 are at highest risk of death from suicide and homicide in which guns are the weapon used. Of particular concern are young people. A survey of 8th and 10th grade students found that almost 7 percent of boys and 2 percent of girls carried knives to school nearly every day.[39]

Information from death certificates is insufficient to categorize firearm-deaths by the type of gun involved (e.g., handgun, assault rifle, or shotgun). Such information is needed in order to target research and prevention efforts to those types of guns that pose the greatest hazard relative to their prevalence in the general population.

7.4 **Reverse to less than 25.2 per 1,000 children the rising incidence of maltreatment of children younger than age 18. (Baseline: 25.2 per 1,000 in 1986)**

Type-Specific Targets

	Incidence of Types of Maltreatment (per 1,000)	1986 Baseline	2000 Target
7.4a	Physical abuse	5.7	<5.7
7.4b	Sexual abuse	2.5	<2.5
7.4c	Emotional abuse	3.4	<3.4
7.4d	Neglect	15.9	<15.9

Baseline data source: Study of the National Incidence of Child Abuse and Neglect, Office of Human Development Services.

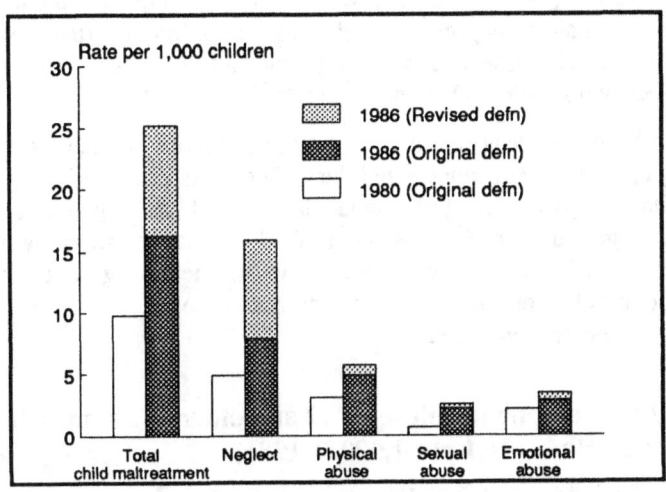

Fig. 7.4 Incidence of child abuse and neglect

The Child Abuse Prevention, Adoption, and Family Services Act of 1988 defines child abuse and neglect as physical or mental injury, sexual abuse or exploitation, negligent treatment, or maltreatment of a child by a person who is responsible for the child's welfare, under circumstances which indicate that the child's health or welfare is harmed or threatened. In 1986, an estimated 1.6 million children nationwide experienced some form of abuse or neglect. Physical abuse accounted for the greatest portion of abuse incidents, followed by emotional and then sexual abuse. Educational neglect was the most frequent category of neglect, followed by physical and then emotional neglect. When compared to 1980 data, increases had occurred in all forms of child abuse and physical and educational neglect. Only moderately severe injuries associated with child abuse were found to decrease.[229]

The targets for this set of objectives are stated as reversing increasing trends rather than achieving specific reductions because of the difficulties in obtaining valid and reliable measurement of child maltreatment. National data are based on incidents that come to the attention of child protection agencies, other investigatory agencies, or professionals in schools, hospitals, or other health or social service agencies. Reported increases may, in fact, reflect greater public awareness and the improved ability of professionals to recognize maltreatment than actual increases in occurrence of maltreatment.

7.5 **Reduce physical abuse directed at women by male partners to no more than 27 per 1,000 couples. (Baseline: 30 per 1,000 in 1985)**

Baseline data source: National Family Violence Survey, ADAMHA.

Studies suggest that between 2 million and 4 million women are physically battered each year by partners including husbands, former husbands, boyfriends, and lovers.[230] Approximately half of these women are single, separated, or divorced. Between 21 and 30 percent of all women in this country have been beaten by a partner at least once.[231]

Women are more often assaulted and raped by a male partner than by a stranger. In addition, women are often battered by their partners during pregnancy. Although male partners are also abused, women appear to be at greater risk of injury from abuse and are likely to attack their partners in self-defense.[553] Once physical violence has occurred in a relationship, it tends to recur and become more severe over time. More than 1 million women seek medical assistance for injuries caused by battering each year, and the vast majority of domestic homicides are preceded by episodes of violence.[232,233]

Domestic violence is a major context for suicide attempts, substance abuse, and mental illness among women and 45 percent of the mothers of abused children are themselves battered women. Programs aimed at prevention of and intervention in partner abuse can also contribute to prevention in these areas and can provide a framework to ensure optimal safety and advocacy for both mother and child.[234,235]

The baseline rate for this objective is an estimate of severe violence, defined as acts that have a relatively high probability of causing an injury. Such acts include kicking, biting, punching, hitting with an object, beating up, threatening with a knife or gun, or using a knife or gun. Efforts to measure partner abuse are limited by what people are willing to reveal to interviewers as well as by inadequate techniques for measuring violent behavior. Improved methods for routinely collecting information on partner abuse and other forms of domestic violence are needed.

7.6 **Reduce assault injuries among people aged 12 and older to no more than 10 per 1,000 people. (Baseline: 11.1 per 1,000 in 1986)**

Baseline data source: National Crime Survey, U.S. Department of Justice.

An assault injury is defined as any physical or bodily harm occurring during the course of a rape, robbery, or any other type of attack upon a person. Each year between 1979 and 1986 more than 2.2 million people suffered nonfatal injuries from violent and abusive behavior. Of these injured victims, 1 million received medical care and 500,000 were treated by emergency medical facilities.[236] Even these figures, however, underestimate the true extent of nonfatal assaultive injury in the United States.

An estimated 28 percent of violent crime victims suffered injuries; more than 13 percent had injuries serious enough to require medical attention; for 7 percent the injury was serious enough to require hospital care and for 1 percent a hospital stay was necessary. Among those victims injured in violent events, an estimated 1 percent received gunshot wounds, 3 percent received knife wounds, and 6 percent suffered broken bones or lost teeth. Rates of injury from violent and abusive behavior were highest for males, blacks, people aged 19 to 24, people who were separated or divorced, those earning less than

$10,000 per year, and residents of central cities. When injured, black victims and elderly victims were substantially more likely than others to require overnight hospitalization.[236]

More than 25 percent of the Nation's 10,000 to 15,000 spinal cord injuries each year are the result of assaultive violence. The proportion of permanent disabling injuries that results from violent behavior varies considerably among geographic areas and population groups and is even higher in urban areas. In Detroit, 40 percent of all traumatic spinal cord injury results from gunshot wounds.[237] This proportion is particularly high among adolescents. In Northern California and Florida, 12 percent and 15.2 percent, respectively, of all spinal cord injuries are caused by violent and unintentional misuse of firearms.[238,239] Even in predominantly rural States such as Arkansas and Oklahoma, gunshot, stabbing, and assault injuries result in between 8.6 and 9.2 percent of all spinal cord disability.[240,241]

The National Crime Survey used to monitor this objective may drastically underreport injuries resulting from the abuse of women because abused women frequently fear reprisals if outsiders are informed and they do not generally regard these events as crimes.[242] In addition, its sampling and interviewing techniques may fail to reach the groups at highest risk for serious injury from assault, and it treats "series" victimizations (i.e., three or more violent events that are similar in nature and experienced by individuals who are unable to identify separately the details of each act) as single incidents.

7.7   **Reduce rape and attempted rape of women aged 12 and older to no more than 108 per 100,000 women. (Baseline: 120 per 100,000 in 1986)**

Special Population Target

Incidence of Rape and Attempted Rape (per 100,000)	1986 Baseline	2000 Target
7.7a Women aged 12-34	250	225

Baseline data source: National Crime Survey, U.S. Department of Justice.

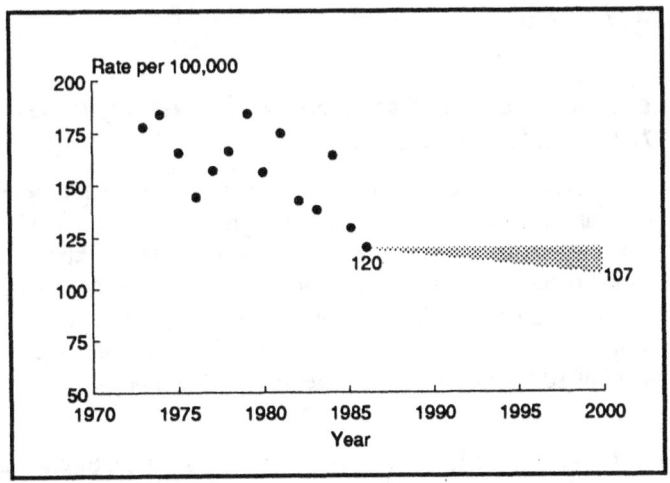

Fig. 7.7

Rate of rape and attempted rape of women aged 12 and older

Young, unmarried, and low-income women are the most frequent victims of rape and rape attempts. Women between the ages of 12 and 34 are particularly vulnerable, with victimization rates more than twice as high as women in other age categories.[243] Most rapists are unarmed and operate alone. Reported offenders are usually strangers to the victim, but this may reflect the reluctance of victims of acquaintance and date rape to report their experiences. Most sexual assaults occur at night and are attempts rather than completed rapes.

The rate of attempted and completed rape is difficult to measure accurately because only about half the victims contact law enforcement officials to report the crime.[243] An advantage of the National Crime Survey for monitoring the incidence of sexual assault is that it detects unreported crimes. However, women may still not report rapes when they are questioned in a context of crime[242] because victims of acquaintance and date rape and other rapes that do not meet common stereotypes often fail to define their experience as rape.

A number of widely accepted false beliefs exist about sexual assault (e.g., rape is always a violent crime and one cannot be raped by someone familiar). One such false belief—that forced kissing, fondling, or sexual intercourse is acceptable behavior in the context of dating relationships—is an important factor underlying sexual assault in our society. A survey of students in the sixth to ninth grades in Rhode Island found that 65 percent of boys and 57 percent of girls believed it was acceptable for a man to force a woman to have sex if they have been dating for more than 6 months. Similarly, 51 percent of boys and 41 percent of girls believed it was acceptable for a man to force a woman to have sex if he had spent a lot of money on her.[244]

Sexual assault awareness programs for adolescents should be initiated to change or modify beliefs that condone sexual assault. The effectiveness of these programs in modifying such beliefs and in subsequently reducing sexually assaultive behavior in dating relationships should also be evaluated.

7.8*   **Reduce by 15 percent the incidence of injurious suicide attempts among adolescents aged 14 through 17. (Baseline data available in 1991)**

* * *

* This objective also appears in the *Mental Health and Mental Disorders* priority area as Objective 6.2.

Risk Reduction Objectives

7.9   **Reduce by 20 percent the incidence of physical fighting among adolescents aged 14 through 17. (Baseline data available in 1991)**

Physical fighting among adolescents is often considered a normal and sometimes even necessary part of growing up. Fighting, however, results in hundreds of homicides and uncounted numbers of nonfatal injuries among adolescents each year. Fighting is the most immediate antecedent behavior for a great proportion of the homicides that occur in this age group and in many instances may be considered a necessary, if not a sufficient, cause. Estimates from the National Adolescent Study Health Survey indicate that 44 percent of 8th and 34 percent of 10th grade students were involved in a physical fight in 1987.[39]

Homicide rates increase by a factor of 15 during adolescence, from a negligible rate of 0.9 per 100,000 at age 10 to 13.9 per 100,000 by age 20.[245] This is proportionately the largest increase in the homicide rate in any decade of life.

A reduction in the incidence of physical fighting may prove extremely important in disrupting the causal mechanisms of homicide and assaultive injury. A variety of professionals have advocated teaching conflict resolution skills to adolescents to decrease their risk of homicide victimization and perpetration.[246] If adolescents can be taught to eschew violence as a way of solving problems, alternative nonviolent patterns of behavior might be carried through life, potentially leading to decreases in other forms of violence and violent injury such as partner abuse.

The Center for Chronic Disease Prevention and Health Promotion (Centers for Disease Control) will initiate a surveillance system of youth risk behaviors that will provide baseline data and track this objective beginning in 1991.

7.10 **Reduce by 20 percent the incidence of weapon-carrying by adolescents aged 14 through 17. (Baseline data available in 1991)**

Approximately 6 out of 10 homicide victims in the United States are killed with firearms; 9 out of 10 are killed with a weapon of some type, such as a gun, knife, or club. Although many people are killed in the course of being robbed or raped, most homicide victims are killed in the context of an argument, often by persons they know.[216] The immediate accessibility of a firearm or other lethal weapon is considered by many to be the factor that turns a violent altercation into a lethal event.[247]

Although the question of restricting firearm ownership and usage is contentious in American society, few argue that adolescents should have unsupervised access to firearms or other lethal weapons. Fewer still argue that adolescents should be permitted to carry loaded firearms or other lethal weapons at school or on city streets. Yet such weapons are routinely confiscated from adolescents by police or school officials across the Nation.[248] Estimates from the National Adolescent Student Health Survey indicate that 14 percent of 8th and 15 percent of 10th grade students carried a knife at school during 1987. This objective seeks to reduce and monitor the incidence of this high-risk behavior.[39]

The Center for Chronic Disease Prevention and Health Promotion (Centers for Disease Control) will initiate a surveillance system of youth risk behaviors that will provide baseline data and track this objective beginning in 1991.

7.11 **Reduce by 20 percent the proportion of people who possess weapons that are inappropriately stored and therefore dangerously available. (Baseline data available in 1992)**

The impulsive nature of many homicides and suicides suggests that a substantial portion of those events might be prevented if immediate access to lethal weapons was reduced,[249,250] in particular through appropriate storage of guns and ammunition. More than half of the 20,000 homicide victims in the United States each year are killed by persons they know.[216] In many instances, these homicides are committed impulsively and the perpetrators are immediately remorseful. Similarly, a substantial proportion of the Nation's 30,000 suicides each year are committed impulsively. Impulsive suicide without concomitant clinical depression appears to account for a particularly large proportion of youth suicides.[251] Homicide and suicide attempts are more likely to result in serious injury and death if lethal weapons are used.[252,253] Firearms are both the most lethal and the most common vehicle used for suicide and homicide, accounting for approximately 60 percent of these violent deaths each year.[228]

The controversy over gun control has obscured the fact that a broad range of environmental and behavioral measures may be effective in reducing the immediate access of certain sectors of the population to loaded firearms. ("Immediate access" may be defined as the ability to retrieve a loaded firearm within 10 minutes.) Immediate access to loaded firearms would be reduced if fewer people purchased them, if weapons and ammunition were stored in separate locations, or if parents locked up their weapons and ammunition so that their children could not use them unsupervised. Parents' access to loaded firearms would not be substantially reduced, but their children would not have immediate access to these lethal weapons. Immediate access to loaded firearms would also be reduced if the number of persons illegally carrying loaded firearms in public were decreased. Some jurisdictions have instituted legal measures to ensure waiting periods for purchasing firearms in order to reduce immediate accessibility to firearms by those most likely to misuse them.

Just as different types of environmental and behavioral measures would, if adopted, reduce access to loaded firearms for some segments of the population, strategies are available by which these measures might be achieved. Educational interventions, for example, might be designed to convince parents to take concrete steps to decrease their children's access to loaded firearms. Educational campaigns might also communicate important research findings regarding the relative risks and benefits of keeping firearms in the home, so that the general population can make better informed decisions. Legislative measures, such as those on waiting periods or prescribing mandatory jail terms for illegally carrying firearms, might be viable strategies, since these measures exact relatively minor costs on individual citizens.

By focusing on reducing immediate access to loaded firearms, this objective is meant to allow great flexibility for States and localities to define which mix of outcomes and strategies will best achieve the objective, given their particular resources and social environment. No particular method for achieving the objective is prescribed so that each locality may choose which of the various strategies is most appropriate and acceptable to its particular population. The Centers for Disease Control plans to establish baseline data and track this objective.

Services and Protection Objectives

7.12 **Extend protocols for routinely identifying, treating, and properly referring suicide attempters, victims of sexual assault, and victims of spouse, elder, and child abuse to at least 90 percent of hospital emergency departments. (Baseline data available in 1992)**

Hospital emergency departments are a key point of contact with victims of violent and abusive behavior. These departments should adopt standard protocols to facilitate and routinize early recognition of such victims and timely referral for appropriate intervention and treatment. Such efforts can be reasonably expected to lower the death and injury rate due to violent and abusive behavior (including the emotional consequences that are frequently associated with repeated exposure to violent and abusive behavior) for individuals who live in an environment where they are likely to be victimized repeatedly.[254,255]

Standard protocols have proven useful in the identification of battered women among female trauma patients in emergency departments. One large metropolitan hospital found that 21 percent of women who used the emergency surgical service were battered and almost half of all injuries presented by women to the emergency surgical service occurred through abuse. However, only 1 battered woman in 25 was diagnosed as such by medical personnel.[234] In another example, the percentage of women identified as battered in the emergency department of the Medical College of Pennsylvania increased from 5.6 percent to 30 percent following staff training and the introduction of a standard protocol.[256]

Protocols for identifying, treating, and referring victims of violent and abusive behavior are used in many hospital emergency departments across the country. A first step toward achieving this objective would be to review and evaluate existing protocols and, on the

7. Violent and Abusive Behavior

basis of such a review, develop model guidelines for hospitals to adopt in implementing standard protocols. The Center for Environmental Health and Injury Control plans to initiate a surveillance system to establish baseline data and track this objective by 1992.

7.13 Extend to at least 45 States implementation of unexplained child death review systems. (Baseline data available in 1991)

Numerous communities have systems to review unexplained child deaths. These systems are important for accurately identifying child abuse deaths, assuring that living children in families in which child abuse deaths occur are adequately protected, and determining how child abuse death cases could have been managed more effectively by agencies with which the child victims had contact.[257] Comparable to hospital protocols that investigate unexpected patient deaths, such systems hold promise of defining remediable weaknesses in community child protection networks. The Center for Environmental Health and Injury Control (Centers for Disease Control) plans to collaborate with the National Committee for Prevention of Child Abuse to establish a baseline and track this objective in 1991.

7.14 Increase to at least 30 the number of States in which at least 50 percent of children identified as neglected or physically or sexually abused receive physical and mental evaluation with appropriate followup as a means of breaking the intergenerational cycle of abuse. (Baseline data available in 1993)

Being abused or neglected as a child increases one's risk for violent behavior as an adult.[258] The common treatment for the physically or sexually abused child is to modify the child's environment by placement outside of the home or to provide therapeutic treatment for the parents. The abused child's devalued self-image, loss of trust, and distorted view of parent-child relationships are not addressed by either of these strategies.[259] If child abuse is to be prevented, abused children must be treated to improve their future relationships with their own children.

Standard diagnostic protocols are needed and should be administered to children identified as being neglected or physically or sexually abused. These assessments should be used to guide abused children to appropriate therapeutic treatments. A variety of treatment strategies exist which may be valuable for breaking the intergenerational cycle of abuse.[260] Nevertheless, further research into the long-term effects of abuse and neglect on children is needed along with long-term evaluations of the effect of psychotherapy.

The Center for Environmental Health and Injury Control will collaborate with the National Committee for Prevention of Child Abuse to establish baseline data and track this objective by 1993.

7.15 Reduce to less than 10 percent the proportion of battered women and their children turned away from emergency housing due to lack of space. (Baseline: 40 percent in 1987)

Baseline data source: Domestic Violence Statistical Survey.

In 1987, nearly 40 percent of battered women and children in need of emergency housing were turned away because of lack of space. In some States, shelters turn away 2 battered women for every woman who receives services. In 1987, there were 935 shelters available to battered women, 550 safe homes, and 303 nonresidential programs.[261]

The lack of available space for battered women and their children could be partially alleviated if more shelters were available. Also, the demand for emergency housing could be reduced if more nonresidential programs were available. Nonresidential programs can help some women to avoid severe battering by providing them with remedial options early in the battering cycle and, thereby, alleviate the demand for shelter services. Increasing nonresidential programs may also be a practical option in rural areas where support for shelters may be unavailable but where battered women are still in need of services.

7.16 Increase to at least 50 percent the proportion of elementary and secondary schools that teach nonviolent conflict resolution skills, preferably as a part of quality school health education. (Baseline data available in 1991)

Schools provide a strategic setting for the prevention of violent and abusive behavior.[262] They contain a captive audience, many of whose members are at risk of becoming victims or perpetrators of interpersonal violence. Health-related knowledge, attitudes, and behaviors can be positively affected through school health education curricula.[263] Curricula have been developed for various grade levels that seek to change knowledge about and attitudes toward violence and to instill interpersonal skills for resolving conflicts nonviolently.[262] The principles underlying these programs, already successfully applied to the prevention of substance abuse, include providing information about the medical and social consequences of individual behaviors and improving interpersonal and decision making skills.[260,265,267]

A program has been developed to show educators how to teach children social and cognitive skills that enable them to resolve conflicts nonviolently.[268] Another program directly focuses on changing adolescents' behaviors and attitudes toward violence. This 10-session high school curriculum teaches students about the magnitude of the violence problem, their vulnerability to violent injury, the role of anger in human interactions, and strategies for nonviolent forms of conflict resolution.[246]

While studies of the effectiveness of these curricula in reducing violent and abusive behaviors are inconclusive, these curricula seem promising. At least one study has shown that they can be effective in diminishing attitudes that justify violent behavior and in improving social problem-solving abilities.[269]

For a definition of quality school health education, see *Educational and Community-Based Programs*. The Center for Chronic Disease Prevention and Health Promotion will initiate a survey to establish baseline data and track this objective in 1991.

7.17 Extend coordinated, comprehensive violence prevention programs to at least 80 percent of local jurisdictions with populations over 100,000. (Baseline data available in 1993)

A coordinated, comprehensive effort by State and local health, criminal justice, and social service agencies is necessary to maximize resources and ensure the availability of violence prevention strategies and information to all segments of the population. Collaboration across these traditionally disparate agencies is necessary to break down barriers that impede violence prevention and control activities.

Without such collaboration, programs such as target hardening, domestic crisis intervention, and violence prevention education very often are developed without regard to other activities operating in an area and/or without the support of the community in which the program operates. These programs typically approach violence prevention from a singular perspective, not recognizing that successful prevention requires a variety of different disciplines and organizations working together to develop a range of programs tailored to the specific needs of a community.

Comprehensive violence prevention programs should incorporate strategies that are potentially effective for preventing specific types of interpersonal violence. For example, a comprehensive approach to the prevention of child maltreatment might include the following strategies:

- Public awareness programs for citizens about positive parenting, positive family support, and cues to suspect child physical and sexual abuse and how to report it to authorities.

- Prenatal health care and parenting education and support programs for new parents (including home health visitor programs).[270]

- Support services for parents under stress (such as child care, respite care, crisis nurseries, helplines, self-help groups, and other natural helping networks, provisions for linkages and continuity of care and services, housing and other basic necessities, job training).

- School-based age-specific prevention education programs for all school-aged children.

- Therapeutic care for victims and perpetrators of physical and sexual abuse; home-based transition and follow up services for children and their families.[260]

- Projects for the prevention of alcohol- and other drug-related child abuse and neglect including substance abuse as a component of parenting education and curriculum training programs.

- Hospital-based (or related health facility as may be available in a rural area) information and referral services for parents of children with disabilities and children who have been neglected or physically or sexually abused by their parents.

- Multidisciplinary training programs for professionals involved in the planning and implementation of community programs.

Comprehensive efforts to address domestic violence in States and local areas may include the following strategies:

- Public awareness programs that help dispel myths about domestic violence and publicize sources of shelter and support for battered women and their children.

- Coordination among the criminal justice system, domestic violence programs, child protective services, substance abuse programs, mental health centers, and the medical community for referral, intervention, and case management.

- Expansion of court-ordered treatment programs for abusers.

- Expansion of emergency shelter and support services for victims.

- Expansion of transitional and low-income housing resources for victims to help them achieve safety and economic self-sufficiency.

- Training programs for professionals in medical, legal, and social service fields who deal with potential victims and abusers or who are involved in the planning and implementation of prevention programs.

Specific strategies that may be useful components of comprehensive programs exist for other types of violence and abuse such as elder abuse, sexual assault, firearm injuries, and acquaintance violence as well.[262] Although there are creative and promising preventive interventions, little is known about their effectiveness. Consequently, it is important that States and local entities initiating comprehensive programs collect rigorous evaluation evidence to document effectiveness.

The Center for Environmental Health and Injury Control (Centers for Disease Control) will collaborate with the National Center on Child Abuse and Neglect and the National Committee for Prevention of Child Abuse to establish baseline data and track this objective by 1993.

* * *

Research Needs

Understanding of the causes of violent and abusive behavior must be advanced substantially to establish a firm foundation for effective prevention. Research should focus on factors that are amenable to change or that suggest the possibility of preventive intervention. These research needs will be most effectively met through multidisciplinary approaches, including such disciplines as epidemiology, sociology, criminology, psychology, economics, medicine, statistics, law, public health, genetics, neurobiology, and biomechanics. Resources are needed to facilitate a coordinated effort to develop and implement a national research agenda over the next decade. Emphasis must also be given to the evaluation of the impact of current violence prevention policies. This is particularly critical because many unevaluated programs are purported to prevent various dimensions of violent and abusive behavior. In addition, the effectiveness of many publicly mandated treatment programs and laws that are intended to modify potential risk factors for violence remains unknown. Specific research needs for the area of violent and abusive behavior are:

- Epidemiologic investigations focusing on quantifying the risk of injury associated with the possession of firearms and factors that may modify that risk.

- The systematic development, implementation, and rigorous evaluation of comprehensive community-based violence prevention programs.

- Basic research on the biomedical, molecular, and genetic underpinnings of interpersonal violence, suicidal behavior, and related mental and behavioral disorders.

- Research recommendations made in *Injury Prevention: Meeting the Challenge*, by the National Committee for Injury Prevention and Control.[262]

- Research recommendations to be made by the National Academy of Sciences' Panel on the Understanding and Control of Violent Behavior in 1991.

- Research recommendations made in the Report of the Secretary's Task Force on Youth Suicide, U.S. Department of Health and Human Services, in 1989.[196]

- Determination of which childhood exposures and behaviors are most predictive of future violent behavior and what interventions are most effective and developmentally appropriate for reducing the effects of harmful exposures or modifying predictive behaviors.

- Identification of situational factors that increase the risk of violent altercations (e.g., the distribution and use of illicit drugs, gang memberships) and situational factors that increase the risk of injury given the occurrence of violent altercations (e.g., intoxication of the combatants, accessibility of lethal weapons).

* * *

Baseline Data Source References

1987 Domestic Violence Statistical Survey, National Coalition Against Domestic Violence, Washington, DC.

National Crime Survey, Bureau of Crime Statistics, U.S. Department of Justice, Washington, DC.

National Family Violence Survey 1985, National Institute of Mental Health, Alcohol, Drug Abuse, and Mental Health Administration, Public Health Service, U.S. Department of Health and Human Services, Rockville, MD.

National Vital Statistics System, National Center for Health Statistics, Centers for Disease Control, Public Health Service, U.S. Department of Health and Human Services, Hyattsville, MD.

Study of the National Incidence of Child Abuse and Neglect, National Center on Child Abuse and Neglect, Administration for Children, Youth, and Families, Office of Human Development Services, U.S. Department of Health and Human Services, Washington, DC.

Educational and Community-based Programs

8

Contents

* * *

8.2 Completion of high school

8.3 Preschool child development programs

8.4 Quality school health education

* * *

8.9 Family discussion of health issues

* * *

8.14 Effective public health systems

[Research Needs]

8. Educational and Community-Based Programs

* * *

Risk Reduction Objective

8.2 Increase the high school graduation rate to at least 90 percent, thereby reducing risks for multiple problem behaviors and poor mental and physical health. (Baseline: 79 percent of people aged 20 through 21 had graduated from high school with a regular diploma in 1989)

Note: This objective and its target are consistent with the National Education Goal to increase high school graduation rates. The baseline estimate is a proxy. When a measure is chosen to monitor the National Education Goal, the same measure and data source will be used to track this objective.

Baseline data source: Current Population Survey, U.S. Department of Commerce.

Dropping out of school is associated with later unemployment, poverty, and poor health. During adolescence, dropping out of school is associated with multiple social and health problems including substance abuse, delinquency, intentional and unintentional injury, and unintended pregnancy. The antecedents of these problems appear to be highly inter-correlated and may form a constellation of common precursors. Some researchers suggest that the antecedents of drug and alcohol problems, school dropout, delinquency, and a host of other problems can be identified in the early elementary grades, long before the actual problems are manifest. These include low academic achievement and low attachment to school; adverse peer influence; inadequate family management and parental supervision; parental substance abuse; sensation-seeking behavior; early use of tobacco, alcohol, or marijuana; early aggressive or acting-out behavior; and diminished self-efficacy. For example, children who perform poorly in school, are more than a year behind their modal grade, and are chronically truant are more likely to exhibit risk behaviors and experience serious problems in adolescence. Children are also placed at increased risk when their attitudes toward education are negative and their adjustment to school has been difficult. Finally, risk is increased if children fail to form meaningful social bonds to positive adult and peer role models with whom they interact at school or in the community.

Although more research on the risk factors for multiple problem behaviors is needed, sufficient scientific knowledge currently exists to guide public health program planning and policy development. For example, child development programs for low-income preschoolers can foster positive attitudes toward school, enhance school performance, and increase high school graduation rates (see Objective 8.3). Mentor programs that pair disadvantaged youth with caring adults have also been shown to be effective in improving both academic and employment success. By addressing high school dropout rates as part of the Nation's health promotion and disease prevention agenda, it may be possible to reduce unwarranted risk of problem behavior and improve the health of our young people.

The target of 90 percent set for this objective is consistent with the National Education Goal to increase the high school graduation rate to at least 90 percent by the year 2000. A National Education Objective under that goal is to eliminate the gap in high school graduation rates between minority and nonminority students. In 1989, only 54 percent of Hispanic and 76 percent of black youth aged 20 through 21 had graduated from high school with a regular diploma. This compares to a graduation rate of 84 percent for white, non-Hispanic youth.

Services and Protection Objectives

8.3 **Achieve for all disadvantaged children and children with disabilities access to high quality and developmentally appropriate preschool programs that help prepare children for school, thereby improving their prospects with regard to school performance, problem behaviors, and mental and physical health. (Baseline: 47 percent of eligible children aged 4 were afforded the opportunity to enroll in Head Start in 1990)**

Note: This objective and its target are consistent with the National Education Goal to increase school readiness and its objective to increase access to preschool programs for disadvantaged and disabled children. The baseline estimate is an available, but partial, proxy. When a measure is chosen to monitor this National Education Objective, the same measure and data source will be used to track this objective.

Baseline data source: Head Start Bureau, Office of Human Development Services.

High-quality early childhood development programs can improve children's social skills, problem-solving abilities, self-esteem, and long-term school performance by providing a positive introduction to learning that instills the motivation and the basic skills they need to thrive in the classroom, at home, and later in life. Pooling the results of 11 preschool experiments, the Consortium for Longitudinal Studies found that students with preschool experience had much lower rates of subsequent special education placement and grade retention and higher rates of high school graduation than students with no preschool experience. Of the former preschoolers who had reached graduation age, 15 percent had been placed in special education classes compared to 40 percent of the children who had not attended preschool, 33 percent had repeated a grade compared to 50 percent, and 67 percent had completed high school compared to 50 percent. Other long-term followup results have shown that State-funded prekindergarten programs in New York and Maryland improved students' later school performance in comparable ways. Similar advantages have been found for a broad array of child development programs, not just those labeled preschool.

The location of the child development program—day care home, community center, or school—does not necessarily determine program outcome. Quality is the critical variable. The most important standards for a high-quality early childhood program are staff training in early childhood education and high adult to child ratios. The National Association for the Education of Young Children recommends an adult to child ratio of 1:10 for 3- and 4-year-olds. Curricula should emphasize play and discovery, not rote learning, and should be developmentally appropriate. To be effective, programs for at-risk preschoolers must be comprehensive, addressing the child's social, emotional, cognitive, and physical development. Parent involvement is also essential and should be maximized. The program must involve parents and other caretakers in day to day decisions as well as offer them education and support. All programs should meet standards for health and safety.

One of the best known early childhood development programs is Head Start, which has served almost 10 million disadvantaged children since its inception in 1965. However, Head Start is not the only program serving disadvantaged children and children with disabilities. Increasing numbers of States and localities are developing preschool programs for disadvantaged children. In addition, low-income children participate in private preschool programs, such as church-based programs, where fees sometimes are a function of income or public funds may subsidize their participation. Early childhood programs for children with disabilities are offered by a variety of providers and take many forms.

8.4 **Increase to at least 75 percent the proportion of the Nation's elementary and secondary schools that provide planned and sequential kindergarten through 12th grade quality school health education. (Baseline data available in 1991)**

Schools offer the most systematic and efficient means available to improve the health of youth and enable young people to avoid health risks. They provide an avenue for reaching more than 46 million students each year. Planned and sequential quality school health education programs help young people at each appropriate grade to develop the increasingly complex knowledge and skills they will need to avoid important health risks, and to maintain their own health, the health of the families for which they will become responsible, and the health of the communities in which they will reside. The content of the education is determined locally by parents, school boards, and other members of the community.

School health education has been defined by the Education Commission of the States,[271] the National Professional School Health Education Organizations,[272] the World Health Organization,[273] and the Centers for Disease Control. To one extent or another, each of these definitions embraces an educational experience that fosters the development of health-related knowledge, attitudes, and skills on various topics within areas such as community health, environmental health, family life, nutrition, physical activity, personal health practices, injury prevention, and substance use and abuse.

Many studies have shown that properly designed and implemented school health education programs can be effective in preventing risk behaviors. For example, the School Health Education Evaluation, a three-year study of four health education programs, demonstrated that the programs evaluated helped children improve health knowledge, attitudes, and behaviors.[274] The effectiveness of these programs were influenced by the amount of classroom time devoted to the program, the extent to which school administrators supported the program, and the extent to which teachers were prepared and motivated to implement the program.

As of 1989, 25 States had mandated that schools implement school health education programs and another 9 States had recommended that schools implement such programs. However, national data sources give varying estimates regarding the actual proportion of schools currently offering comprehensive school health education curricula. In 1985, a Metropolitan Life survey of public school district superintendents estimated that 34 percent of the Nation's children receive multitopic, multigrade school health education. A 1988 Metropolitan Life survey of public school teachers (grades 3 through 12) found 67 percent reporting that their schools offered multitopic, multigrade curricula. Most experts consider these to be overestimates. The National School Boards Association is currently using the CDC interim definition to assess the extent to which the Nation's 15,000 school districts require broad-based school health education programs.

To attain this objective, all States and school districts should require and support planned and sequential quality school health education for students in kindergarten through 12th grade. To assure the implementation of high-quality school health education programs, States should require health literacy, the health equivalent of basic literacy, as a requirement for graduation.

Other aspects of the school environment are also important to school health. State and local health departments can work with schools to provide a multidimensional program of school health that may include school health education, school-linked or school-based health services designed to prevent, detect, and address health problems, a healthy and safe school environment, physical education, healthful school food service selections,

8. Educational and Community-Based Programs

psychological assessment and counseling to promote child development and emotional health, schoolsite health promotion for faculty and staff, and integrated school and community health promotion efforts.

* * *

8.9 **Increase to at least 75 percent the proportion of people aged 10 and older who have discussed issues related to nutrition, physical activity, sexual behavior, tobacco, alcohol, other drugs, or safety with family members on at least one occasion during the preceding month. (Baseline data available in 1991)**

Note: This objective, which supports family communication on a range of vital personal health issues, will be tracked using the National Health Interview Survey, a continuing, voluntary, national sample survey of adults who report on household characteristics including such items as illnesses, injuries, use of health services, and demographic characteristics.

The World Health Organization characterizes the family as the "primary social agent in the promotion of health and well-being."[275] The family, no matter how loosely defined—even as household—is a place where lifestyle patterns are initiated, maintained, and altered over time. It is where risk factors tend to cluster, and in most cases, members share a genetic history. It is the most basic consumer unit for foods, products, and services that influence health status. It is a major source of stress and social support.

In 1985, a Gallup survey demonstrated the influence of the family upon health-related behavior patterns. Gallup interviewed 1011 adults, asking them how they changed their behavior and who helped them change. They found that a spouse or significant other was more likely to influence a person's health habits than anyone else, including the family doctor. Husbands were twice as likely, for instance, to quit smoking (22 percent versus 11 percent) and more likely to lose weight (42 percent versus 31 percent) than single men.

Research on the family's impact on health provides empiric evidence that family patterns influence such conditions as coronary heart disease, hypertension, diabetes, substance abuse and mental disorders, anorexia nervosa, childhood illnesses, asthma, schizophrenia, and depression.[276]

* * *

8.14 **Increase to at least 90 percent the proportion of people who are served by a local health department that is effectively carrying out the core functions of public health. (Baseline data available in 1992)**

Note: The core functions of public health have been defined as assessment, policy development, and assurance.[277] Local health department refers to any local component of the public health system, defined as an administrative and service unit of local or State government concerned with health and carrying some responsibility for the health of a jurisdiction smaller than a State.

The Institute of Medicine (IOM) Report *The Future of Public Health* acknowledged past public health successes but described in detail problems within the U.S. public health system.[277] The AIDS epidemic, which threatens the health of millions of Americans, has also brought the inadequacies of our public health system into high visibility. That same system is in critical need of improvement if the Nation is to address not only AIDS, but the burden of chronic diseases in our aging population and injuries and violence to our young. Both the Presidential Commission on HIV Infection and the IOM report outline steps necessary to strengthen the public health system and call for a plan of action for improvements. The desired outcome is a public health system effectively performing the core functions of public health agencies, which the IOM report identifies for all levels of government as assessment, policy development, and assurance. Specifically, public health agencies should (1) regularly and systematically collect, assemble, analyze, and make available information on the health of the community (i.e., assessment); (2) exercise their responsibility to serve the public interest in the development of comprehensive public health policies by promoting the use of the scientific knowledge base in decision-making (i.e., policy development); and (3) assure their constituents that services necessary to achieve agreed-upon goals are provided by encouraging actions of others (private and public), requiring action through regulation, or providing services directly (i.e., assurance).

The current public health system is built around governmental agencies—primarily Federal, State, and local health departments. Approximately 94 percent of the population is presently served by a State or local health department, but the number, quality, and effectiveness of the services provided varies greatly. Other critical participants in the system include clinical medicine, voluntary agencies, schools and universities, business and industry, professional associations, community organizations, and third-party payers. A governmental presence is needed at the local level to provide leadership in identifying and prioritizing community health problems and coordinating the efforts of the various private and public sector participants to assure that necessary health promotion and disease prevention services are provided. Consensus must be developed and institutionalized on the appropriate roles, attributes, and standards of effective performance of all parties within the public health system to fully realize the benefits of effective public health practice.

The public health community has recognized these problems and has initiated three landmark actions that have helped focus opinion on the need for definition and consensus with respect to the public health system. In 1979, the publication of *Model Standards: A Guide for Community Preventive Health Services* advanced the concept of a governmental presence at the local level to assure the public's health.[278] In 1987, the National Association of County Health Officials entered into a cooperative agreement with CDC entitled APEX/PH (A Protocol for Excellence in Public Health). This protocol will provide a process by which local health authorities determine their specific community-based roles, assess their internal capacities, and provide direction to their efforts. In 1988, *The Future of Public Health* proposed the core functions of public health.[277]

In addition, the 1990 objectives played a most significant role by providing direction and focus to the health promotion and disease prevention efforts of the public health system. However, the objectives did not specifically address the inadequacies in the system itself that might adversely affect their achievement. A public health system effectively carrying out the core functions will assure that scarce public health resources are directed to address identified health problems of high priority. If achievement of the year 2000 objectives is to be a reality, there must be a public health system with the capacity to carry out the necessary strategies. This cross-cutting objective helps to assure the existence, effectiveness, and appropriate distribution of that capacity.

* * *

Research Needs

High priority research needs in health promotion include:

- Research into the factors influencing health-related behavior change.

- Evaluation of the degree to which health promotion in schools, communities, health care facilities, worksites, and religious institutions changes lifestyle choices, and the consequent changes in health status, health service use, productivity, and economic costs to society.

- Studies to delineate the most effective elements of intervention strategies carried out in schools, worksites, community-based programs, and health care settings.

- Investigation of the ways changes in the external social environment reinforce and/or interact with health promotion and education strategies.

- Research into reasons people change or do not change behavior related to health as a result of exposure to health promotion programs.

- Further research on worksite programs, particularly more studies of programs in new and emerging service industries and small business and programs that use the worksite to reach not only workers but their families, retirees, and the community at large.

- Research in health promotion for special worker populations such as women, older adults, and minority groups who are entering the workforce in increasing numbers. Also, hourly employees who are often passed by in traditional approaches. Research is needed on what encourages hourly workers to heed educational messages and to take part in health-enhancing activities, and how to create a supportive work environment conducive to good health choices.

* * *

- Operational research in local public health (e.g., strategic and capacity-building planning models, specification of core community services, and alternatives for organizing and delivering community programs).

* * *

Baseline Data Source References

Current Population Reports (Series P-20, School Enrollment, Social and Economic Characteristics of Students, no. 222, 303, 362, 392, and 409), Bureau of the Census, U.S. Department of Commerce, Washington, DC.

Head Start Bureau, U.S. Department of Health and Human Services, Washington, DC.

Unintentional Injuries

9

Contents

* * *

- 9.3 Motor vehicle crash-related deaths
- 9.4 Fall-related deaths
- 9.5 Drowning deaths
- 9.6 Residential fire deaths

* * *

- 9.8 Nonfatal poisoning
- 9.9 Nonfatal head injuries
- 9.10 Nonfatal spinal cord injuries
- 9.11 Secondary disabilities associated with head and spinal cord injuries
- 9.12 Motor vehicle occupant protection systems
- 9.13 Helmet use by motorcyclists and bicyclists
- 9.14 Safety belt and helmet use laws
- 9.15 Handgun design to protect children
- 9.16 Fire suppression sprinkler installation
- 9.17 Smoke detectors
- 9.18 Injury prevention instruction in schools
- 9.19 Protective equipment in sporting and recreation events

* * *

- 9.21 Injury prevention counseling by clinicians
- 9.22 Emergency medical services and trauma systems
- [Research Needs]

9. Unintentional Injuries

***

Health Status Objectives

***

9.3 Reduce deaths caused by motor vehicle crashes to no more than 1.9 per 100 million vehicle miles traveled and 16.8 per 100,000 people. (Baseline: 2.4 per 100 million vehicle miles traveled (VMT) and 18.8 per 100,000 people (age adjusted) in 1987)

Special Population Targets

Deaths Caused by Motor Vehicle Crashes (per 100,000)		1987 Baseline	2000 Target
9.3a	Children aged 14 and younger	6.2	5.5
9.3b	Youth aged 15-24	36.9	33

***

Type-Specific Targets

Deaths Caused By Motor Vehicle Crashes		1987 Baseline	2000 Target
9.3e	Motorcyclists	40.9/100 million VMT & 1.7/100,000	33/100 million VMT & 1.5/100,000
9.3f	Pedestrians	3.1/100,000	2.7/100,000

Baseline data sources: Fatal Accident Reporting System (FARS), U.S. Department of Transportation; for American Indians/Alaska Natives, National Vital Statistics System, CDC.

Motor vehicle-related fatalities account for about half of all unintentional injury deaths and are the leading cause of work-related injury deaths. Approximately 46,000 people die each year and more than 3.5 million are injured. Society loses nearly $75 billion annually as the result of motor vehicle crashes.[279]

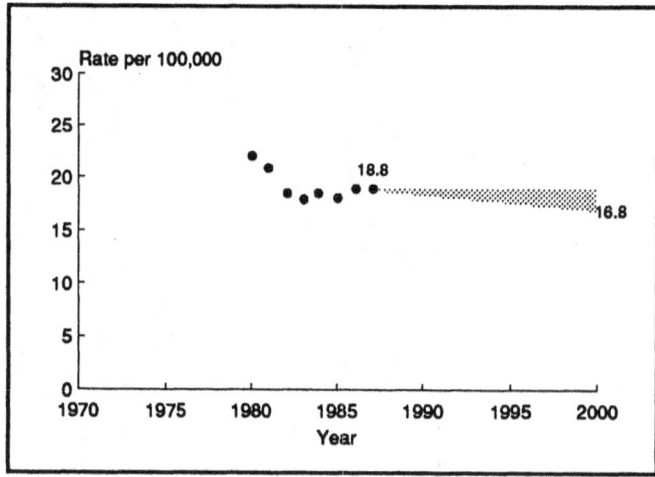

Fig. 9.3i

Motor vehicle crash death rate per 100 million vehicle miles traveled

9. Unintentional Injuries

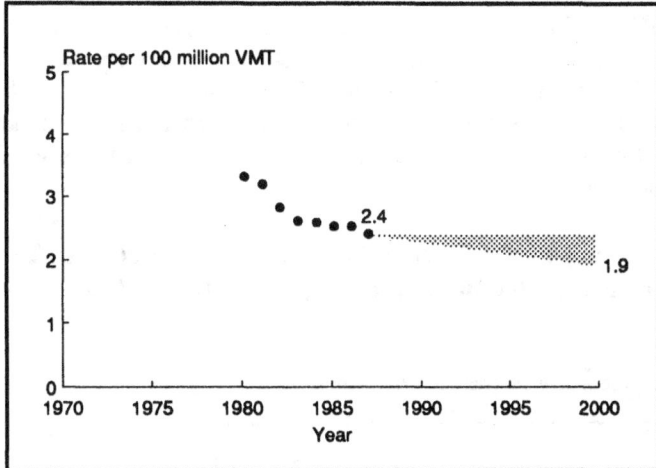

Fig. 9.3ii

Age-adjusted motor vehicle crash death rate per 100,000 people

This objective includes rates for deaths per 100,000 population and deaths per million VMT. Population-based rates can misrepresent the impact of highway safety measures because they do not measure exposure to crash risk. As the number of miles driven increases, the risk of a crash increases. Therefore, the VMT-based death rate provides a more accurate measure of motor vehicle safety. Population rates, however, are important in describing motor vehicle crash injury as a public health problem, particularly for the high-risk groups, such as young adults, for whom VMT rates are not available. Deaths from off-road vehicle (all-terrain vehicles, trail bikes, snowmobiles) crashes are not included in this objective because the hazards encountered on these vehicles are very different from those of on-road vehicles. Furthermore, because registration of off-road vehicles or their riders is not uniformly required, data on VMT or number of users are not routinely available.

The year 2000 target rates were established after considering recent trends in the death rate, the impact of future automatic occupant protection systems, and anticipated demographic changes. Reduction of the overall death rate will depend upon several factors, including use of mass transit, continued reductions in drunk driving, and improvement of pedestrian, motorcycle, and bicycle safety.

Motorcycle, pedestrian, and bicycle casualties account for almost 30 percent of motor vehicle deaths each year. Motorcycle crashes cause approximately 11 percent of all motor vehicle deaths. Many motorcycle crash injuries are due to lack of operator skill, intoxication of the operator, and absence of protective headgear.[280] Countermeasures, including use of motorcycle helmets, are strongly associated with decreased death and injury.[281] An increase in alcohol/drug use prevention and deterrence activities is also associated with decreased death and disability.

Motor vehicle crashes involving pedestrians have steadily declined over the past 50 years to a low of 6,746 deaths in 1987. Nonetheless, pedestrians account for 14.5 percent of all motor vehicle-related fatalities, and alcohol is associated with close to 50 percent of pedestrian deaths.[282] Safety programs directed at youthful pedestrians have been shown to be effective and may be partly responsible for the 24-percent decline in deaths of children less than 15 years old between 1980 and 1986.[105]

* * *

Speed is a fundamental factor in the physical forces involved in crashes.[283] Highway speed enforcement efforts have generated significant yearly increases in speeding citations, yet speed continues to rise. Law enforcement agencies have not been able to keep pace with the increased demands of traffic. In the future, law enforcement needs a comprehensive approach, including improved public information and education efforts, expanded public and private support, and new strategies such as the legal prohibition of radar detectors, as well as carefully monitored speed limits. Improved motor vehicle technology, such as antilock braking systems, side impact protection, and modification of the highway environment by the elimination of roadside and roadway hazards also offers important preventive measures.[284]

9.4 **Reduce deaths from falls and fall-related injuries to no more than 2.3 per 100,000 people. (Age-adjusted baseline: 2.7 per 100,000 in 1987)**

* * *

Baseline data source: National Vital Statistics System, CDC.

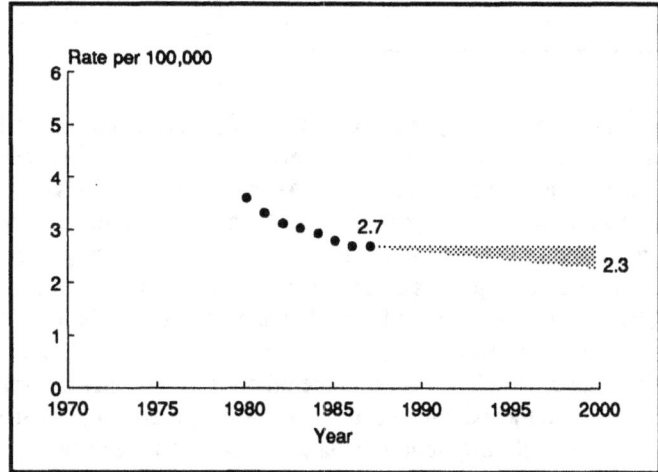

Fig. 9.4

Age-adjusted death rate from falls and fall-related injuries

Falls and fall-related injuries occur at every age. . . .

While fall-related death rates for children are relatively low in comparison with rates for older adults, fall-related disability is a significant problem in childhood.[285,286] Prevention strategies, including safe playground equipment and protective bars on upper story windows, have proven effective for reducing falls at the youngest ages.[287,288]

* * *

9.5 **Reduce drowning deaths to no more than 1.3 per 100,000 people. (Age-adjusted baseline: 2.1 per 100,000 in 1987)**

Special Population Targets

	Drowning Deaths (per 100,000)	*1987 Baseline*	*2000 Target*
9.5a	Children aged 4 and younger	4.2	2.3
9.5b	Men aged 15-34	4.5	2.5
9.5c	Black males	6.6	3.6

Baseline data source: National Vital Statistics System, CDC.

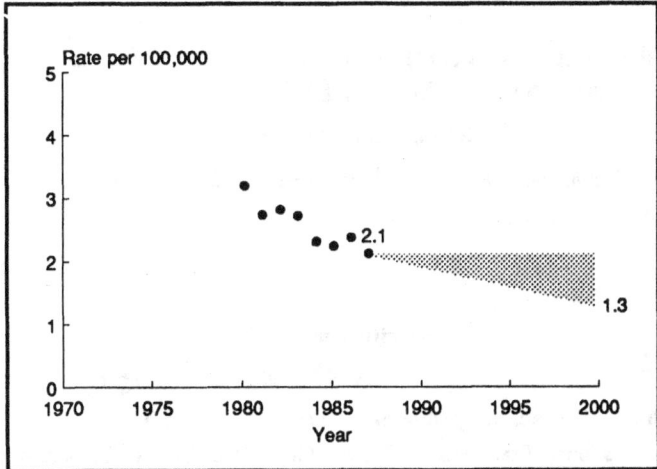

Fig. 9.5
Age-adjusted drowning death rate

Drowning rates dropped considerably between 1979 and 1987, when 5,100 people drowned in the United States, placing it second among unintentional injuries in years of potential life lost. Those at highest risk include males, children less than 5 years old, blacks, American Indians, and some occupational groups.[289] The highest drowning rates are among children aged 4 and younger and men aged 15 through 34.[290] Rates are consistently higher among black men than among white men.[289]

The causes of the remarkably high rate of drowning by black males are unknown and virtually unstudied. Epidemiologic research and surveillance should be attempted to improve understanding of the causes and mechanisms of drowning by black males so that appropriate interventions can be developed and evaluated. The projected 45-percent reduction of drowning in this group assumes that feasible interventions will be identified.

Causes of drowning for men aged 15 through 34 are multiple, but appear to center around boating and water activities and alcohol use combined with these activities. All States and territories currently have laws to prohibit operating a boat under the influence of alcohol or drugs, but stronger regulations and enforcement are needed to reduce the deaths in this age group. Public awareness of the importance of encouraging safe operating practices and discouraging alcohol use are also potentially effective measures.

This objective is based on a projected reduction of 50 percent from drowning in swimming pools and a reduction of 33 percent from boating activities.[291,292] Potentially effective strategies, such as four-sided fencing, alarms, properly designed pool covers, and safety regulations are available to prevent pool drowning by preschool children. These strategies are difficult to implement and monitor because of the more than 40,000 local jurisdictions.

Reductions in drowning rates between 1979 and 1987 may represent an increased number of near-drowning victims. The rates of near drowning where victims are left with permanent neurologic damage are unknown. Epidemiologic surveillance and followup of near-drowning cases are needed to determine the true magnitude of the problem. Although intervention strategies have been developed to decrease drowning deaths, research is needed to evaluate the effectiveness of such strategies, including widespread cardiopulmonary resuscitation (CPR) training, expanded implementation of emergency medical services (EMS) protocols, and expanded availability of regional intensive care facilities.

9.6 Reduce residential fire deaths to no more than 1.2 per 100,000 people. (Age-adjusted baseline: 1.5 per 100,000 in 1987)

Special Population Targets

Residential Fire Deaths (per 100,000)	1987 Baseline	2000 Target
9.6a Children aged 4 and younger	4.4	3.3

* * *

Type-Specific Target

	1983 Baseline	2000 Target
9.6e Residential fire deaths caused by smoking	17%	5%

Baseline data sources: National Vital Statistics System, CDC; National Fire Incident Reporting System, Federal Emergency Management Agency.

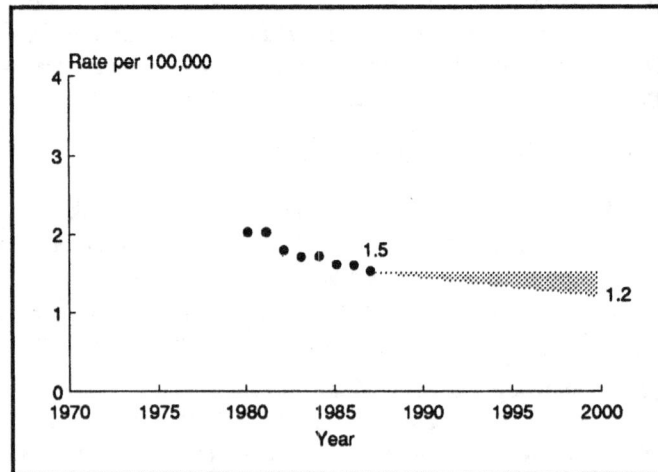

Fig. 9.6

Age-adjusted residential fire death rate

Residential fires account for 75 to 80 percent of all fire deaths and are the fourth leading cause of unintentional injury deaths. Direct causes of fire-related death include burns, asphyxiation, and traumatic injuries sustained by firefighters. Subsequent infection of a burn injury is an indirect cause of fire death. Fire-related injuries, particularly burns, are complex to treat, carry higher risks, and require longer hospitalization than other types of injuries. Burn injuries also cause more intense and more prolonged suffering than other traumas.

Residential fires claimed 4,274 people in 1987. Children aged 4 and younger and people aged 65 and older have unusually high death rates, and higher rates are also observed for men, blacks, American Indians, and the poor.[293] Those who live in substandard housing without smoke detectors are often at the highest risk of fire death. Cigarette-ignited fires cause about 7 percent of all residential fires but 17 percent of the fatal fires. Many fires start when cigarettes continue to burn after being dropped or set down and ignite upholstery, bedding, or clothing. Strategies to reduce smoking and alcohol abuse will contribute to achieving this objective, as would the introduction of cigarettes designed not to ignite furnishings and child-resistant cigarette lighters, technologies that have been tested and found feasible.[294] Improved public awareness of home fire safety measures, including functional smoke detectors and home evacuation plans, and greater fire safety of products can contribute to reduced home fire deaths and disabilities.

* * *

9. Unintentional Injuries

9.8 **Reduce nonfatal poisoning to no more than 88 emergency department treatments per 100,000 people. (Baseline: 103 per 100,000 in 1986)**

Special Population Target

Nonfatal Poisoning (per 100,000)	1986 Baseline	2000 Target
9.8a Among children aged 4 and younger	650	520

Baseline data source: National Electronic Injury Surveillance System, Consumer Product Safety Commission.

Poisoning by solids and liquids and poisoning by gases are two distinct subcategories within the category of poisoning. The recent histories of these two subcategories are very different. The very young have been the subject of extensive poison prevention activities for solids and liquids, but deaths from solids and liquids have increased in recent years to a 1987 age-adjusted rate of approximately 1.7 per 100,000 people. At the same time, deaths from gases have been declining and reached an all-time low in 1987 of 0.4 per 100,000 population.[287]

Men aged 25 through 44 appear to be most responsible for the increase in poisoning by solids and liquids, with a substantial number of deaths as a result of poisoning from illicit drugs (see *Alcohol and Other Drugs*).

While mortality associated with poisoning of children less than 5 years old has declined and is quite low, morbidity is still alarmingly high. In 1987, there were over 107,000 children under 5 years of age treated in hospital emergency departments for poisoning. Approximately 700,000 poison exposures involving children in this age group were reported to poison control centers during the same year.[295]

Past actions such as the Poison Prevention Packaging Act (PPPA), the annual poison prevention week, the shift to less toxic fuels (natural gas and LP gas) for cooking and heating, and safety standards for products that release combustion byproducts have all helped to reduce the risk of poisoning.

Prescription drugs and some other hazardous materials are sold primarily in child resistant containers as required by the PPPA. Improved enforcement of PPPA provisions on dispensing of medicines by pharmacists and physicians involving State, local, and Federal authorities should help to improve enforcement and reduce poisoning morbidity. Improvements in child resistant containers should be sought so they can be more readily used by older people than current containers.

* * *

The public needs to be informed of the potential for household poisoning, especially when children visit households where poisons have not been adequately secured. Broader dissemination of poison prevention messages and development of new poison prevention strategies are needed.

9.9 **Reduce nonfatal head injuries so that hospitalizations for this condition are no more than 106 per 100,000 people. (Baseline: 125 per 100,000 in 1988)**

Baseline data source: National Hospital Discharge Survey, CDC.

Head injuries are the most common severe disabling injuries in the United States. Approximately 500,000 new cases occur annually. Local studies report rates between 180 and 500 per 100,000 people requiring hospitalization because of head injuries. The physical and emotional toll associated with these injuries can be enormous for the survivors and their families. People with existing disabilities from head injuries are at high risk for further secondary disabilities.[296] Prevention efforts should target motor vehicle crashes, falls, diving and water safety, and violence (suicide and assault), which are the most common underlying causes.[297]

Serious limitations in head injury data have been a barrier to prevention efforts. These include complex problems of defining injury criteria, outcome measures, and severity scaling. To adequately measure this objective, standardized definitions and data elements are needed.

9.10 **Reduce nonfatal spinal cord injuries so that hospitalizations for this condition are no more than 5 per 100,000 people. (Baseline: 5.9 per 100,000 in 1988)**

Special Population Target

Nonfatal Spinal Cord Injuries (per 100,000)	1988 Baseline	2000 Target
9.10a Males	8.9	7.1

Baseline data source: National Hospital Discharge Survey, CDC.

Spinal cord injuries are catastrophic health events resulting in enormous human and economic costs. Estimates of spinal cord injury in the United States range from 2.8 to 5 per 100,000 people. Approximately 40 percent of spinal cord injuries are fatal, but data on spinal cord injuries in people dying prior to receiving treatment are inadequate.[298] Males sustain about 80 percent of spinal cord injuries. Adolescents and young adults (aged 15 through 24) are at highest risk of spinal cord injuries, which result in lifelong needs for special services and reduced potential for employment.[299]

Motor vehicle crashes are the primary cause of spinal cord injuries in the United States, accounting for about 50 percent of the cases.[300] Falls are the second leading cause,[301] followed by diving. In some urban settings, firearms and assaults are the major causes.[237]

The development, implementation, and evaluation of effective prevention strategies have been limited by a lack of adequate data. To accurately measure this objective, a standardized case definition and a minimum data set are needed for public health surveillance. States can make spinal cord injuries a reportable health condition.

Some spinal cord injuries occur after contact with the health care system. Appropriate handling of injured persons by medical care personnel will reduce the incidence of these injuries. Proper handling will also avoid more severe injury to those already injured. Increasing the awareness of emergency medical service personnel and others should be a priority for training programs and other injury prevention programs.

9.11 **Reduce the incidence of secondary disabilities associated with injuries of the head and spinal cord to no more than 16 and 2.6 per 100,000 people, respectively. (Baseline: 20 per 100,000 for serious head injuries and 3.2 per 100,000 for spinal cord injuries in 1986)**

Baseline data source: National Head and Spinal Cord Injury Survey, CDC.

Note: Secondary disabilities are defined as those medical conditions secondary to traumatic head or spinal cord injury that impair independent and productive lifestyles.

Injuries to the central nervous system, such as spinal cord injury and traumatic brain injury, are often associated with significant physical, neuropsychological, and psychosocial impairments that result in long-term disability and the need for extensive treatment and rehabilitation. Nearly all of the estimated 8,000 people with spinal cord injuries and 10 percent of the 500,000 people with traumatic brain injuries that occur annually experience secondary complications and disability as a result of their injuries.[302]

9. Unintentional Injuries

Secondary complications of spinal cord and traumatic brain injuries include bladder and urinary tract infections, pressure sores (decubitus ulcers), and respiratory tract problems. While these secondary disabilities are not usually fatal, they impair independent living and are costly to treat. For instance, each decubitus ulcer may result in treatment costs of over $58,000.[303]

Strategies to prevent the occurrence of secondary disabilities and to reduce their severity can be implemented in organized systems of care that include nonhospital settings, such as outpatient clinics or homes. People with spinal cord injuries treated in hospitals that are part of organized systems of treatment and rehabilitation have a lower incidence of complications than those treated in hospitals that are not part of such a system.[304] Similar reductions of the incidence of secondary disability in people with traumatic brain injuries are anticipated when they are treated in similar systems of care.

Prevention of complications secondary to spinal cord injuries and traumatic brain injuries should be a joint priority between clinical and public health providers. Each person with such injuries should be evaluated to determine the likelihood of complications secondary to the primary injury and should be followed in a longitudinal system that consists of patient education and provision of appropriate care.

Risk Reduction Objectives

9.12 Increase use of occupant protection systems, such as safety belts, inflatable safety restraints, and child safety seats, to at least 85 percent of motor vehicle occupants. (Baseline: 42 percent in 1988)

Special Population Target

Use of Occupant Protection Systems	1988 Baseline	2000 Target
9.12a Children aged 4 and younger	84%	95%

Baseline data sources: National Highway Traffic Safety Administration and Fatal Accident Reporting System (FARS), U.S. Department of Transportation.

Achievement of the 85-percent use goal will depend on a number of factors, including the design of occupant protection systems provided by auto makers in coming years and the number of States with mandatory safety belt use laws. Beginning with the 1990 models, automobile manufacturers are required to equip all of their passenger cars with automatic crash protection. Most of the manufacturers are providing automatic safety

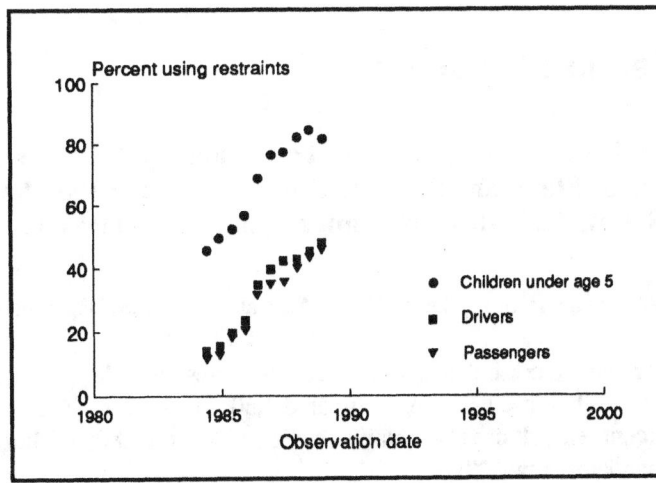

Fig. 9.12

Occupant restraint use by drivers, passengers, and children aged 4 and younger belts and some are offering air bag systems to meet the new Federal requirement. The restraint systems themselves will need to be constantly improved to keep abreast of advancing technology and to make them convenient and comfortable to use.

Based on current usage rates for automatic and manual belt systems, achievement of this objective is not unreasonable. However, the 17 States without mandatory belt use laws in 1989 will need to enact such laws, and several States with weak laws will need to strengthen them. The law enforcement community and the public at large must be convinced that these laws are important enough to warrant vigorous enforcement and public acceptance of that enforcement. In addition, the correct use of belts for all automobile occupants, including occupants of heavy trucks, should be promoted.

The special population target for passengers under 5 years old relates especially to the correct use of safety seats. It has been observed that child safety seats are often attached to the car incorrectly or not at all. Both safety seat manufacturers and automobile makers need to make proper installation and use of the seats easier for parents. Also, parents need to be aware that use of the seats is vital for all children under 5, not just infants. Instructions on the proper use of infant safety seats should be given to all parents of newborn infants.

9.13 **Increase use of helmets to at least 80 percent of motorcyclists and at least 50 percent of bicyclists. (Baseline: 60 percent of motorcyclists in 1988 and an estimated 8 percent of bicyclists in 1984)**

Baseline data sources: For motorcyclists, National Highway Traffic Safety Administration 19 Cities Survey, U.S. Department of Transportation; for bicyclists, R.C. Wasserman et al. 1988.

Head injury is the leading cause of death in motorcycle and bicycle crashes. Compared with motorcycle riders wearing helmets, unhelmeted riders are 2 times more likely to incur a fatal head injury and 3 times more likely to incur a nonfatal head injury.[305] The risk of head injury for unhelmeted bicyclists is more than 6½ times greater than for helmeted bicyclists.[306]

This objective reflects an expectation that gains made in motorcycle safety during the next 10 years will offset the dramatic setbacks in prevention of motorcycle crash-related injuries of the past 10 years and that more States will pass helmet use laws. For bicycling, the attitudes of children must be changed so they accept helmet use as a part of bicycling, just as professional athletes use them for sports. Achievement of this two-part objective will require major campaigns to raise the public awareness on motorcycle and bicycle safety issues and the importance of helmets.

Services and Protection Objectives

9.14 **Extend to 50 States laws requiring safety belt and motorcycle helmet use for all ages. (Baseline: 33 States and the District of Columbia in 1989 for automobiles; 22 States, the District of Columbia, and Puerto Rico for motorcycles)**

Baseline data source: National Highway Traffic Safety Administration, U.S. Department of Transportation.

Examination of motor vehicle crash deaths has proven that rates are reduced in those States with mandatory seatbelt use laws. An estimated 4,500 lives were saved in 1988 as a result of the 45-percent seatbelt use rate obtained nationwide, and 3,800 of those were in States that have mandatory laws.[307]

Between 1976 and 1980, State laws requiring helmet use were weakened or repealed in 28 States. In those States between 1975 (the year before repeals began) and 1980, motorcycle fatalities increased 56 percent while motorcycle registrations increased only 1 percent. Currently only 22 States, the District of Columbia, and Puerto Rico require helmet use by all motorcyclists; 24 States require use by motorcyclists below a certain age, usually 18. Four States have no requirement at all.[308] A recent study suggests that the rate of motorcycle-related deaths associated with head injury between 1979 and 1986 was almost twice as high in States with partial or no motorcycle helmet-use laws than in States with comprehensive helmet-use laws.[309]

9.15 **Enact in 50 States laws requiring that new handguns be designed to minimize the likelihood of discharge by children. (Baseline: 0 States in 1989)**

Baseline data source: Center for Environmental Health and Injury Control, CDC.

In 1987, 3,416 people under the age of 20 died from gunshot wounds. Although the death rate from firearm injuries generally is lower among children than young and middle-aged adults, opportunities for preventing firearm-related deaths may be greatest among children. One strategy is to modify the design of all newly manufactured handguns to prevent their discharge by children. Handguns that are more difficult for children to discharge may prevent a portion of both the unintentional and intentional discharges of handguns associated with firearm injuries in children.

9.16 **Extend to 2,000 local jurisdictions the number whose codes address the installation of fire suppression sprinkler systems in those residences at highest risk for fires. (Baseline data available in 1991)**

Residential sprinklers, particularly when used in combination with smoke detectors, provide a high level of protection from fire. While smoke detectors are capable of preventing more than half of the nearly 4,500 annual residential fire deaths, home sprinkler systems could save another 30 percent.[310] Sprinklers would have a much greater effect, however, than detectors on preventing injuries and property damage. The effect of sprinklers and detectors used in combination would be much greater than either one alone.

Requiring sprinklers for new construction is the most cost-effective and feasible approach to introducing residential sprinklers into U.S. housing. Retrofitting homes is possible but may not occur frequently because of the high cost involved. Because many small jurisdictions in the United States do not have building codes, the introduction of the requirements in the areas likely to be at highest risk—poor, rural, and minority communities—may be hampered without concerted efforts to promulgate new building codes. Requiring sprinklers in new manufactured housing (mobile homes) would be another important measure, since the risk of fire death in manufactured housing is twice the risk in other settings.[311]

9.17 **Increase the presence of functional smoke detectors to at least one on each habitable floor of all inhabited residential dwellings. (Baseline: 81 percent of residential dwellings in 1989)**

Baseline data source: International Association of Fire Chiefs.

The risk of dying in homes without detectors is approximately twice that of dying in homes protected with detectors. Those who are less likely to possess smoke detectors—the elderly and the poor—are also at higher risk of fire death.

To achieve the fire death objectives, high priority must be given to placing detectors in homes that are not protected. Even though detectors are extremely reliable, most detectors are powered by batteries that must be replaced periodically. One study of detectors and fatal fires found that dead batteries were to blame in about two-thirds of the instances of detector failure.[312]

9.18 **Provide academic instruction on injury prevention and control, preferably as part of quality school health education, in at least 50 percent of public school systems (grades K through 12). (Baseline data available in 1991)**

A large number of school-age children suffer disabling and fatal injuries each year. As educational programs for school children are developed and proven effective in preventing injuries, they should be included in quality health education curricula at the appropriate grade level. Education should aim not only at reducing risks of injury directly but also at preparing children to be knowledgeable members of the adult community. For a definition of quality school health education, see *Educational and Community-Based Programs*. The Center for Chronic Disease Prevention and Health Promotion will initiate a survey to establish baseline data and track this objective in 1991.

9.19* **Extend requirement of the use of effective head, face, eye, and mouth protection to all organizations, agencies, and institutions sponsoring sporting and recreation events that pose risks of injury. (Baseline: Only National Collegiate Athletic Association football, hockey, and lacrosse; high school football; amateur boxing; and amateur ice hockey in 1988)**

Baseline data source: Center for Prevention Services, CDC.

Trauma to the head, face, eyes, and mouth is an all-too-frequent occurrence in athletic competition. Organizations with recreation and sports programs, as well as those that provide space, equipment, or facilities for sports, can reduce traumas by requiring the use of appropriate protective gear. In 1962, the use of mouth guards became mandatory for high school football. In 1974, the NCAA made mouth protectors and face guards mandatory for football, hockey, and lacrosse. Few organized leagues and intramural sports require protective gear. The exceptions are football, boxing (which requires mouth guards), and collegiate and under-18 ice hockey, which require players to wear face guards, helmets, and mouth guards.

Regulations requiring the use of protective headgear could considerably reduce injuries among those involved in professional and amateur sports, including basketball, football, ice hockey, field hockey, baseball, softball, lacrosse, soccer, squash, racquetball, wrestling, boxing, and gymnastics. For example, the use of mouth protectors and face guards in organized football reduced the incidence of mouth and face injuries from 50 percent of all football injuries during the 1950s to about 0.4 percent today. In contrast, 10 percent of baseball and 13 percent of ice hockey injuries are to the mouth and face. Mouth protectors and face guards are not currently required in these sports.

* This objective also appears as Objective 13.16 in *Oral Health*.

* * *

9.21 **Increase to at least 50 percent the proportion of primary care providers who routinely provide age-appropriate counseling on safety precautions to prevent unintentional injury. (Baseline data available in 1992)**

The opportunities for physician intervention in unintentional injury prevention are plentiful. In 1987, the average American had 5.4 contacts with a physician. In addition, three-fourths of all Americans had at least one contact with their physician during the previous year. Although behavioral risk factor counseling from a variety of sources—nurses, nurse practitioners, physician assistants, health educators—is beneficial, patients continue to view physicians as the most credible source of health information. Yet physicians do not always seize the opportunity to counsel patients about the prevention of unintentional injuries. Fewer than half the respondents in families with children under 5 years of age reported that a doctor had discussed the importance of using car safety seats for their children.[313]

Health care providers should urge all patients to use federally approved occupant restraints (e.g., safety belts and child safety seats) for themselves and others, to wear safety helmets when riding motorcycles, and to avoid driving under the influence of alcohol or other drugs. Counseling is particularly urged for individuals at increased risk of motor vehicle injury—adolescents and young adults, alcohol and other drug users, and patients whose medical conditions may diminish motor vehicle safety. Patients should be told not to drink alcohol or use other drugs when swimming, boating, bicycling, or handling firearms. Smokers should be told not to smoke near upholstery or in bed. Adult patients should be urged to install and periodically check smoke detectors in their homes and to set hot water heaters at 120 degrees Fahrenheit.

All patients with children in the home should be counseled to place all medications, toxic substances, matches, and firearms out of reach of children, to have a 1 oz bottle of syrup of ipecac available, and to display the telephone number of the nearest poison control center. To prevent falls in children, adults should be advised to have collapsible gates or other barriers at stairway entrances, to install 4-foot fences with latch-gates around swimming pools, and to place window guards in high-rise buildings.

Bicyclists and parents of children who ride bicycles should be made aware of the importance of wearing safety helmets and avoiding riding in heavy traffic. To prevent falls among older people, health care providers should suggest modifications to their home environments, test their visual acuity periodically, monitor their use of drugs, counsel them on medical conditions affecting mobility, and when appropriate, recommend physical exercise to maintain and improve flexibility and mobility.

The Office of Disease Prevention and Health Promotion in the Public Health Service will initiate a survey to gather baseline data and begin tracking of this objective in 1991.

9.22 **Extend to 50 States emergency medical services and trauma systems linking prehospital, hospital, and rehabilitation services in order to prevent trauma deaths and long-term disability. (Baseline: 2 States in 1987)**

Baseline data source: Center for Environmental Health and Injury Control, CDC.

Prevention of death and disability following injury requires easy and timely access to high-level prehospital emergency medical services (EMS). Prevention of adverse outcomes also requires that prehospital personnel transport people with life-threatening injuries directly to trauma center hospitals. Approximately one-third of hospital deaths occurring after injury victims have been transported to the nearest hospital were preventable if treatment had been altered.[314]

Although prehospital care provided by personnel trained in basic life support is adequate for most injuries, personnel trained in advanced life support are preferable for care of more severely injured patients.[315] In each State, a variety of public and private entities, such as cities, counties, fire departments, ambulance companies, volunteer groups, and hospitals provide prehospital personnel and services.[316] For the purpose of evaluating the public's ease of access to EMS and the type of services rendered, States collect data from the various entities that provide prehospital care.[317] States differ, however, in their capacity to gather and analyze these data, and in some States the scope of EMS evaluation is limited because the data are sparse or not readily available through computerized systems. The number of ambulance and rescue services and the level of care they provide when accessed by residents of specified communities are key structural characteristics of EMS that bear on patient outcomes.

Preventable hospital trauma deaths usually are due to failure to promptly diagnose and treat life-threatening injuries. When prehospital personnel deliver patients with severe injuries to hospitals incapable of caring for them, preventable deaths may result from inadequate care or from delays caused by the need to transfer the patients to another hospital. A solution to this problem is for States to foster the development of regional trauma systems.[318] In those systems, patients with life-threatening injuries are transported directly to designated trauma centers that are staffed and equipped to treat severely injured patients on a 24-hour basis.

Highly structured and integrated rehabilitation services begin immediately in the acute care hospital so that each injured patient recovers as completely as possible and has the best opportunity to return to productive status. In the Maryland trauma system, for example, a team of rehabilitation specialists initiates their care while patients are still hospitalized at the Shock Trauma Center in Baltimore. The same team continues to provide services when patients are transferred to the nearby trauma rehabilitation center.[319]

Although trauma systems can prevent death and long- and short-term disability, fewer than half the States have initiated trauma center designation and even fewer have implemented all the components of trauma systems.[320] Documenting the magnitude of the local trauma problem is an important first step in overcoming barriers to implementation of trauma systems. Trauma registries can serve as the principal tool for ongoing evaluation of trauma care, regardless of the status of regional trauma system development.[554] For a comprehensive evaluation of State or regional trauma care, registries must include data from all acute care hospitals and data on prehospital deaths. Linkage of data from the acute care phase of treatment with outcome data from rehabilitation services is fundamental for analysis of the effectiveness of trauma care.

* * *

Research Needs

Injury control in the United States will depend on the ability to identify and document the magnitude of the problem, understand the mechanisms of injury, and establish strategies and programs that are effective in addressing specific problems. Evaluation research on the effectiveness of interventions is required to make the public policy and resource allocation decisions needed to reduce injuries. Research on injury prevention will require the coordinated efforts of investigators in epidemiology, biomechanics and engineering, medicine, statistics, health economics, social science, behavioral science, criminal justice, law, occupational health, public health and others. Attention should be given in the next decade to the specific research recommendations [relating to children] in:

- *Injury in America: A Continuing Public Health Problem*, a report of the Committee on Trauma Research of the Institute of Medicine.[314]

- *Injury Control, A Review of the Status and Progress of the Injury Control Program at the Centers for Disease Control.*

- *Cost of Injury in the United States: A Report to Congress*[300]

* * *

9. Unintentional Injuries

Data Source References

National Vital Statistics, National Center for Health Statistics, Centers for Disease Control, Public Health Service, U.S. Department of Health and Human Services, Hyattsville, MD.

Federal Accident Reporting System, Federal Highway Administration, Department of Transportation, Washington, DC.

National Fire Incident Reporting System, U.S. Fire Administration, Federal Emergency Management Agency, Washington, DC.

National Electronic Injury Surveillance System, U.S. Consumer Product Safety Commission, Washington, DC.

National Hospital Discharge Survey, National Center for Health Statistics, Centers for Disease Control, Public Health Service, U.S. Department of Health and Human Services, Hyattsville, MD.

National Head and Spinal Cord Injury Survey, Center for Environmental Health and Injury Control, Centers for Disease Control, Public Health Service, U.S. Department of Health and Human Services, Atlanta, GA.

National Highway Traffic Safety Administration's 19 Cities Survey, Department of Transportation, Washington, DC.

Wasserman, R.C.; et al. "Bicyclists, Helmets and Head Injuries: A Rider-Based Study of Helmet Use and Effectiveness," *American Journal of Public Health*, 78(9):1220-1221, 1988.

International Association of Fire Chiefs, Washington, DC.

Center for Environmental Health and Injury Control, Centers for Disease Control, Public Health Service, U.S. Department of Health and Human Services, Atlanta, GA.

Center for Prevention Services, Centers for Disease Control, Public Health Service, U.S. Department of Health and Human Services, Atlanta, GA.

Environmental Health

11

Contents

11.1	Asthma hospitalizations
	* * *
11.4	Blood lead levels
	* * *
11.6	Radon testing
	* * *
11.11	Home testing for lead-based paint
	* * *
	[Research Needs]

11. Environmental Health

* * *

Health Status Objectives

11.1 Reduce asthma morbidity, as measured by a reduction in asthma hospitalizations to no more than 160 per 100,000 people. (Baseline: 188 per 100,000 in 1987)

Special Population Targets

Asthma Hospitalizations (per 100,000)	1987 Baseline	2000 Target

* * *

11.1b Children	284[†]	225

[†]*Children aged 14 and younger*

Baseline data source: National Hospital Discharge Survey, CDC.

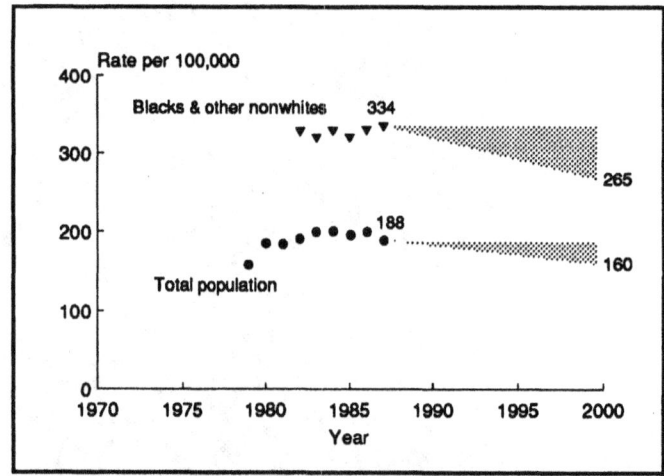

Fig. 11.1

Asthma hospitalization rates

Asthma is a serious chronic condition that affects approximately 10 million Americans. People with asthma experience over 100 million days of restricted activity annually, and costs for asthma exceed $4 billion each year. Asthma is much more common among children than adults. For example, in 1987, 5.2 percent of people under age 17 had asthma, compared to 3.9 percent of people aged 65 and older. There is no difference in asthma prevalence by gender. Although hospitalizations for asthma are more common among blacks, the proportion of blacks with asthma is only slightly higher than whites (4.4 percent versus 4 percent, respectively).[321]

The reported prevalence of asthma is increasing. Between 1979 and 1987, the percent of the population with asthma increased by about one-third; increases in asthma have been reported in all age, race, and sex groups. In 1987, there were over 450,000 hospitalizations for asthma, with rates rising especially fast among children. Between 1979 and 1987, the hospitalizations rose by 43 percent among children aged 15 and younger, from 198 to 284 discharges per 100,000 children.[321] Environmental factors, such as ozone and other air pollutants, may have contributed to rising morbidity and mortality. In addition, indoor air pollutants, particularly biological pollutants, formaldehyde, and combustion-related pollutants are associated with increased morbidity among people with asthma.

11. Environmental Health

The death rate from asthma among blacks is 3 times as high as the rate among whites. Reasons for the discrepancy are unclear, although some evidence suggests that they may be related both to the level of health care services and to environmental factors (e.g. residing in urban areas where air pollution may be more prevalent). Given recent advances in treating asthma and technological developments in toxic agent control, many asthma deaths should be preventable.

The National Heart, Lung, and Blood Institute of the National Institutes of Health, and other professional and private organizations (e.g., the American Lung Association and the American Thoracic Society) have targeted asthma for major efforts to reduce morbidity and mortality. Primary prevention through identification and reduction or elimination of environmental risk factors is a critical part of their efforts. National progress in reducing air pollution should contribute to reductions in asthma hospitalizations.

* * *

11.4   Reduce the prevalence of blood lead levels exceeding 15 µg/dL and 25 µg/dL among children aged 6 months through 5 years to no more than 500,000 and zero, respectively. (Baseline: An estimated 3 million children had levels exceeding 15 µg/dL, and 234,000 had levels exceeding 25 µg/dL, in 1984)

Special Population Target

Prevalence of Blood Lead Levels Exceeding 15 µg/dL & 25 µg/dL	1984 Baseline	2000 Target
11.4a Inner-city low-income black children (annual family income <$6,000 in 1984 dollars)	234,900 & 36,700	75,000 & 0

Baseline data sources: National Health and Nutrition Examination Survey, CDC; Agency for Toxic Substances and Disease Registry.

High blood lead levels are among the most prevalent childhood conditions and the most prevalent environmental threat to the health of children in the United States. Childhood lead poisoning is totally preventable. Judging by progress since 1978, the year 2000 objective should be considered an interim step toward a year 2010 objective of eliminating elevated blood lead levels in the United States. Decreased levels of lead in gasoline, air, food, and releases from industrial sources have resulted in lower mean blood lead levels. However, lead in paint, dust, and soil in inner-city urban areas has been reduced only to a limited extent. Lead in the home environment is the major remaining source of human lead exposure in the United States.

The 1988 Agency for Toxic Substances and Disease Registry report on the extent of lead poisoning in the United States estimated that, based on projections from the National Health and Nutrition Examination Survey (NHANES) II, in 1984, in standard metropolitan statistical areas, there were 2.4 million white and black children aged 6 months through 5 years with blood levels above 15 µg/dL and 200,000 children above 25 µg/dL. This would correspond to approximately 3 million and 250,000, respectively, for all children six months through five years in the total U.S. population. Of the approximately 350,000 inner-city black children aged 6 months through 5 years, with annual family incomes of less than $6,000, more than two-thirds were estimated to have blood lead levels above 15 µg/dL, and 36,700 (10.6 percent) to have blood lead levels above 25 µg/dL.[322] Blood lead levels indicating cause for concern when found in children have been lowered over the past several decades because of new health information.

Health effects of highly elevated lead levels include coma, convulsions, profound irreversible mental retardation and seizures, and death. Even low levels of exposure can result in persistent impairments in central nervous system function, especially in children, including delayed cognitive development, reduced I.Q. scores, impaired hearing, adverse impacts on blood production, vitamin D, and calcium metabolism (which have far-reaching physiological effects), and growth deficits. There may also be significant adverse effects on fetuses through prenatal exposure. In adults, lead in the blood may interfere with hearing, increase blood pressure and, at high levels, cause kidney damage and anemia.[322]

Cooperative efforts with agencies outside the Department of Health and Human Services, such as EPA, the Department of Housing and Urban Development, and State and local childhood lead poisoning prevention programs are critical to achieving this objective. Further, close working efforts must be established with occupational health authorities to assure that the removal of lead-based paint from homes is performed in a safe fashion, protecting both residents and the workers performing the removal. A national strategy to eliminate exposure is critical to achieving this objective.

Risk Reduction Objectives

* * *

11.6   Increase to at least 40 percent the proportion of homes in which homeowners/occupants have tested for radon concentrations and that have either been found to pose minimal risk or have been modified to reduce risk to health. (Baseline: Less than 5 percent of homes had been tested in 1989)

Special Population Targets

Testing and Modification As Necessary	Baseline	2000 Target
* * *		
11.6b Homes with children	—	50%

Baseline data sources: Office of Radiation Programs, EPA; Center for Environmental Health and Injury Control, CDC.

Radon is a unique environmental problem because it occurs naturally. Most indoor radon comes from the rock and soil beneath buildings and enters structures through cracks or openings in foundations or basements. When inhaled, radon decay products release ionizing radiation that can damage lung tissue and lead to lung cancer. EPA estimates that up to eight million homes may have radon levels exceeding four picocuries per liter of air, the level at which EPA recommends corrective action.[323] Knowledge about the effects of radon as an indoor air hazard has developed rapidly in recent years; radon now leads a growing list of indoor air hazards, including tobacco smoke, formaldehyde, asbestos, and organic chemicals.

EPA estimates that approximately 20,000 cases per year of lung cancer occur as a result of radon exposure. The National Academy of Sciences has noted that cigarette smoke acts synergistically with radon gas in causing lung cancer, amplifying the effects of cigarette smoke on lung cancer rates.[324] A special population target to increase testing in the homes of smokers and former smokers is included to give particular emphasis to reducing radon exposure among cigarette smokers.

Households with children also should be targeted for radon testing and mitigation. Children may be at higher risk than adults from indoor radon because they receive a higher dose per unit of exposure than adults. Further, children tend to be more sensitive to the carcinogenic effects of radiation. According to the International Commission of Radiologic Protection, those aged 20 and younger who are exposed to radon appear to

11. Environmental Health

have a higher risk of developing lung cancer than those exposed later in life.[325] As with smoking, the risk of lung cancer may decrease over time once exposure is eliminated. If excess radon exposure is eliminated in childhood, individual risk of lung cancer may be substantially reduced before middle age when lung cancer tends to occur.

Although the objective targets dramatic increases in the proportions of homes tested for radon and modified to reduce risk, the objective is thought to be attainable because of: (1) the low cost and ease of radon testing ($15 to $40 per test kit; no special training needed to perform the test); (2) the relative ease of mitigation; and (3) the increasing number of new homes with low radon levels due to installation of radon-resisting features.

***

Services and Protection Objectives

11.11 Perform testing for lead-based paint in at least 50 percent of homes built before 1950. (Baseline data available in 1991)

There are a number of sources of environmental lead exposure, including contaminated air and water supplies. A very important route of exposure in children is the ingestion of lead-based paint chips, lead-impregnated plaster, or contaminated dust or dirt found in dilapidated homes, particularly those built before 1950.[326] These building conditions are found most commonly in low-income neighborhoods. As a result, about 19 percent of black children who are poor or who live in the center of large American cities have lead levels above 30 $\mu g/dL$.[326] When lead exposure estimates are stratified according to national socioeconomic and demographic variables, no economic or racial subgroup of children is exempt from the risk of having lead exposure that is sufficiently high to cause adverse health effects. Nevertheless, the prevalence of elevated lead levels in inner-city, underprivileged children remains the highest among the various strata.

Compared to other sources of environmental exposure, the home environment is the least regulated and the most dependent upon individual awareness and initiative. Specific knowledge possessed by people is essential to corrective action. Active participation and intervention by residents and homeowners is a necessary component of lead exposure abatement. However, some homeowners are unable to afford extensive home repair or renovation to reduce lead exposure. Lead paint abatement can be costly, with costs ranging from $3,000 to $15,000 per home.[327] Thus, to reduce lead toxicity among children, it may be necessary for governments to perform lead-based paint testing and abate lead hazards.

A related issue is lead in drinking water. The primary source of lead in drinking water is corrosion of plumbing materials, such as lead service lines and lead solders, in water distribution systems and in houses and larger buildings. Virtually all public water systems serve households with lead solders of varying ages, and most faucets are made of materials that can contribute some lead to drinking water. . . .

***

Research Needs

Although objectives for basic and applied biomedical research in the environmental health sciences are not included in the year 2000 objectives, such studies should be given high priority. [Delineated needs may have particular relevance for maternal and child populations, e.g. pregnant women (environmental contaminants), adolescents and youth (recreational noise).] PHS is committed to supporting a sustained program of basic and applied toxicological, biomedical, and epidemiological research in environmental health.

- There is an urgent need for reliable information on the health effects of environmental contaminants. The National Academy of Sciences reported in 1984 that 82 percent of major industrial chemicals have not been tested for their toxic properties.

Scientific data are a critical part of the base for risk management decisions, for cost-effectiveness and cost-benefit analyses of various regulatory actions, and for use by health agencies and medical care providers in response to human exposure. Too little is known about the mechanisms by which chemical and physical agents harm human health. Methods to detect human exposure to many chemicals have not been developed. Distribution and detection of subtle effects of environmental chemicals in human organs are essentially unknown.

Laboratory-based toxicologic studies and basic biomedical research provide the foundation for effective environmental health programs. However, better models to extrapolate findings from laboratory studies to humans are needed. Research should be linked to sensitive new environmental monitoring and disease surveillance systems to help guide progress toward meeting the environmental health objectives for the year 2000.

Public perceptions of risk from exposure to hazardous materials do not compare well to scientific estimates of risk. Additional research is needed into how the public forms opinions of risk and how these opinions change in response to new information.

- Nationwide efforts to delineate the extent and possible human health effects of atmospheric warming and ozone depletion are needed.

Current research suggests an atmospheric warming trend over the past century, that if continued, could have severe public health effects. For example, total daily mortality rates in some United States cities increase 30 to 50 percent during prolonged heat waves.[328] Data have evolved over the past century, and the conclusion that the earth is warming is not universally shared, but the weight of scientific opinion favors this conclusion. Although it is impossible to predict or quantify the exact impact of global warming trends accurately, quick response requires that programs be put in place to monitor early changes and assess potential risks.

Depletion of stratospheric ozone also presents potentially significant health risks. The ozone layer, a thin blanket of gas about six miles above the earth's surface, filters out a portion of the sun's ultraviolet radiation. The ozone layer has been affected by release of chlorofluorocarbons (CFCs) into the atmosphere. In the lower atmosphere, CFCs trap heat, but higher up in the atmosphere these compounds destroy ozone. At the South Pole, up to 50 percent of the ozone is destroyed each spring over an area the size of the United States. Similar, but less severe losses occur over the Arctic. Were greater levels of ultraviolet rays to reach the earth's surface, the incidence of skin cancer and cataracts would be expected to increase.

Several agencies, including EPA, the Department of Energy, the National Oceanic and Atmospheric Administration, and the National Aeronautics and Space Administration have already allocated substantial resources to the problem of global climate change. However, atmospheric warming and ozone depletion trends will not be reversed overnight. Implementation of measures to counteract these trends will require extensive coordination among numerous nations as well as health and environmental agencies within the United States. A fuller understanding of the potentially enormous impact of global warming and ozone depletion on human health will require much further research, including a substantial contribution from the public health system.

11. Environmental Health

- More information is needed on prevalent and potentially harmful environmental conditions including excessive noise and low-level ionizing radiation.

Over 21 million Americans suffer hearing impairment. In 1988, 90.8 per 1,000 people had hearing impairments and 7.5 per 1,000 were deaf in both ears.[410] There are approximately 28 million people in the United States with impaired hearing. Approximately 10 million of these cases are associated with loud noise. For many of these individuals, exposure to occupational and recreational noise has caused irreversible damage to the inner ear. However, it is unclear whether the incidence of hearing impairment has risen in recent years, because few studies of noise induced hearing loss have been conducted. Additional research on the prevalence and severity of environmental noise pollution is needed so that appropriate public health protections can be implemented.

Exposure to large doses of ionizing radiation is known to increase the incidence of many types of cancer, but dose-incidence relationships have not been well defined. As a result, cancer risk associated with low-level radiation can only be estimated through uncertain extrapolations from higher dose data. Several studies suggest that there may be no safe threshold for exposure to ionizing radiation. This possibility has prompted repeated attempts to measure the effect of low-level radiation among populations living in areas of high background radiation, populations exposed occupationally to low-level radiation, and populations receiving small doses from other natural and man-made sources. Such studies have not conclusively demonstrated carcinogenic effects.[329] However, this may be due to methodological limitations. Further research is needed to clarify the relationship between low-level radiation and cancer.

* * *

Baseline Data Source References

Agency for Toxic Substances and Disease Registry, Public Health Service, U.S. Department of Health and Human Services, Atlanta, GA.

Center for Environmental Health and Injury Control, Centers for Disease Control, Public Health Service, U.S. Department of Health and Human Services, Atlanta, GA.

National Health and Nutrition Examination Survey, National Center for Health Statistics, Centers for Disease Control, Public Health Service, U.S. Department of Health and Human Services, Hyattsville, MD.

National Hospital Discharge Survey, National Center for Health Statistics, Centers for Disease Control, Public Health Service, U.S. Department of Health and Human Services, Hyattsville, MD.

Office of Air and Radiation, Environmental Protection Agency, Washington, DC.

Office of Radiation Programs, Environmental Protection Agency, Washington, DC.

Oral Health

13

Contents

13.1 Dental caries

13.2 Untreated dental caries

***

13.8 Protective sealants

13.9 Water fluoridation

13.10 Topical and systemic fluorides

13.11 Baby bottle tooth decay

13.12 Oral health screening, referral, and followup

***

13.15 Oral health care for infants with cleft lip and/or palate

13.16 Protective equipment in sporting and recreation events

[Research Needs]

13. Oral Health

* * *

Health Status Objectives

13.1 Reduce dental caries (cavities) so that the proportion of children with one or more caries (in permanent or primary teeth) is no more than 35 percent among children aged 6 through 8 and no more than 60 percent among adolescents aged 15. (Baseline: 53 percent of children aged 6 through 8 in 1986-87; 78 percent of adolescents aged 15 in 1986-87)

Special Population Targets

	Dental Caries Prevalence	*1986-87 Baseline*	*2000 Target*
13.1a	Children aged 6-8 whose parents have less than high school education	70%	45%
13.1b	American Indian/Alaska Native children aged 6-8	92%[†] 52%[‡]	45%
13.1c	Black children aged 6-8	61%	40%
13.1d	American Indian/Alaska Native adolescents aged 15	93%[‡]	70%

[†]*In primary teeth in 1983-84*
[‡]*In permanent teeth in 1983-84*

Baseline data sources: *Oral Health in United States Children*, NIH; for children whose parents have less than a high school education, North Carolina Oral Health School Survey; Indian Health Service.

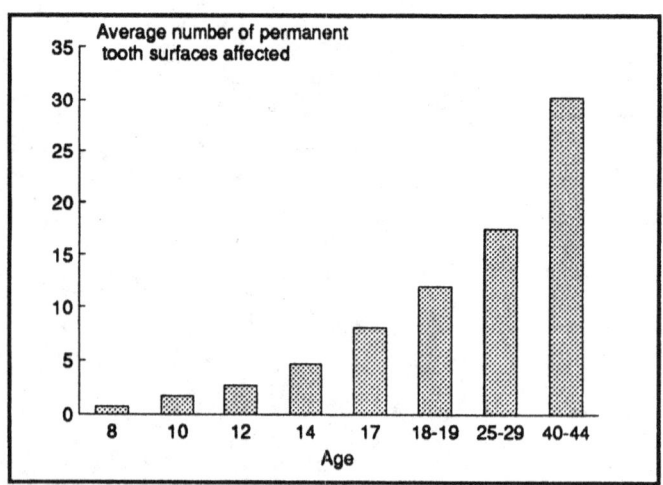

Fig. 13.1

Cumulative caries experience

Dental caries is perhaps the most prevalent disease known. Except in its early stages, it is irreversible and cumulative. Children aged 6 through 8 are at an important stage of dental development; they have a complement of primary teeth as well as their permanent first molars and incisors. The importance of optimal oral health for these children cannot be overemphasized; it is critical not only to their current oral functioning, but also for long-term health. Separate targets are set for adolescents because the prevalence of dental caries is so much higher among adolescents than young children. Moreover, an objective targeted at teenagers will better reflect the cumulative caries experience of children during the 1990s.

Community water fluoridation and use of preventive services, such as sealants and topical fluoride treatments, along with appropriate oral health behaviors, decrease the chances that children and adolescents will develop caries. Many young children, particularly those in high-risk groups, do not receive adequate fluoride exposure or adhesive sealants, regular professional care, or oral hygiene instruction. Unfortunately, many physicians do not conduct even a rudimentary examination of young patients' mouths or provide children or their parents with oral health counseling or referral for care.[45] For children from low-income families, a significant hurdle is paying for services.

13.2   Reduce untreated dental caries so that the proportion of children with untreated caries (in permanent or primary teeth) is no more than 20 percent among children aged 6 through 8 and no more than 15 percent among adolescents aged 15. (Baseline: 27 percent of children aged 6 through 8 in 1986; 23 percent of adolescents aged 15 in 1986-87)

Special Population Targets

Untreated Dental Caries:		1986-87 Baseline	2000 Target
Among Children—			
13.2a	Children aged 6-8 whose parents have less than high school education	43%	30%
13.2b	American Indian/Alaska Native children aged 6-8	64%[†]	35%
13.2c	Black children aged 6-8	38%	25%
13.2d	Hispanic children aged 6-8	36%[‡]	25%
Among Adolescents—			
13.2a	Adolescents aged 15 whose parents have less than a high school education	41%	25%
13.2b	American Indian/Alaska Native adolescents aged 15	84%[†]	40%
13.2c	Black adolescents aged 15	38%	20%
13.2d	Hispanic adolescents aged 15	31-47%[‡]	25%

[†]*1983-84 baseline*
[‡]*1982-84 baseline*

Baseline data sources: *Oral Health in United States Children*, NIH; Indian Health Service; Hispanic Health and Nutrition Examination Survey (Hispanic HANES), CDC; for children and adolescents whose parents have less than a high school education, North Carolina Oral Health School Survey.

Early diagnosis and timely treatment of caries can halt tooth destruction and prevent tooth loss. Yet in 1986-87 the proportions of children aged 6, 7, and 8 with untreated decay in primary teeth were 32, 27, and 25 percent, respectively; in permanent teeth 39, 32, and 24 percent of children had decay that had not been treated.[330]

Surveys have shown that, because of inadequate receipt of routine dental care, certain populations experience higher rates of untreated caries. For example, the prevalence of untreated decay may be higher among the children of migrant workers than the total population; migrant workers' use of dental services is well below the national average.[331]

Healthy Children 2000

Dental caries is a unique microbial infection. Once established, it is progressive, does not heal without treatment, and leaves visible evidence of past infection. Because early diagnosis and prompt treatment of caries can halt tooth destruction and prevent tooth loss, low prevalence of untreated caries should be attainable. Financial, cultural, psychological, social, and geographic barriers contribute to lack of treatment.

***

Risk Reduction Objectives

13.8 **Increase to at least 50 percent the proportion of children who have received protective sealants on the occlusal (chewing) surfaces of permanent molar teeth. (Baseline: 11 percent of children aged 8 and 8 percent of adolescents aged 14 in 1986-87)**

Note: Progress toward this objective will be monitored based on prevalence of sealants in children at age 8 and at age 14, when the majority of first and second molars, respectively, are erupted.
Baseline data source: *Oral Health of United States Children*, NIH.

Since the early 1970s, childhood dental caries on smooth tooth surfaces has declined markedly. In 1986-87, approximately 90 percent of the decay in children's teeth occurred in pits and fissures, and almost two-thirds was found on the chewing surfaces alone.[330] Pit-and-fissure sealants—plastic coatings that are applied to susceptible tooth surfaces—have existed for many years. If sealants were applied routinely to susceptible tooth surfaces, most incremental tooth decay among American children could be prevented.

Sealants are most effective when they are applied to teeth just after eruption of the first and second molars—when children are approximately aged 6 through 8 (for first molars) and when they are aged 12 through 14 (for second molars). When applied properly, sealants are exceptionally safe, highly effective, and long lasting.

13.9 **Increase to at least 75 percent the proportion of people served by community water systems providing optimal levels of fluoride. (Baseline: 62 percent in 1989)**

Note: Optimal levels of fluoride are determined by the mean maximum daily air temperature over a 5-year period and range between 0.7 and 1.2 parts of fluoride per one million parts of water (ppm).
Baseline data source: Fluoridation Census, CDC.

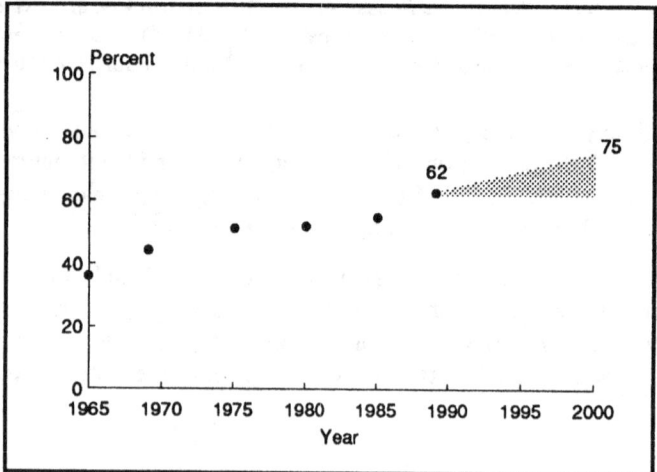

Fig. 13.9

Percentage of people served by community water systems with optimal levels of fluoride

Community water fluoridation is the single most effective and efficient means of preventing dental caries in children and adults, regardless of race or income level.[332] Widespread exposure to fluorides through drinking water and dental products appears to be the primary cause of the declining prevalence of dental caries in the school-age population. While a nationwide decline in caries has occurred in both fluoridated and nonfluoridated communities, caries prevalence is still significantly lower among children in fluoridated areas.

This objective is challenging. The proportion of people served by fluoridated water supplies increased only 8 percent during the 1980s. A concerted national effort will be necessary to reach this target.

13.10 **Increase use of professionally or self-administered topical or systemic (dietary) fluorides to at least 85 percent of people not receiving optimally fluoridated public water. (Baseline: An estimated 50 percent in 1989)**

Baseline data source: National Health Interview Survey, CDC.

A substantial proportion of the population receives drinking water from nonfluoridated individual sources or nonfluoridated community water systems.[333] Children in these nonfluoridated areas should be exposed to one systemic form of fluoride while tooth enamel is forming; adults in these nonfluoridated areas should be exposed to a topical form of fluoride at optimal levels throughout life. Examples of fluoride treatments include professionally applied topical fluoride, fluoride dentifrice, and fluoride mouth rinses, all of which can prevent initial decay and promote the repair of early-stage caries. Systemic forms include fluoride tablets or drops, vitamin/fluoride combinations, and school water supplies.

Studies are underway to determine the optimal level of aggregate fluoride exposure necessary to prevent tooth decay.

13.11* **Increase to at least 75 percent the proportion of parents and caregivers who use feeding practices that prevent baby bottle tooth decay. (Baseline data available in 1991)**

Special Population Targets

Appropriate Feeding Practices	Baseline	2000 Target
13.11a **Parents and caregivers with less than high school education**	—	65%
13.11b **American Indian/Alaska Native parents and caregivers**	—	65%

Baby bottle tooth decay is a severe form of dental caries in toddlers that can lead to destruction of primary teeth. It is caused by frequent or prolonged use of nursing bottles that contain milk, sugared water, fruit juice, or other sugary beverages during the day or night. Continual use of a sweetened pacifier and/or breastfeeding at will throughout the night can also cause baby bottle tooth decay.

The prevalence of baby bottle tooth decay has been estimated at 53 percent among American Indian and Alaska Native Head Start children. Prevalence in the urban population has been estimated at 1 to 11 percent.[334,335] Preventing baby bottle tooth decay will require efforts by many segments of the community, including dental professionals and those who interact with parents and caregivers (e.g., nurses, physicians, preschool teachers). Success in primary prevention has been achieved in American Indian and Alaska Native communities using a comprehensive, multidiciplinary program.

*This objective also appears as Objective 2.12 in *Nutrition*.

Services and Protection Objectives

13.12 Increase to at least 90 percent the proportion of all children entering school programs for the first time who have received an oral health screening, referral, and followup for necessary diagnostic, preventive, and treatment services. (Baseline: 66 percent of children aged 5 visited a dentist during the previous year in 1986)

Note: School programs include Head Start, prekindergarten, kindergarten, and 1st grade.
Baseline data source: National Health Interview Survey, CDC.

Despite dramatic success in the reduction of caries in children over the past 20 years, many oral diseases still appear in young children. Early dental care is an opportunity to educate parents about effective techniques for preventing oral diseases. Since not all children benefit from primary prevention, secondary preventive services, including early diagnosis and prompt treatment, can eliminate pain, infection, and progressive oral diseases.

Unfortunately, early and regular dental care among children is far from universal. In 1986 only 25 percent of children aged 2 had ever visited a dentist; by ages 5 and 7, the proportions increased to 75 percent and 89 percent, respectively.[336] Achievement of this objective could be linked to other medical requirements for children entering school. Special efforts should be made to reach developmentally disabled children, as well as children with other disabling conditions.

* * *

13.15 Increase to at least 40 the number of States that have an effective system for recording and referring infants with cleft lips and/or palates to craniofacial anomaly teams. (Baseline: In 1988, approximately 25 States had a central recording mechanism for cleft lip and/or palate and approximately 25 States had an organized referral system to craniofacial anomaly teams)

Baseline data source: Illinois State Health Department.

Cleft lip and palate are reported in 760 to 930 per 100,000 live births and isolated cleft palate is reported in 470 to 570 per 100,000 live births; however, several national and regional studies have found that the incidence of both is underreported.[337] In Illinois, for example, birth certificate data from 1986 to 1988 show underreporting of 35 percent. Improper case ascertainment and undiscovered cases are the primary reasons for underreporting.[337]

Physicians and nurses in hospital nurseries are usually the first to examine newborns and are responsible for noting congenital anomalies and describing them on the medical record. Therefore, hospital personnel must clearly understand the definitions of congenital defects and abnormalities of the lips and palate, properly examine newborns, and record correctly any malformations.

Newborns with cleft lip/palate should be referred immediately to an interdisciplinary team for intervention to minimize the physical and psychosocial trauma that can be associated with eating, drinking, speech, and hearing disorders. Although surgical repair of the lips can be performed soon after birth, repair of the palate should often be delayed several years to allow facial growth and arch development. Prompt professional attention to cleft lip and cleft palate can help prevent these conditions from affecting sound child development.

13.16* Extend requirement of the use of effective head, face, eye, and mouth protection to all organizations, agencies, and institutions sponsoring sporting and recreation events that pose risks of injury. (Baseline: Only National Collegiate Athletic Association football, hockey, and lacrosse; high school football; amateur boxing; and amateur ice hockey in 1988)

Baseline data source: Center for Prevention Services, CDC.

*For commentary, see Objective 9.19 in *Unintentional Injuries*.

* * *

Research Needs

High priority research needs include:

- Better methods of predicting who will experience caries and periodontal diseases by different levels of severity are needed. Oral diseases affect populations and individuals in unique ways and at different rates.

* * *

- Clinical decision-making practices of dentists so that dental practice can be improved.

- Characteristics of populations lacking dental insurance. Because of the importance of clinically based primary and secondary prevention services for oral health, and thus the importance of dental insurance coverage, studies are needed to describe the characteristics of people who are not covered by dental insurance.

- The effectiveness of dental providers in counseling patients to quit tobacco use needs further evaluation. Tobacco is a primary risk factor for a broad range of oral conditions.

- The specific etiologies of periodontal diseases and patterns of progression.

- Improved screening and diagnostic capabilities for diagnosing, preventing, and controlling all oral diseases at both patient and population levels.

* * *

- Expanded knowledge of optimal use of fluorides both in drinking water and in dental products to ensure maximum benefits while minimizing the risk of dental fluorosis.

* * *

Baseline Data Source References

Center for Prevention Services, Centers for Disease Control, Public Health Service, U.S. Department of Health and Human Services, Atlanta, GA.

Hispanic Health and Nutrition Examination Survey, National Center for Health Statistics, Centers for Disease Control, Public Health Service, U.S. Department of Health and Human Services, Hyattsville, MD.

Illinois State Health Department, Springfield, IL.

Indian Health Service, Public Health Service, U.S. Department of Health and Human Services, Rockville, MD.

National Health Interview Survey, National Center for Health Statistics, Centers for Disease Control, Public Health Service, U.S. Department of Health and Human Services, Hyattsville, MD.

North Carolina Oral Health School Survey, North Carolina Division of Dental Health, Raleigh, NC, and the University of North Carolina School of Public Health, Chapel Hill, NC.

Oral Health in United States Children, National Institute of Dental Research, National Institutes of Health, Public Health Service, U.S. Department of Health and Human Services, Bethesda, MD.

Maternal and Infant Health

Contents

14.1 Infant mortality

14.2 Fetal deaths

14.3 Maternal mortality

14.4 Fetal alcohol syndrome

14.5 Low birth weight

14.6 Weight gain during pregnancy

14.7 Severe complications of pregnancy

14.8 Cesarean delivery

14.9 Breastfeeding

14.10 Alcohol, tobacco, and drug use during pregnancy

14.11 Prenatal care

14.12 Age-appropriate preconception counseling by clinicians

14.13 Counseling on detection of fetal abnormalities

14.14 Risk-appropriate care

14.15 Newborn screening and followup

14.16 Primary care for babies

[Research Needs]

14. Maternal and Infant Health

* * *

Health Status Objectives

14.1 Reduce the infant mortality rate to no more than 7 per 1,000 live births. (Baseline: 10.1 per 1,000 live births in 1987)

Special Population Targets

Infant Mortality (per 1,000 live births)		1987 Baseline	2000 Target
14.1a	Blacks	17.9	11
14.1b	American Indians/Alaska Natives	12.5†	8.5
14.1c	Puerto Ricans	12.9†	8

Type-Specific Targets

Neonatal and Postneonatal Mortality (per 1,000 live births)		1987 Baseline	2000 Target
14.1d	Neonatal mortality	6.5	4.5
14.1e	Neonatal mortality among blacks	11.7	7
14.1f	Neonatal mortality among Puerto Ricans	8.6†	5.2
14.1g	Postneonatal mortality	3.6	2.5
14.1h	Postneonatal mortality among blacks	6.1	4
14.1i	Postneonatal mortality among American Indians/Alaska Natives	6.5†	4
14.1j	Postneonatal mortality among Puerto Ricans	4.3†	2.8

†1984 baseline

Note: Infant mortality is deaths of infants under 1 year; neonatal mortality is deaths of infants under 28 days; and postneonatal mortality is deaths of infants aged 28 days up to 1 year.
Baseline data sources: National Vital Statistics System, CDC; Linked Birth and Infant Death Data Set, CDC.

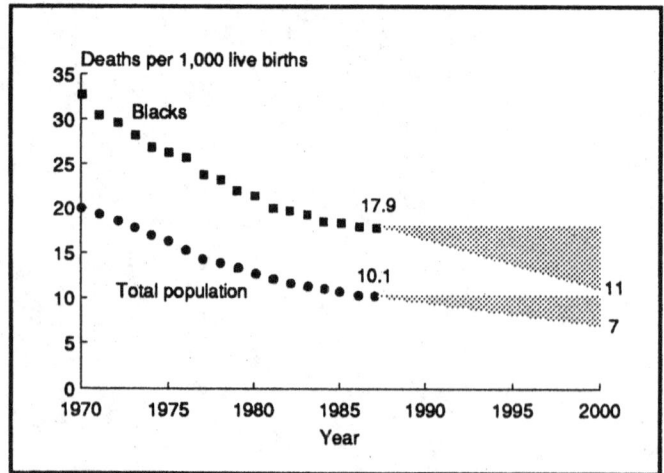

Fig. 14.1

Infant mortality rates

The infant mortality rate has declined steadily over the last quarter century reaching 10.1 in 1987, the lowest rate ever recorded in the United States. The rate of decline, however, has slowed from 4.7 percent per year during the 1970s to 2.8 percent per year during the 1980s. Maintenance of the 2.8 percent decline experienced during the 1980s would result in an infant mortality rate of 7 by the year 2000. This is a formidable target, especially since the most recent provisional data from 1987-89 show an average annual decline of 1.5 percent.

The decline in infant mortality during the 1970s is largely attributable to advances in neonatal intensive care and the dissemination of these advances throughout the Nation causing a marked reduction in birth-weight-specific mortality.[338] The percentage of low weight births declined slightly during the 1970s, but during the 1980s the birth weight distribution remained essentially constant.

Infant mortality rates are usually calculated by dividing the number of infant deaths in a given year (obtained from death certificates) by the number of live births in the same year (obtained from birth certificates). Race-specific infant mortality rates calculated in this way are valid only when the coding of race on both birth and death certificates is comparable. However, results from the 1983 and 1984 Linked Birth and Infant Death Data Set show that the coding for races other than white or black are not comparable. In studies based on these files, which were done for this document, it was possible to compare the race of child on the birth certificate (used as the denominator of the usual infant mortality rate) with race of child on the death certificate (used as the numerator of the usual infant mortality rate) for all infant deaths. Although the race coding for whites and blacks differed by less than 2 percent, from 25 to 40 percent of infant deaths among American Indians and Asian Americans were coded to a different race on the death certificate. For this reason, infant mortality rates for minorities other than blacks should be tracked using the Linked Birth and Infant Death Data Set, which is currently available only for 1983 and 1984, but will be available annually for 1985 and later. The infant mortality rates based on these linked files (using the child's race as reported on the birth certificate) are as follows:

	1983	1984
All races	10.9	10.4
White	9.3	8.9
Black	18.9	17.9
American Indian	14.4	12.5
Asian	8.4	8.8

Infant mortality rates are also available for Hispanics in the 23 States and the District of Columbia where Hispanic origin of the mother was coded on the birth certificate. Infant mortality rates based on the linked files are as follows:

	1983	1984
Non-Hispanic White	9.2	8.6
Non-Hispanic Black	18.8	17.8
Hispanic	9.5	9.3
Mexican	9.1	8.9
Puerto Rican	12.9	12.9
Cuban	7.5	8.1
Central & South American	8.5	8.3
Other & Unknown Hispanic	10.6	9.6

Only blacks, American Indians, and Puerto Ricans have infant mortality rates substantially higher than the United States average. Unfortunately there are no long-term trend data available to assess the potential for further reductions. For example, the unusually large decline between 1983 and 1984 in American Indian infant mortality may reflect a short-term fluctuation rather than real progress. In the absence of trend data, the infant mortality objectives for these groups are derived from the objectives for neonatal and postneonatal mortality (see below) and set at 8.5 per 1,000 live births for American Indians and at 8.0 per 1,000 live births for Puerto Ricans.

Infant mortality rates vary substantially among and within racial and ethnic groups. The overall American Indian rate does not reflect the diversity among Indian communities, some of which have infant mortality rates approaching twice the national rate. The rate for black infants (17.9 per 1,000 live births in 1987) continues to be twice that of white infants (8.6 per 1,000 live births). Black women are twice as likely as white women to experience prematurity, low birth weight, and infant and fetal death. Blacks are also more likely to be affected by a variety of risk factors related to prolonged social and economic deprivation. Among these are young maternal age, high birth order, less education, and inadequate prenatal care. However, these conditions do not entirely explain the black-white disparity.[339]

A recent study estimated that more than 10 percent of infant deaths could be prevented by effective family planning.[340] Because black women are 2.5 times more likely to have an unplanned birth than white women, effective pregnancy planning is an important intervention in reducing racial differences in pregnancy outcomes.[341]

The annual decline in black infant mortality rates slowed from 4.1 percent per year during the 1970s to 2.2 percent per year in 1981 through 1986, in part, due to an increase in the incidence of live births under 1,500 grams. A target of 11 infant deaths per 1,000 live births among black women implies a 3.5 percent annual decline in mortality rates from 1986 levels. Even if the objectives for low birth weight and very low birth weight are achieved, approximately 3 percent per year declines in birth-weight-specific infant mortality rates will be required to achieve the black infant mortality target. If the birth weight distribution remains unchanged, 4 percent per year declines in weight-specific mortality will be necessary to achieve the target.

Neonatal Mortality

Between 1970 and 1981 the neonatal mortality rate declined by 5.7 percent per year but the decline slowed to 3.5 percent per year between 1981 and 1986. Improvements in infant mortality rates due to neonatal intensive care were especially pronounced in the neonatal period and accounted for much, if not all, of the decrease. Analysis of the 1983 Linked Birth and Infant Death Data Set indicates that there is much greater variation in postneonatal than neonatal birth-weight-specific mortality rates by maternal risk groups. This suggests that improvements in neonatal mortality are less feasible than in postneonatal mortality. For these reasons, the objective of 4.5 deaths per 1,000, a slight slowdown in the annual rate of decline (to 2.8 percent per year), was selected as consistent with what would be feasible over the next decade.

The leading causes of death in the neonatal period are congenital anomalies, respiratory distress syndrome, disorders relating to short gestation, and effects of maternal complications.[342] Survival during the neonatal period is sensitive to improvement in perinatal services, including the technology of newborn intensive care units, high quality prenatal care, and use of obstetric technologies. Further reduction in the neonatal mortality rate requires concentrated attention to reducing low birth weight and congenital anomalies.

As blacks have the highest neonatal mortality rate, achievement of the overall neonatal mortality target will be determined in large part by reductions in neonatal mortality among blacks. Between 1970 and 1981, the neonatal mortality rate among blacks declined by 4.6 percent per year but the decline slowed to 2.7 percent per year between 1981 and 1986. Acceleration in the decline among blacks to 3.6 percent per year is necessary to reach the target. The neonatal mortality rate among ethnic groups other than blacks should be tracked using the Linked Birth and Infant Death Data Set. Results from those files for 1983 and 1984 show the following neonatal mortality rates:

	1983	1984
All races	7.1	6.8
White	6.1	5.9
Black	12.3	11.7
Indian	7.0	6.1
Asian	5.0	5.6

Neonatal mortality rates based on the linked files for Hispanics in the 23 States and the District of Columbia where Hispanic origin of the mother was coded on the birth certificate are as follows:

	1983	1984
Non-Hispanic White	6.0	5.7
Non-Hispanic Black	11.9	11.3
Hispanic	6.2	6.2
Mexican	5.9	5.8
Puerto Rican	8.7	8.6
Cuban	5.0	6.4
Central & South American	5.8	5.9
Other & Unknown Hispanic	6.4	6.5

Only blacks and Puerto Ricans have neonatal mortality rates substantially higher than the United States average. Unfortunately there are no long-term trend data available prior to 1983 to assess the potential for further reductions among Puerto Ricans. However, the ratio of the black to the overall neonatal mortality rate was 1.72 in 1984 and the year 2000 target reduces this ratio by 9 percent, to 1.56. In 1984, the ratio of the Puerto Rican to the overall neonatal rate was 1.26. If the 9 percent reduction targeted for blacks is applied to this ratio, the result is a ratio of 1.15, so the target for Puerto Ricans is set at 5.2 per 1,000 live births.

Postneonatal Mortality

During the 1970s and 1980s, postneonatal mortality has declined more slowly than neonatal mortality. A partial explanation may be that the reduction in neonatal mortality led to a higher risk profile for the cohort of infants surviving to the postneonatal period.[343] Achievement of the postneonatal targets implies an increase in the rate of decline to 2.8 percent per year. Data from the 1983 Linked Birth and Infant Death Data Set suggests that this is possible. If all infants had achieved the birth-weight-specific postneonatal mortality rate experienced by the lowest risk maternal subgroup (married women in their twenties with 13 or more years education), the overall postneonatal mortality rate would have been about 30 percent lower.

The four leading causes of death in this period are sudden infant death syndrome (SIDS), congenital anomalies, injuries, and infection.[342] SIDS accounts for slightly more than one-third of deaths. The etiology of SIDS has not been identified, although a number of risk factors are known, including maternal smoking and drug use, teenage birth, and infections late in pregnancy. Infants born to families who have experienced a previous SIDS death are also at risk. Improvement in postneonatal mortality requires better knowledge about SIDS and congenital anomalies and improved receipt of services by infants, especially vulnerable infants. Injuries and infections are the most amenable to prevention.

Blacks have a higher postneonatal mortality rate than whites. Between 1970 and 1981, the postneonatal mortality rate among blacks declined by 3.1 percent per year but the rate of decline slowed to 1.3 percent per year between 1981 and 1986. Achievement of the target would require an acceleration in the black rate of decline to 3.2 percent per year. Data from the 1983 Linked Birth and Infant Death Data Set suggest that this is a realistic goal. If all black infants had achieved the birth-weight-specific postneonatal mortality rate experienced by the lowest risk maternal group among blacks (married women in their twenties with 13 or more years of education), the overall postneonatal mortality rate among blacks would have been about 40 percent lower.

The postneonatal mortality rate among ethnic groups other than blacks should be tracked using the Linked Birth and Infant Death Data Set. Results from those files for 1983 and 1984 show the following postneonatal mortality rates:

	1983	1984
All races	3.8	3.6
White	3.2	3.1
Black	6.6	6.2
Indian	7.3	6.5
Asian	3.3	3.1

Postneonatal mortality rates based on the linked file for Hispanics in the 23 States and the District of Columbia where Hispanic origin of the mother was coded on the birth certificate are as follows:

	1983	1984
Non-Hispanic White	3.2	3.0
Non-Hispanic Black	6.9	6.5
Hispanic	3.3	3.1
Mexican	3.2	3.2
Puerto Rican	4.2	4.3
Cuban	2.5	1.7
Central & South American	2.6	2.4
Other & Unknown Hispanic	4.1	3.1

Of these racial and ethnic groups, only American Indians, blacks, and Puerto Ricans have postneonatal mortality rates substantially higher than the United States average. As before, there are no long-term trend data available prior to 1983 except for blacks to assess the potential for further reductions. However, postneonatal mortality rates for blacks and American Indians are about equal, so the same target can be used for both groups. The ratio of the black to the overall postneonatal mortality rate was 1.72 in 1984 and the year 2000 target reduces this ratio by 7 percent, to 1.6. In 1984, the ratio of the Puerto Rican to the overall postneonatal rate was 1.19. If the 7 percent reduction targeted for blacks is applied to this ratio, the result is a ratio of 1.11. Thus, the target for Puerto Ricans is set at 2.8 per 1,000 live births.

14.2 **Reduce the fetal death rate (20 or more weeks of gestation) to no more than 5 per 1,000 live births plus fetal deaths. (Baseline: 7.6 per 1,000 live births plus fetal deaths in 1987)**

Special Population Target

Fetal Deaths	1987 Baseline	2000 Target
14.2a Blacks	12.8†	7.5†

†*Per 1,000 live births plus fetal deaths*

Baseline data source: National Vital Statistics System, CDC.

Between 1970 and 1981, the fetal death rate declined by 4.1 percent per year, but the decline slowed to 3.2 percent per year between 1981 and 1986. Maintenance of this decline would result in a fetal death rate of 5 per 1,000 in the year 2000. Monitoring this objective will be complicated by reporting problems. There is evidence that fetal deaths, especially those near the 20-week gestational age cutoff, are underreported.[344] Attempts are now being made to improve reporting. If reporting is improved, the real rate of decline in the fetal death rate will be understated.

Fetal death is associated with pregnancies complicated by maternal factors such as Rh sensitization and diabetes.[345] Improvements in clinical management of such conditions has contributed to reductions in fetal deaths. Sustained clinical management prior to and/or throughout such high-risk pregnancies is needed. Early, comprehensive, risk-appropriate care is of particular importance.

Blacks have the highest fetal death rate of any minority group, so achievement of this objective will be determined in large part by reductions in fetal deaths among blacks. Between 1970 and 1981, the fetal death rate among blacks declined by 4.5 percent per year, but the decline slowed to 2.3 percent per year between 1981 and 1986. Achieving this objective would require an acceleration in the black rate of decline to 3.6 percent per year.

14.3   Reduce the maternal mortality rate to no more than 3.3 per 100,000 live births. (Baseline: 6.6 per 100,000 in 1987)

Special Population Target

	Maternal Mortality	*1987 Baseline*	*2000 Target*
14.3a	Blacks	14.2[†]	5[†]

[†]*Per 100,000 live births*

Note: The objective uses the maternal mortality rate as defined by the National Center for Health Statistics. However, if other sources of maternal mortality data are used, a 50-percent reduction in maternal mortality is the intended target.

Baseline data sources: National Vital Statistics System, CDC; Maternal Mortality Surveillance System, CDC.

In 1987, 251 maternal deaths were reported by the National Center for Health Statistics. While this number of deaths is small, maternal mortality remains significant because a high proportion of the deaths are preventable. Additionally, there is an unacceptable racial differential, with black women dying at three times the rate of white women. Achievement of this objective and special population target would reduce the gap between whites and blacks by more than 50 percent. In 1987, black women had a maternal mortality rate of 14.2 per 100,000 live births compared with a rate of 5.1 for white women.

Statistics on maternal mortality are available from national vital statistics published by the National Center for Health Statistics. Counts are based entirely on the physician's certification of cause of death on the death certificate, which the National Center for Health Statistics processes and tabulates according to the classification system, definitions, and rules for selecting underlying cause of death specified by the World Health Organization (WHO) in the International Classification of Diseases, Ninth Revision (ICD-9). According to WHO, "a maternal death is defined as the death of a woman while pregnant or within 42 days of termination of pregnancy, irrespective of the duration and the site of the pregnancy, from any cause related to or aggravated by the pregnancy or its management but not from accidental or incidental causes."[346]

National vital statistics are not designed for studying maternal deaths, and independent studies have found that up to 40 percent of maternal deaths have been misclassified as nonmaternal in State and national vital statistics. Most independent studies of maternal mortality report rates that are higher than those reported by the National Center for Health Statistics. For example, a study of maternal deaths by CDC for 1974 through 1978 revealed that the number of deaths classified by national vital statistics as maternal was 20 percent less than the number classified by State vital statistics.[347] For deaths occurring in 1980 through 1985, selected maternal mortality committees reported 39 percent more deaths than State vital statistics. One study found that the maternal mortality rate for all races was 14.1 per 100,000 live births; for whites the rate was 10.0 and for black and other minority women the rate was 26.7 per 100,000 live births.[348]

Differing sources of information will therefore influence the rate to be achieved by the year 2000. An absolute rate of 3.3 should be the target only if national vital statistics figures are used. If other sources of information are used, a 50 percent reduction in the 1987 rate is a preferable target. The use of a percentage change will allow the use of any source of reporting.

Review of maternal deaths by maternal mortality review committees in some States, and studies of maternal deaths at the hospital, local, and State level have contributed to our understanding of the risk factors of maternal death, as well as to the evaluation and improvement of the quality of care. However, the very small numbers of maternal deaths in hospitals, even State-wide, make it impossible to make conclusions based on findings from hospital and State based data. A surveillance system has been developed and implemented by CDC to identify, study, and determine causes of maternal death using national aggregated data.

14.4 **Reduce the incidence of fetal alcohol syndrome to no more than 0.12 per 1,000 live births. (Baseline: 0.22 per 1,000 live births in 1987)**

Special Population Targets

Fetal Alcohol Syndrome (per 1,000 live births)		1987 Baseline	2000 Target
14.4a	American Indians/Alaska Natives	4	2
14.4b	Blacks	0.8	0.4

Baseline data source: Birth Defects Monitoring System, CDC.

Heavy alcohol consumption during pregnancy is known to cause alcohol-related defects among infants and fetal alcohol syndrome, which is characterized by growth retardation, facial malformations, and central nervous system dysfunctions including mental retardation.[349] Although the lower limit of safe alcohol consumption during pregnancy has not been documented, it is clear that most known adverse effects in infants are associated with heavy maternal alcohol use. One study found that infants born to mothers who reported consuming two or more drinks each day during pregnancy had, on average, a 7-point decrement in I.Q. at age 7.[350]

American Indians on reservations and blacks seem to bear a disproportionate share of fetal alcohol syndrome-related morbidity.[351] Using data for the period 1981 through 1986 from the CDC birth defects monitoring program, it appears that the rates of fetal alcohol syndrome among American Indians/Alaska Natives and blacks were 33 and 7 times higher than whites, respectively.

In American Indians and Alaska Natives, the incidence of fetal alcohol syndrome varies considerably among tribal group. Baseline and study data for American Indians and Alaska Natives are averages and do not indicate the wide range in incidence experienced from region to region.

Since fetal alcohol syndrome is directly related to alcohol consumption during pregnancy, it is entirely preventable. Thus a relatively ambitious target, a 50-percent reduction, has been set. It should be noted that surveillance for fetal alcohol syndrome is expected to improve over the coming decade. Legislation enacted in 1989 requires State health departments to begin annual reporting on the incidence of fetal alcohol syndrome as part of their responsibilities under the Maternal and Child Health Block Grant. As a result, the incidence of the condition may appear to increase.

Preventive interventions to reduce maternal use of alcohol include health education to increase awareness of the hazards of alcohol use and identification of alcohol abuse or addiction prior to conception or in early pregnancy.

Risk Reduction Objectives

14.5 Reduce low birth weight to an incidence of no more than 5 percent of live births and very low birth weight to no more than 1 percent of live births. (Baseline: 6.9 and 1.2 percent, respectively, in 1987)

Special Population Target

		1987 Baseline	2000 Target
Low Birth Weight			
14.5a	Blacks	12.7%	9%
Very Low Birth Weight			
	Blacks	2.7%	2%

Note: Low birth weight is weight at birth of less than 2,500 grams; very low birth weight is weight at birth of less than 1,500 grams.
Baseline data source: National Vital Statistics System, CDC.

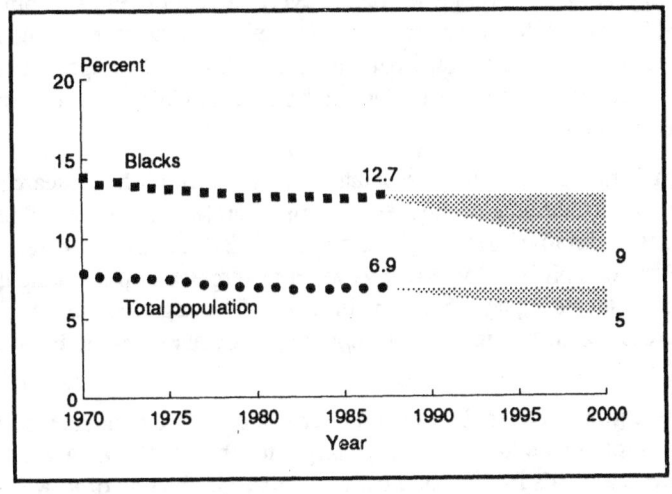

Fig. 14.5

Incidence of low birth weight

From 1970 to 1981, low birth weight declined 1.3 percent per year. The rate was stagnant from 1981 through 1986. Low-birth-weight infants include newborns who are born too early and those whose intrauterine growth is retarded. About two-thirds of the decline in low birth weight during the 1970s was due to a reduction in intrauterine growth retardation and only one-third to reductions in preterm births.[352] A number of risk factors for low birth weight have been identified, including younger and older maternal age, high parity, poor reproductive history (especially history of low birth weight), low socioeconomic status, low level of education, late entry into prenatal care, low pregnancy weight gain and/or low prepregnancy weight, smoking, and substance abuse.[353]

Smoking has been linked to low birth weight and is estimated to be associated with from 20 to 30 percent of all low-birth-weight births in this country.[354] Other behaviors, such as alcohol consumption and illicit drug use are also associated with low birth weight, although the evidence, particularly for alcohol consumption, is less complete than for smoking.[355,356] Certain medical conditions, such as placenta previa and premature rupture of the membranes, are also associated with low birth weight.

A number of recent studies have examined the effects of illicit drug use on pregnancy outcomes, including impaired fetal growth.[357] Infants born to mothers with positive urine assays for either marijuana or cocaine were significantly smaller than the infants of nonusers. Women addicted to cocaine and/or marijuana are also likely to be alcohol and tobacco users.[358]

Available data on disabilities among low-birth-weight infants consider the rate and severity of disability within the different weight categories. In studies of births between 1975 and 1985, 303 children (26 percent) out of 1,169 survivors with birth weights less than 1,500 grams had moderate or severe disabilities. Moderate or severe disabilities are I.Q.s below 80, cerebral palsy, major seizure disorders, and blindness. Among infants with birth weights of less than 2,500 grams, disability rate estimates vary between two percent and 4.5 percent.[359]

Recent trends for blacks for the years 1981 through 1986 show essentially no change in the percentage of infants with low birth weight. The trend must be substantially changed if blacks are to meet the year 2000 low-birth-weight target. Several of the known risk factors for low birth weight, such as maternal cigarette smoking, are more prevalent among black mothers. In addition, there are still disparities in receipt of comprehensive prenatal care between whites and blacks.

Data show an average decline in very low birth weight of about 0.1 percent for the years 1970 to 1981. For the years 1981 through 1986, however, the rate of very low birth weight has *increased* by about 0.9 percent per year. Therefore, given recent trends, it is unlikely that the objective of no more than 1 percent of very low birth weight infants by the year 2000 will be met without a vigorous commitment to providing high quality prenatal care to at-risk women.

Very low birth weight births are primarily associated with preterm birth. Research should focus on better understanding of the mechanisms of preterm delivery and its associated risk factors. As with low birth weight, the use of illicit drugs may increase the risk of very low birth weight births. Specific interventions targeted at preventing drug use among women of childbearing age should be initiated. The negative effects of external factors such as stress and strenuous work during pregnancy also need additional consideration.

For all racial and ethnic groups except blacks and Puerto Ricans, the incidence of very low birth weight is lower than the total population target for the year 2000 target of 1 percent of live births. Recent trends for blacks show an increase in the rate of very low birth weight for the years 1981 through 1986 of about 1.6 percent per year.

14.6 **Increase to at least 85 percent the proportion of mothers who achieve the minimum recommended weight gain during their pregnancies. (Baseline: 67 percent of married women in 1980)**

Note: Recommended weight gain is pregnancy weight gain recommended in the 1990 National Academy of Science's report, Nutrition During Pregnancy.[360]

Baseline data source: National Natality Survey, CDC.

An infant's birth weight is a major determinant of his or her potential for survival and future development. A strong relationship between pregnancy weight gain and birth weight has been demonstrated consistently, and low maternal weight gain is considered a risk factor that may be susceptible to intervention.[361,362] In 1980, the proportion of low weight births declined from 13.9 percent when weight gain was less than 16 pounds to 6.1 percent for gains of 21 to 25 pounds, and to 4 percent when mothers gained 36 pounds or more.[363]

A low prepregnancy weight combined with a small pregnancy weight gain is associated with a very high incidence of low birth weight. The incidence, however, declines sharply as weight gain rises, regardless of prepregnancy weight.[363]

Approximately one-third of all mothers gain inadequate weight during their pregnancies. Two groups particularly at risk for having low-birth-weight infants and other adverse outcomes of pregnancy, teenagers and black women, both tend to gain less weight during pregnancy than the population as a whole. Higher weight gain for these and other at-risk groups of women, e.g., smokers, is associated with a lower incidence of adverse outcomes.[360]

Caloric intake is associated with pregnancy weight gain and pregnancy outcome. Although a pregnant woman can gain adequate weight regardless of the nutritional quality of her diet, the goal is to promote desired weight gain through sound dietary practices and a nutritionally adequate diet. Factors other than nutritional intake that influence pregnancy weight gain, such as smoking, strenuous physical work, and chronic illness must be taken into account for nutritional management during pregnancy.

14.7 **Reduce severe complications of pregnancy to no more than 15 per 100 deliveries. (Baseline: 22 hospitalizations (prior to delivery) per 100 deliveries in 1987)**

Note: Severe complications of pregnancy will be measured using hospitalizations due to pregnancy-related complications.
Baseline data source: National Hospital Discharge Survey, CDC.

Complications of pregnancy are associated with maternal mortality and perinatal morbidity and mortality, as well as chronic conditions for both mothers and their babies. In addition, complications of pregnancy lead to a loss of productivity, generate substantial hospital costs, and cause emotional distress among families.

In 1987, approximately 860,000 hospitalizations were for pregnancy-related complications not associated with delivery. Of these admissions, approximately 27 percent involved preterm labor; 9 percent, spontaneous abortion; 8 percent, genitourinary infection; 8 percent, hemorrhage during early pregnancy; 7 percent, vomiting; 6 percent, pregnancy-induced hypertension; 5 percent, diabetes mellitus; and 4 percent, missed abortion.

Achieving this objective will require greater attention to determining the etiology of, and effective interventions for, serious complications, with reductions varying by type of complication. This objective targets reductions in all pregnancy related complications. However, complications treated without hospitalization are very difficult to track. Hospitalizations are used as a proxy for all severe complications of pregnancy. The objective should not be interpreted as advocating reductions in hospitalization per se. In many instances, hospitalization is necessary for treatment.

14.8 Reduce the cesarean delivery rate to no more than 15 per 100 deliveries. (Baseline: 24.4 per 100 deliveries in 1987)

Type-Specific Targets

Cesarean Delivery (per 100 deliveries)	*1987 Baseline*	*2000 Target*
14.8a Primary (first time) cesarean delivery	17.4	12
14.8b Repeat cesarean deliveries	91.2†	65†

†*Among women who had a previous cesarean delivery*

Baseline data source: National Hospital Discharge Survey, CDC.

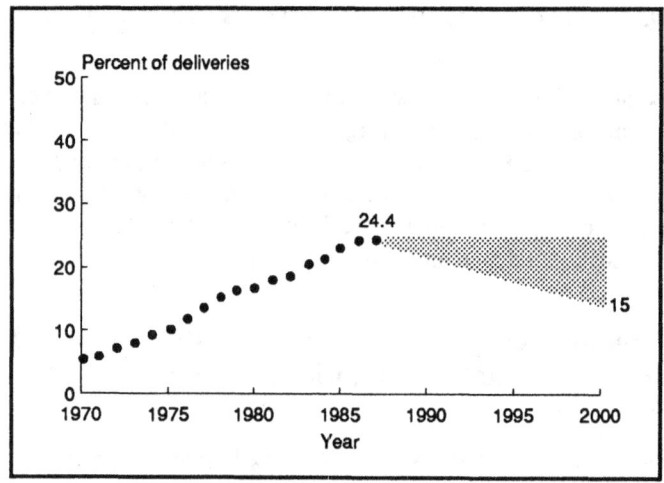

Fig.14.8 Cesarean delivery rate

Cesarean delivery rates in the United States have increased each year since 1965. Yet, there is no evidence that maternal and child health has improved as a result of this increase. Cesarean delivery carries an increased risk of maternal mortality and morbidity, as well as an increased risk of perinatal morbidity.[364] Maternal mortality rates associated with cesarean deliveries have been reported to range from 2 to 26 times that associated with vaginal delivery, and, in 1986, the average length of hospital stay for cesarean deliveries was 6 days compared with 3 for vaginal deliveries.[365,366,367] The increased mortality risk may, however, be partially due to the lack of adjustments for conditions causing the cesarean delivery. If rates continued rising at the current pace, cesarean deliveries would account for 29 percent of all deliveries in 1990, and 40 percent in the year 2000. However, recent estimates for 1987 indicate that the rates of cesarean delivery may be reaching a plateau.

To reduce the cesarean delivery rate, one hospital recently evaluated the effect of selected clinical criteria and review mechanisms (e.g., requiring a second opinion, recognizing vaginal birth after previous cesarean delivery as the preferred method, instituting a peer review process).[368] Findings indicated a decrease in the rate from 17.5 percent of total deliveries in 1985 to 11.5 percent in 1987. It should be noted that this decrease occurred at a time when national rates were rising.

Other recommendations for decreasing cesarean delivery rates include: eliminating incentives for physicians and hospitals such as equalizing reimbursement for vaginal and cesarean deliveries; public dissemination of physician- and hospital-specific cesarean delivery rates to increase public awareness of differences in practice; and addressing malpractice concerns, which may be a strong driving force behind the increasing rates of cesarean delivery.

From 1980 to 1985, 48 percent of the increase in the cesarean delivery rate was due to repeat cesarean deliveries. The American College of Obstetricians and Gynecologists (ACOG) issued guidelines in October 1988 on repeat cesarean deliveries based on a finding that "a trial of labor [is] successful in 50 to 80 percent of patients who had low transverse uterine incisions from previous deliveries and who were selected candidates for vaginal birth in subsequent pregnancies."[369] ACOG recommended that each hospital develop its own protocol for management of patients with previous cesarean delivery. These guidelines recommend that in the absence of a contraindication, women with one previous cesarean delivery with a low transverse incision should be counseled and encouraged to attempt labor in their current pregnancy.

14.9* **Increase to at least 75 percent the proportion of mothers who breastfeed their babies in the early postpartum period and to at least 50 percent the proportion who continue breastfeeding until their babies are 5 to 6 months old. (Baseline: 54 percent at discharge from birth site and 21 percent at 5 to 6 months in 1988)**

Special Population Targets

	Mothers Breastfeeding Their Babies:	1988 Baseline	2000 Target
	During Early Postpartum Period —		
14.9a	Low-income mothers	32%	75%
14.9b	Black mothers	25%	75%
14.9c	Hispanic mothers	51%	75%
14.9d	American Indian/Alaska Native mothers	47%	75%
	At Age 5-6 Months —		
14.9a	Low-income mothers	9%	50%
14.9b	Black mothers	8%	50%
14.9c	Hispanic mothers	16%	50%
14.9d	American Indian/Alaska Native mothers	28%	50%

Baseline data sources: Ross Laboratories Mothers Survey; for American Indians and Alaska Natives, Pediatric Nutrition Surveillance System, CDC.

Breastfeeding is the optimal way of nurturing full-term infants while simultaneously benefiting the lactating mother. The advantages of breastfeeding range from biochemical, immunologic, enzymatic, and endocrinologic to psychosocial, developmental, hygienic, and economic. Human milk contains the ideal balance of nutrients, enzymes, immunoglobulin, anti-infective and anti-inflammatory substances, hormones, and growth factors.[370] Further, breast milk changes to match the changing needs of the infant. Breast-feeding provides a time of intense maternal-infant interaction. Lactation also facilitates the physiologic return to the prepregnant state for the mother while suppressing ovulation for many.[371]

Although breastfeeding is strongly recommended, it is not appropriate for babies whose mothers use drugs such as cocaine, PCP, or marijuana, take more than minimal amounts of alcohol, or who receive certain therapeutic or diagnostic agents such as radioactive elements and cancer chemotherapy. Women who are HIV positive should also avoid breastfeeding.

Analysis of data from the Ross Laboratories Mothers Survey indicates that breastfeeding rates continue to be highest among women who are older, well-educated, relatively affluent, and/or who live in the western United States (71 percent at discharge from birth site and 31 percent at 5 to 6 months). Among those least likely to breastfeed are women who are low-income, black, less than age 20, and/or who live in the southeastern United

States. Low-income and black women should receive special attention because they have low rates of breastfeeding and are a significant proportion of all new mothers (approximately 25 percent and 17 percent, respectively).[372]

An important barrier to achieving this objective is the general absence of work policies and facilities that support lactating women. Given the large percentage of mothers of young children who work outside the home, efforts to increase breastfeeding should focus on convincing employers to provide assistance such as extended maternity leave, part-time employment, provision of facilities for pumping breast milk or breastfeeding, and on-site child care. Another important barrier is portrayal of bottle rather than breastfeeding as the norm in American society and the absence of breastfeeding incentives and support for low-income women. Overcoming these barriers will require public and professional education, improved support from health care providers and employers, and the involvement of culturally sensitive social, religious, and professional groups. The media can play an important role by more frequently portraying breastfeeding as the norm.

*This objective also appears as Objective 2.11 in *Nutrition*.

14.10 **Increase abstinence from tobacco use by pregnant women to at least 90 percent and increase abstinence from alcohol, cocaine, and marijuana by pregnant women by at least 20 percent. (Baseline: 75 percent of pregnant women abstained from tobacco use in 1985)**

Note: Data for alcohol, cocaine, and marijuana use by pregnant women will be available from the National Maternal and Infant Health Survey, CDC, in 1991.

Baseline data sources: For cigarette smoking, National Health Interview Survey, CDC.

Poor pregnancy outcomes due to maternal smoking, alcohol, and/or illicit drug use are well documented. Smoking is closely associated with low birth weight.[354] Heavy alcohol consumption is associated with fetal alcohol syndrome which is characterized by growth retardation, facial malformations, and central nervous system dysfunctions including mental retardation.[349] Illicit drug use, most notably the use of cocaine by women, is associated with fetal distress and impaired fetal growth,[355,357] and may result in ongoing developmental problems during and after infancy.[373]

In 1985, 25 percent of pregnant women used tobacco. Warning labels on cigarette packages now alert users to the danger to the fetus. Warning labels on alcoholic beverages concerning the dangers of alcohol use during pregnancy may reduce consumption of alcoholic beverages during pregnancy. Ideally, abstention from alcohol use by women who are pregnant or who anticipate becoming pregnant, would become the norm among American women. Preconception counseling by health care providers, especially nurse midwives and obstetricians, could reinforce public awareness messages on tobacco products and alcoholic beverages.

Services and Protection Objectives

14.11 Increase to at least 90 percent the proportion of all pregnant women who receive prenatal care in the first trimester of pregnancy. (Baseline: 76 percent of live births in 1987)

Special Population Targets

Proportion of Pregnant Women Receiving Early Prenatal Care	1987 Baseline	2000 Target
14.11a Black women	61.1†	90†
14.11b American Indian/Alaska Native women	60.2†	90†
14.11c Hispanic women	61.0†	90†

†*Percent of live births*

Baseline data source: National Vital Statistics System, CDC.

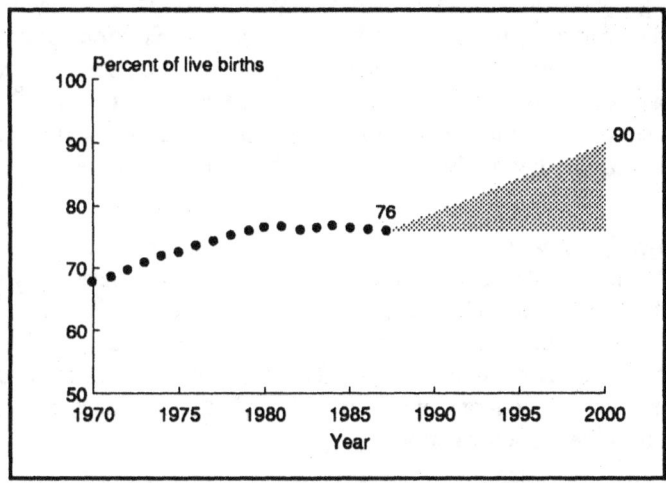

Fig. 14.11

Percentage of pregnant women receiving first trimester prenatal care

Early, high-quality prenatal care is critical to improving pregnancy outcomes. Prenatal care is especially important for women at increased medical and/or social risk. For example, women who are substance abusers are unlikely to get prenatal care.[374] Maternal characteristics associated with receiving late or no prenatal care include low income, less than a high school education, teenage pregnancy, and a large number of children.[375]

Low income has been consistently correlated with lack of early and sufficient care. More than 14 million women of reproductive age have no insurance to cover maternity care.[376] Recent Congressional mandates expanding Medicaid have resulted in more women being eligible for prenatal and postpartum care, but difficulties remain in getting eligible women into care. In addition, there is a growing shortage of obstetrical providers, often attributed to rising malpractice insurance rates.[148] Expanding the number of maternity providers through increased use of certified nurse midwives and nurse practitioners could help alleviate this problem.

Between 1970 and 1980, there was a significant trend toward increasing early entry into prenatal care. Increases were especially large for the groups with the lowest levels of care. Since 1980, however, the proportion of women who begin prenatal care in the first trimester of pregnancy has reached a plateau among all racial and ethnic groups. Of special concern is the increase between 1982 and 1987 in the proportions of women not receiving care until their third trimester or receiving no care. Because of the lack of progress in this area, the target proposed for the year 2000 is the same as the target set for 1990.

14.12* **Increase to at least 60 percent the proportion of primary care providers who provide age-appropriate preconception care and counseling. (Baseline data available in 1992)**

The purpose of providing preconception care and information is to ensure that women are healthy prior to beginning pregnancy, thereby reducing the risk of adverse pregnancy outcomes. Such care should be available to all women desiring pregnancy and their partners. Many medical conditions, personal behaviors, and environmental conditions associated with poor pregnancy outcomes can be identified and modified or treated prior to conception.

Awareness of illness or conditions such as diabetes, which should be controlled before pregnancy, is beneficial in planning pregnancy. Strict glucose control before conception and throughout gestation, coupled with close management, can be effective in reducing adverse outcomes among offspring of women with diabetes. One and a half million women of childbearing age are diabetic. In diabetic women, infection occurs with greater frequency and severity; the likelihood of hypertension increases fourfold; injury to the birth canal is more common because of the tendency to larger babies; cesarean sections are required more frequently; and hemorrhage after delivery is more likely.[368] Intervention in other illnesses or conditions prior to pregnancy, such as poor nutrition or phenylketonuria which require diet modification, would be beneficial, as would counseling concerning HIV.

Preconception identification of women with medical illness or unhealthy behaviors and couples at risk for offspring with genetic disorders provides the opportunity to inform and counsel on the hazards of unhealthy behaviors, appropriate treatment, the risks of genetic disorders in their offspring, pregnancy planning, early entry into prenatal care, or avoidance of pregnancy. Family planning services and education must be an integral part of preconception care to reduce the large number of unintended pregnancies in this country and to assure adequate spacing between pregnancies.[377]

Identification of, and intervention to modify, maternal behaviors such as smoking and alcohol use and/or use of illicit drugs should occur prior to pregnancy. As damage to the fetus from drug and/or alcohol use can occur early in pregnancy, intervention to modify or eliminate the behavior(s) prior to pregnancy is crucial. Counseling regarding drug use must also include use of prescription medications during pregnancy, since some drugs have been documented as powerful teratogens. For example, about 25 percent of human fetuses exposed to isotretin during the first trimester are affected with severe congenital abnormalities and other developmental disabilities.[378]

Primary care providers should not limit counseling to maternal behavior. The behaviors of other household members can also affect pregnancy outcome. For example, recent reports suggest that exposure to environmental tobacco smoke during pregnancy may be associated with low birth weight.[70]

*This objective also appears as Objective 5.10 in *Family Planning*.

14.13 **Increase to at least 90 percent the proportion of women enrolled in prenatal care who are offered screening and counseling on prenatal detection of fetal abnormalities. (Baseline data available in 1991)**

Note: This objective will be measured by tracking use of maternal serum alpha-fetoprotein screening tests.

Prenatal screening can be used to identify serious disorders which have long term consequences for infants and their families. The purpose of such screening is to allow for initiation of interventions to ameliorate the consequences of the disorders through counseling and specialized obstetric and neonatal care.

Maternal serum alpha-fetoprotein (MSAFP) testing was initially employed in the early 1970s as a screening test to detect neural tube defects in fetuses. As experience with the test grew, it became evident that an abnormal level of MSAFP was an indicator of several other conditions such as twin pregnancy, ventral wall defects, Down Syndrome, and fetal demise.[379,380]

MSAFP screening carried out at 15 to 18 weeks of pregnancy is now the standard of care for women enrolling in early prenatal care. The test is not informative at other stages of pregnancy. Abnormal levels of MSAFP indicate a need for further tests such as ultrasonography and amniocentesis. In the event of a fetal abnormality, testing and counseling early in pregnancy provides an opportunity for families to prepare to care for a disabled infant, and increasingly, for medical interventions to correct some problems *in utero*. Women should be informed about the availability of this screening technique at their initial prenatal care visit.

After licensure of a commercially produced test kit by the Food and Drug Administration, the American College of Obstetricians and Gynecologists (ACOG) issued an alert to its members in 1985, strongly recommending that every prenatal patient be advised of the availability of this test.[381] Current ACOG standards recommend that MSAFP screening be offered to all patients.[382] Since 1986, California has required that the test be offered to all pregnant women who register for care before the end of the period in which the test is effective.

14.14 **Increase to at least 90 percent the proportion of pregnant women and infants who receive risk-appropriate care. (Baseline data available in 1991)**

Note: This objective will be measured by tracking the proportion of very low birth weight infants (less than 1,500 grams) born in facilities covered by a neonatologist 24 hours a day.

The course of pregnancy is a dynamic process in which a woman's risk status can change at any point. Therefore, comprehensive and coordinated mechanisms should be in place to match the intensity of health care to the pregnant woman's and infant's degree of risk.

Implementing coordinated systems of perinatal care and assuring receipt of risk-appropriate care have been inhibited by changing circumstances in health care delivery, in spite of established standards by professional organizations. These inhibiting factors include increased competition and changes in financing mechanisms, advances in medical technology, changing patterns of medical practice and care delivery, legal and liability issues, and diffusion of specialists.[383]

The quality assurance mechanisms needed to measure this objective (e.g., chart audits) are not feasible for obtaining national data estimates. However, a proxy measure, such as the percentage of very low birth weight infants referred for delivery to a facility that provides high-risk care for mothers and infants, would be indicative of risk-responsive care.

14.15 **Increase to at least 95 percent the proportion of newborns screened by State-sponsored programs for genetic disorders and other disabling conditions and to 90 percent the proportion of newborns testing positive for disease who receive appropriate treatment. (Baseline: For sickle cell anemia, with 20 States reporting, approximately 33 percent of live births screened (57 percent of black infants); for galactosemia, with 38 States reporting, approximately 70 percent of live births screened)**

Note: As measured by the proportion of infants served by programs for sickle cell anemia and galactosemia. Screening programs should be appropriate for State demographic characteristics.
Baseline data source: Council of Regional Networks for Genetic Services.

Virtually all States screen infants for genetic and metabolic disorders and treat or refer for treatment those with a confirmed diagnosis. However, some disorders are more uniformly screened for than others, and followup testing and early initiation of preventive treatment is uneven. It is crucial that State commitment to screening is accompanied by commitment to treatment of affected newborns discovered through screening. States should screen for additional conditions only when they are committed to treating newborns discovered to have disease. Further, States should add only those screening tests which are efficient and effective, e.g., accurate (they detect the disorder in question); reliable (do not produce excessive false positives or false negatives; useful (treatment is available for the disorder); and affordable.

Screening for PKU and congenital hypothyroidism is virtually universal, although reporting is not. While it is important to continue screening and appropriate followup for these disorders and to improve reporting, it is the intent of this objective to focus on two disorders for which screening and followup has been less consistent, sickle cell anemia and galactosemia.

Sickle cell diseases affect 1 in every 400 black newborns. These and other hemoglobinopathies are common in people of African, Asian, Mediterranean, Caribbean, and South and Central American origins.[384] While universal screening for sickle cell is recommended, States with negligible at-risk populations may choose to target their testing programs.

Significant mortality and morbidity are associated with sickle cell because of increased susceptibility to severe bacterial infections. Meningitis, pneumonia, and septicemia are major causes of death among children with the disorder.[385] Early diagnosis and immediate entry into programs of comprehensive care, including the initiation of penicillin prophylaxis, has been found to reduce the morbidity and mortality associated with sickle cell.[385]

The inherited disorder of galactosemia leads to an increased risk of death from overwhelming infection in early infancy, with failure to thrive, vomiting, liver disease, and mental retardation in untreated survivors. A galactose-free diet should be begun as soon as possible and continued throughout life.[386] Treatment should be initiated within the first week of life to avoid early death, but 1988 data indicated that only 37 percent of the cases reported met this criterion.[387]

14.16 **Increase to at least 90 percent the proportion of babies aged 18 months and younger who receive recommended primary care services at the appropriate intervals. (Baseline data available in 1992)**

Assuring that infants receive appropriate primary care will help reduce infant mortality and childhood disease through prevention and early identification of health problems, including developmental and emotional problems. Achievement of this objective requires resolution of the issues of financing of care and acceptability of care. Barriers to achievement include a lack of knowledge about the value of preventive services (by both providers and parents), inability to pay for care, and geographic and personnel limitations.

Another important challenge for the delivery of primary care services is the fragmentation that often characterizes health care services delivery. If primary care is to reduce infant mortality and childhood morbidity, primary care providers must be linked to providers of specialty care. To establish these crucial links, primary care providers must identify children who need specialized attention, know suitable specialty resources, make appropriate and timely referrals, and work collaboratively with those providing care.

Only a few studies have examined the receipt of sets of services. One study found that although 93 percent of newborns had received at least one well-care examination, only 44 percent had received three or more doses of diphtheria-pertussis-tetanus (DPT) vaccine and three or more doses of polio vaccine by age 18 months. An ambulatory care quality assurance study also found well-baby care inadequate in delivering complete sets of preventive services.

Two sets of recommendations could be used to track progress toward this objective. The American Academy of Pediatric's Committee on Practice and Ambulatory Medicine publishes a recommended set of preventive services for infants in its *Guidelines for Health Supervision*.[388] Another useful set is the U.S. Preventive Services Task Force recommendations for infants contained in its *Guide to Clinical Preventive Services*.[45]

* * *

Research Needs

Priorities include investigation of:

- The etiology of preterm birth generally, and very low birth weight specifically, including investigations into the physiology of uterine activity and the physiology and chemical events that influence fetal growth and development.

- Reasons for the exceedingly high rate of low birth weight among blacks.

- Effective methods for modifying unhealthy behavior among pregnant women (e.g., tobacco, alcohol, and/or drug use).

- Methods of improving prenatal and perinatal care services for high-risk populations and increasing acceptability and use of services.

- Factors associated with care-seeking behaviors and effective methods for improving use of prenatal care.

- The etiology and prevention of congenital anomalies and sudden infant death syndrome.

- The etiology and preventive management of severe complications of pregnancy, such as vomiting and pregnancy-induced hypertension.

* * *

Baseline Data Source References

Birth Defects Monitoring System, Center for Environmental Health and Injury Control, Centers for Disease Control, Public Health Service, U.S. Department of Health and Human Services, Atlanta, GA.

Council of Regional Networks for Genetic Services, Phoenix, AZ.

Maternal Mortality Surveillance System, Center for Chronic Disease Prevention and Health Promotion, Centers for Disease Control, Public Health Service, U.S. Department of Health and Human Services, Atlanta, GA.

National Health Interview Survey, National Center for Health Statistics, Centers for Disease Control, Public Health Service, U.S. Department of Health and Human Services, Hyattsville, MD.

National Hospital Discharge Survey, National Center for Health Statistics, Centers for Disease Control, Public Health Service, U.S. Department of Health and Human Services, Hyattsville, MD.

Linked Birth and Infant Death Data Set, National Center for Health Statistics, Centers for Disease Control, Public Health Service, U.S. Department of Health and Human Services, Hyattsville, MD.

National Maternal and Infant Health Survey, National Center for Health Statistics, Centers for Disease Control, Public Health Service, U.S. Department of Health and Human Services, Hyattsville, MD.

National Vital Statistics System, National Center for Health Statistics, Centers for Disease Control, Public Health Service, U.S. Department of Health and Human Services, Hyattsville, MD.

Pediatric Nutrition Surveillance System, Center for Chronic Disease Prevention and Health Promotion, Centers for Disease Control, Public Health Service, U.S. Department of Health and Human Services, Atlanta, GA.

Ross Laboratories Mothers Survey, Ross Laboratories, Columbia, Ohio.

Cancer

16

Contents

* * *

16.4 Cervical cancer

* * *

16.9 Actions to reduce sun exposure

* * *

16.12 Pap tests

* * *

16.15 Pap test quality

* * *

[Research Needs]

16. Cancer

* * *

Health Status Objectives

* * *

16.4 Reduce deaths from cancer of the uterine cervix to no more than 1.3 per 100,000 women. (Age-adjusted baseline: 2.8 per 100,000 in 1987)

Note: In its publications, the National Cancer Institute age adjusts cancer death rates to the 1970 U.S. population. Using the 1970 standard, the equivalent baseline and target values for this objective would be 3.2 and 1.5 per 100,000, respectively.

Baseline data source: National Vital Statistics System, CDC.

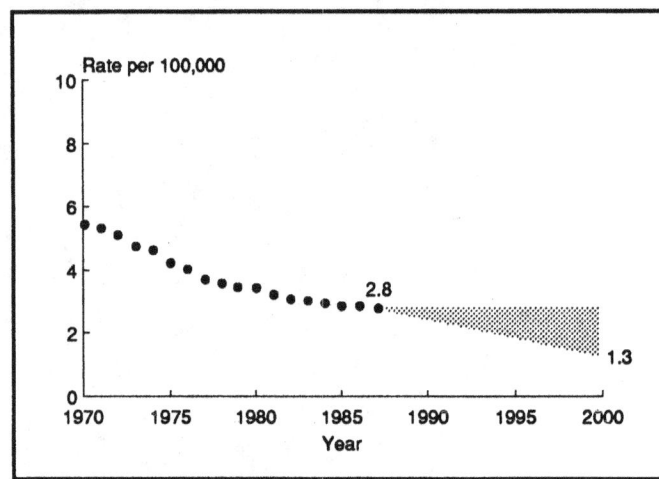

Fig. 16.4

Age-adjusted cervical cancer death rate

Cancer of the uterine cervix is one of the most commonly occurring cancers for women. More than 50,000 cases of carcinoma in situ of the uterine cervix are detected annually. In 1990, approximately 13,500 new cases of invasive cancer of the uterine cervix will be diagnosed, and about 6,000 women will die from cervical cancer.[389]

Use of the Pap test to screen for cervical cancer greatly reduces the risk of death from invasive cervical cancer. The decline in cervical cancer mortality in the 1970s and 1980s is thought to be due primarily to the widespread use of the Pap test for early detection of cervical cancer. The most recent National Health Interview Survey suggests that a significant proportion of women are not receiving Pap tests regularly and that the women at greatest risk of cervical cancer mortality (older women) are least likely to have been screened.[390]

Increasing Pap test utilization has the potential to reduce mortality from cancer of the uterine cervix between the years 1990 and 2000. Data from the International Agency for Research on Cancer (IARC) indicate the impact of recency of Pap test utilization on the incidence of invasive cervical cancer.[391] Furthermore, increased utilization of Pap tests may produce a shift toward earlier stage disease, with its attendant improved survival rate.[392] Realizing the full potential for risk reduction due to Pap tests will also require efforts to ensure the quality of specimen collection and laboratory analysis (see Objective 16.15).

To set a target value for this objective, the age-adjusted death rate for cervical cancer was projected to the year 2000 assuming a logarithmic trend. The estimated reduction in cervical cancer deaths was developed using the CAN*TROL computer model[393] and then applied to the expected value. The CAN*TROL model calculates the effect of specified cancer control activities on cancer incidence, prevalence, and mortality. The model calculations included the following data inputs: (1) the estimated 1985 U.S. female population, (2) incidence rates for cancer of the uterine cervix among women, (3) stage distributions for women receiving and not receiving annual Pap test screening, and (4) stage-specific survival rates.

For the purposes of this modeling effort, it was assumed that women aged 20 through 85 would receive the stage-shift benefit from increased cervical cancer screening. Increased utilization of Pap tests was assumed to occur in three increments. The proportion of women aged 20 and older annually receiving Pap tests was set at 62 percent between 1990 and 1995, 69 percent between 1996 and 1998, and 75 percent between 1999 and 2000. These figures compare with the 1987 estimate of 56 percent of women aged 18 and older who received a Pap test in the previous year.[390]

Given these parameters, the CAN*TROL model estimates that the age-adjusted death rate for cancer of the uterine cervix will decline by 12 percent from a projected rate in the year 2000 of 1.5 per 100,000 to 1.3 per 100,000 women.

* * *

Risk Reduction Objectives

* * *

16.9 **Increase to at least 60 percent the proportion of people of all ages who limit sun exposure, use sunscreens and protective clothing when exposed to sunlight, and avoid artificial sources of ultraviolet light (e.g., sun lamps, tanning booths). (Baseline data available in 1992)**

Skin cancer is the most common form of cancer in the United States, accounting for about 600,000 new cases annually or roughly one-third of all new cancer cases.[389] Most skin cancers are basal cell and squamous cell carcinomas that are highly treatable and rarely metastasize. Of the two, basal cell cancer is more common. Squamous cell is more invasive and accounts for three-fourths of nonmelanoma skin cancer deaths. However, both types will account for only about 2,500 deaths in 1990.[389] The most serious form of skin cancer is malignant melanoma. It is far rarer but also far more lethal and accounts for 74 percent of all skin cancer deaths. The incidence of melanoma is increasing more rapidly than any other cancer, and the number of deaths from melanoma has surpassed that for cancer of the cervix. Between 1973-74 and 1985-86, the death rate for melanoma rose from 1.7 per 100,000 people to 2.2 per 100,000.[394] An estimated 27,600 new cases of malignant melanoma will occur in 1990, and 6,300 people will die of this disease.[389]

Exposure to nonionizing solar radiation appears to be the chief risk factor for nonmelanoma skin cancer and may be responsible for more than 90 percent of skin cancer cases.[395] The carcinogenic effects appear to be produced by ultraviolet-B (UV-B) radiation in the 290 to 320 nanometer range, the same range that produces tanning and burning in human skin. Data indicate that nonmelanoma skin cancer is related to annual cumulative exposure. The association is strongest for squamous cell carcinoma but is also strong for basal cell carcinoma. Solar radiation may be responsible for more than 90 percent of nonmelanoma skin cancer cases. Solar radiation has also been linked to skin melanoma incidence but the association is less certain. Skin melanoma may be related to exposure to high intensity UV radiation (e.g., sunburns) or exposure at young ages rather than cumulative exposure.

The incidence of nonmelanoma skin cancer varies directly with exposure to ultraviolet light and indirectly with the degree of skin pigmentation. Skin cancer rates are highest for whites, lower for Asians, and lowest for blacks. In 1977-87, the incidence for blacks was only 3.4 per 100,000 compared to 232.6 per 100,000 for whites.[395] Compared to white women, white men experience 1½ to 2 times the incidence of basal cell cancer and 2 to 3 times the incidence of squamous cell cancer. Both types occur most often on the face, head, and neck. Women have higher rates than men for both types of cancers on the legs. Men have more squamous cell cancer of the lip.

Numerous authorities have recommended that people of all ages, and especially those with light complexions, limit sun exposure. Parents and caregivers should limit sun exposure for infants and children. Special care should be taken to limit sun exposure in warmer climates, at higher altitudes, during the summer months, and during midday. Time of day and time of year are important determinants of exposure to UV-B radiation. The greatest amount of UV-B radiation occurs during the summer months, and one-third of a day's total amount occurs between the hours of 11 a.m. and 1 p.m. (or 12 noon and 2 p.m. Daylight Savings Time).[395] Although latitude or distance from the equator generally determines amount of UV-B radiation in a given location, amount of ozone in the atmosphere, altitude, and sky cover are also determining factors.

Sunscreen agents can block carcinogenic UV rays[396] and can reduce the incidence of skin tumors in laboratory animals.[397,398] Hence, many authorities advocate the use of sunscreen preparations rated 15 SPF (Sun Protective Factor) or more during sun exposure. In addition, individuals should avoid unnecessary UV exposure from artificial sources like sunlamps and tanning booths.

Specific baseline data for this objective are not available. However, a survey found that 30 percent of adults and 50 percent of adolescents engage in sun tanning.[399] Fully 23 percent of adults and 33 percent of adolescents fail to use protective measures while sun tanning.

Efforts to educate the public about the hazards of sun exposure and the value of protective actions may facilitate attainment of this objective. In 1987, only 54 percent of adults and 37 percent of adolescents were aware of the risks of sun exposure.[399] Employers of outdoor workers should consider sun exposure when establishing work schedules and should encourage the use of sunblocks and protective clothing. School playgrounds and outdoor recreation areas should ensure the availability of adequate shade.

Services and Protection Objectives

* * *

16.12 Increase to at least 95 percent the proportion of women aged 18 and older with uterine cervix who have ever received a Pap test, and to at least 85 percent those who received a Pap test within the preceding 1 to 3 years. (Baseline: 88 percent "ever" and 75 percent "within the preceding 3 years" in 1987)

Special Population Targets

Pap Test:	1987 Baseline	2000 Target
Ever Received—		
16.12a Hispanic women aged 18 and older	75%	95%
* * *		
16.12c Women aged 18 and older with less than high school education	79%	95%
16.12d Low-income women aged 18 and older (annual family income <$10,000)	80%	95%
Received Within Preceding 3 Years—		
16.12a Hispanic women aged 18 and older	66%	80%
* * *		
16.12c Women aged 18 and older with less than high school education	58%	75%
16.12d Low-income women aged 18 and older (annual family income <$10,000)	64%	80%

Baseline data source: National Health Interview Survey, CDC.

A number of studies have found that the Pap test is effective in screening for cancer of the uterine cervix, reducing mortality from the disease by as much as 75 percent.[391,400,401,402,403,404] The decline in cervical cancer mortality in the 1970s and 1980s is thought by many experts to be due primarily to widespread use of the Pap test for early detection of cervical cancer.

A variety of recommendations have been made regarding the age at which screening for cervical cancer should begin and the frequency with which it should occur. In the United States, current recommendations of various government and professional groups leave the frequency of screening to the discretion of the physician, though all organizations suggest an interval of 1 to 3 years.[405] Examination of results of ongoing screening programs in Europe and North America indicate that the greatest protection against cervical cancer is provided in the 5 years following a negative smear, but the effect virtually disappears after 10 years.[391,555] A recent case control study conducted in the United States indicates an increasing risk of cervical cancer if the screening interval exceeds 2 years.[406]

Age influences both cervical cancer incidence and survival. While younger women are more frequently diagnosed with cervical cancer, older women are more often diagnosed at later stages of the disease and are more likely to die from it than younger women. Although the benefit of Pap testing after age 65 has been questioned if repeated tests have been normal, a significant number of older women have not received regular screening. Thus, further screening of this age group is important and is likely to extend substantial health benefits to older women.[405]

Low income, low education, and advancing age are all associated with a decreased likelihood of receiving Pap tests....

* * *

16.15 Ensure that Pap tests meet quality standards by monitoring and certifying all cytology laboratories. (Baseline data available in 1991)

The accuracy of the Pap test is dependent on adequate collection, correct preparation and staining, and accurate interpretation. The diagnostic value of the specimen will be seriously compromised if any of these components is inadequate. Recently, there has been much coverage in the press regarding the reliability of the Pap test, especially pertaining to false negative results. A wide range of false negative results is reported in the literature, though comparison between reports is difficult because of differences in sample collection, range of lesions assessed, and methods used to calculate results.[407] Regardless of the percentage of false negatives, it is clear that the error rate of cytologic screening is substantial and that remedial actions are needed.[408]

No national systems are currently in place to ensure the quality of cytology laboratories. However, the Clinical Laboratory Improvement Amendments of 1988 propose a set of requirements that laboratories will have to meet in order to qualify for Medicare reimbursement. The legislation requires certification, accreditation, and inspection of Pap smear cytology laboratories and will regulate the number of cytology slides any individual may screen in a 24-hour period. Furthermore, laboratory reports to physicians will have to identify inadequate smears, as well as provide detailed descriptions of abnormal smears and recommendations for followup.[405] The recent promulgation of the 1988 Bethesda System for reporting cervical and vaginal cytologic diagnosis,[409] which modifies the original Papanicolaou classification, should help to reduce errors in communicating results to physicians.

While the effective implementation of the Clinical Laboratory Improvement Amendments of 1988 may reduce the false negative rate for Pap tests, this legislation also has implications for the availability and cost of services. Limiting the number of slides that can be read per day will increase the need for cytotechnologists. A perceived shortage of these professionals already exists. In addition, Medicare coverage of routine Pap tests will probably increase the demand for both screening services and cytotechnologists. This may result in increased costs as well as increased lag times between sampling and evaluation.[405]

* * *

Research Needs

High priority research needs include:

Cancer Control Science

- The behavioral and environmental determinants of cancer. For example, do socioeconomic characteristics fully determine group differences in cancer prevention and control behavior or are there ethnic, cultural, and institutional determinants?

- Effective channels and techniques for cancer prevention and control interventions. For example, effective approaches to cancer prevention and control through health care professionals, schools, mass media, public health departments, community coalitions, marketing channels, and microcomputer-telephone networks.

- The determinants of initiation of tobacco use in young consumers and development of effective interventions to prevent early initiation of tobacco use.

- The development and testing of cancer prevention and control interventions for special populations, including youth, older adults, blacks, Hispanics, Asians and Pacific Islanders, and American Indians and Alaska Natives.

- The implications of interventions for the public, professionals, industry, and society.

- Why cancer incidence and death rates differ with advancing age.

- Ways to improve access to state-of-the-art cancer care for all populations.

- Ways to reduce the differences in cancer survival and mortality between populations at lower risk of death due to cancer and those at higher risk (e.g., blacks, low-socioeconomic status populations).

- Which early detection tests are efficacious and effective for specific age and risk groups. For example, is flexible sigmoidoscopy efficacious and effective for asymptomatic populations over the age of 50?

- Cost-effective methods for the delivery of early detection services.

- New early detection technology, such as blood serum markers.

- New statistical methods to evaluate screening in control trial and uncontrolled settings.

- Ways to improve the quality of early detection and screening services.

Cancer Prevention

- The relationship between food intake, biochemical levels of nutritional compounds, and cancer incidence. For example, what are the potential roles of fiber and vitamins in dietary cancer prevention?

- The relative importance of cancer risk factors and the temporal relationships between risk factor reduction, cancer incidence, cancer survival, and cancer mortality.

- The efficacy of potential chemoprevention agents.

- Identification of foods and dietary factors that alter risks for specific cancers and elucidation of the underlying mechanisms.

- Quantification of dietary macro- and micro-constituents.

- Identification of biologic and biochemical markers of dietary exposure.

Applied Research

- Expanded and improved computerized simulation models of the determinants of temporal paths of cancer incidence, survival, and mortality.

- A reliable data base of the economic costs of cancer and cancer treatment.

- The economic determinants of the supply and efficient organization of cancer prevention and control services and the financial and insurance aspects of access to such services.

- Dissemination of research on effective channels and techniques for cancer prevention and control interventions.

- Dissemination of information about the determinants of initiation of tobacco use in young consumers and effective interventions to prevent early initiation of tobacco use.

- Dissemination of results of research on cancer prevention and control interventions for special populations, including youth, older adults, blacks, Hispanics, Asians and Pacific Islanders, and American Indians and Alaska Natives.

* * *

Baseline Data Source References

National Health Interview Survey, National Center for Health Statistics, Centers for Disease Control, Public Health Service, U.S. Department of Health and Human Services, Hyattsville, MD.

National Vital Statistics System, National Center for Health Statistics, Centers for Disease Control, Public Health Service, U.S. Department of Health and Human Services, Hyattsville, MD.

Diabetes and Chronic Disabling Conditions

17

Contents

***

17.2 Disability due to chronic conditions

***

17.4 Activity limitation due to asthma

***

17.6 Hearing impairment

17.7 Vision impairment

17.8 Mental retardation

***

17.10 Diabetes-related complications

17.11 Diabetes incidence and prevalence

17.12 Overweight

17.13 Moderate physical activity

17.14 Patient education for chronic and disabling conditions

17.15 Clinician assessment of child development

17.16 Earlier detection of hearing impairment in children

***

17.20 Service systems for children with or at risk of chronic and disabling conditions

[Research Needs]

17. Diabetes and Chronic Disabling Conditions

* * *

Health Status Objectives

Chronic Disabling Conditions

* * *

17.2 Reduce to no more than 8 percent the proportion of people who experience a limitation in major activity due to chronic conditions. (Baseline: 9.4 percent in 1988)

* * *

Note: Major activity refers to the usual activity for one's age-gender group whether it is working, keeping house, going to school, or living independently. Chronic conditions are defined as conditions that either (1) were first noticed 3 or more months ago, or (2) belong to a group of conditions such as heart disease and diabetes, which are considered chronic regardless of when they began.
Baseline data source: National Health Interview Survey, CDC.

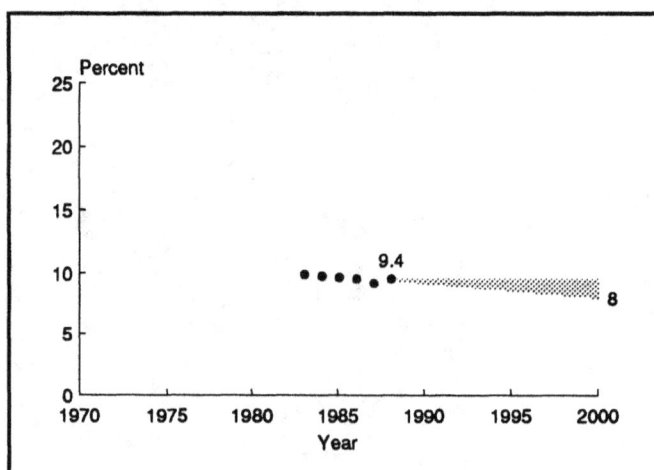

Fig. 17.2

Prevalence of limitation of major activity

Difficulty in fulfilling one's role as an employee, student, homemaker, or independent older adult is one measure of disability. In 1988, 9.4 percent of the population suffered a limitation in major activity due to chronic conditions. About 4.0 percent were unable to carry on a major activity, such as working or keeping house, and an additional 5.4 percent were limited in the amount or kind of major activity they could perform.[410]

Limitation in major activity rises sharply with advancing age. In 1988, the prevalence of disability so defined was 3.9 and 5.9 percent for people younger than age 18 and people aged 18 through 44, respectively. However, 16.9 percent of people aged 45 through 64 and 22.6 percent of people aged 65 and older suffered a limitation in major activity. The prevalence of limitation in major activity also increases markedly as family income declines. Overall, Native Americans and blacks are more likely to report limitation in major activity than whites. For blacks, the difference is largely explained by income differences.[410] Hispanics are less likely to experience limitation in major activity: 6.6 percent in 1986-88. This may be due in part to the young age distribution of the Hispanic population. Rates for older Hispanics are slightly higher than those for whites and the population overall.

The prevalence of limitation in major activity decreased steadily from 9.9 percent in 1983 to 9.2 percent in 1987, then rose to 9.4 in 1988. The target of 8 percent, if achieved, will represent a 15-percent reduction in disability between 1988 and the year 2000.

* * *

17.4 Reduce to no more than 10 percent the proportion of people with asthma who experience activity limitation. (Baseline: Average of 19.4 percent during 1986-88)

Note: Activity limitation refers to any self-reported limitation in activity attributed to asthma.
Baseline data source: National Health Interview Survey, CDC.

Asthma is a serious chronic condition that affects approximately 10 million Americans. Nearly 20 percent of people with asthma suffer some limitation in their daily activities due to their disease. In 1983-85, asthma accounted for 4.3 percent of the prevalence of activity limitation due to chronic conditions for people of all ages, and 18 percent of that experienced by people younger than age 18.[411] People with asthma experience well over 100 million days of restricted activity annually. Asthma is the leading cause of school absenteeism among children. Costs for asthma care exceed $4 billion a year.

Asthma is much more common among children than adults and is the most common chronic disorder among youth. In 1987, the prevalence of asthma among people younger than age 18 was 5.2 percent, compared with 3.9 percent among adults aged 65 and older. There is no difference in asthma prevalence by gender. The proportion of blacks with asthma is slightly higher than whites, 4.4 percent versus 4.0 percent, respectively. Increases in the prevalence of asthma have been reported for all age, race, and gender groups. Between 1979 and 1987, the percent of the population with asthma increased by about one-third.

In 1987, there were over 450,000 hospitalizations for which asthma was the first-listed diagnosis. Hospitalizations for asthma have been increasing among children. From 1979 to 1987, the hospital discharge rate with asthma as the first-listed diagnosis rose 43 percent among children younger than age 15, from 198 to 284 discharges per 100,000 population (see Objective 11.1 in *Environmental Health*).

In 1988, 4,580 people died from asthma in the United States. Between 1979 and 1986, the age-adjusted death rate from asthma increased from 0.9 per 100,000 to 1.2 per 100,000, a 33-percent increase. The greatest increase in asthma death rates has occurred among minorities and people aged 65 and older. Whereas blacks were twice as likely to die from asthma as their white counterparts in 1979, blacks were three times as likely to die from asthma as whites in 1987. For some age groups, the death rate is six times greater among blacks. Populations at particularly high risk for experiencing asthma-related morbidity and mortality include inner city and economically disadvantaged populations.

Reducing asthma-related morbidity and mortality will require more effective management of this condition by health care providers and by the people and families of people with asthma. Patient education programs can help to decrease asthma morbidity and mortality and enhance the quality of life for people with asthma (see Objective 17.14). To promote the use of optimal therapeutic and management strategies by health professionals, guidelines for the management of asthma are being formulated by the National

Asthma Education Program. These guidelines emphasize the importance of the cooperative management of asthma by health professionals and patients.

* * *

17.6 Reduce significant hearing impairment to a prevalence of no more than 82 per 1,000 people. (Baseline: Average of 88.9 per 1,000 during 1986-88)

* * *

Note: Hearing impairment covers the range of hearing deficits from mild loss in one ear to profound loss in both ears. Generally, inability to hear sounds at levels softer (less intense) than 20 decibels (dB) constitutes abnormal hearing. Significant hearing impairment is defined as having hearing thresholds for speech poorer than 25 dB. However, for this objective, self-reported hearing impairment (i.e., deafness in one or both ears or any trouble hearing in one or both ears) will be used as a proxy measure for significant hearing impairment.

Baseline data source: National Health Interview Survey, CDC.

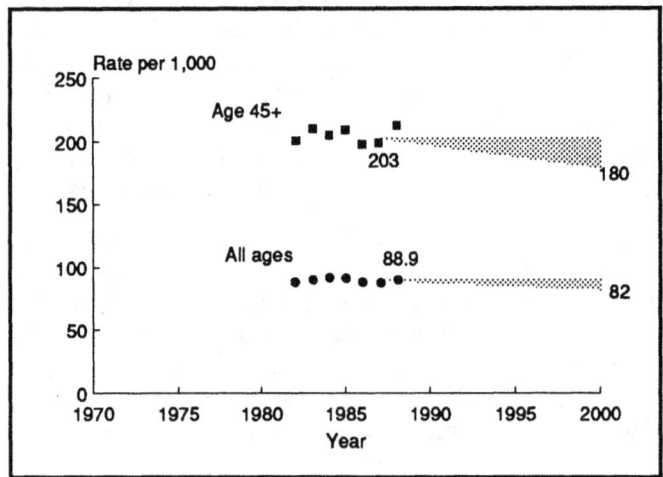

Fig. 17.6

Prevalence of hearing impairment

Disability due to hearing impairment is far reaching and can affect many aspects of life. The ramifications of auditory handicaps are seen in developmental, educational, cognitive, emotional, and social aspects of human life, and vary greatly with the type, timing, and severity of the hearing impairment, and whether or not the impairment is associated with abnormalities in any other organ system. Language delay, poor speech intelligibility, and poor understanding of spoken speech are invisible barriers that can be insurmountable for people with hearing impairments without early diagnosis and without the proper support services. Inadequate early identification, education, and vocational planning, together with indifference by the public and health care providers, limit educational and occupational opportunities for people with hearing impairment.[412,413,414] People with hearing impairment often have less desirable jobs and housing and lower incomes than those without hearing impairment.[415,416] It is estimated that the annual loss of earnings to people with hearing impairment, as a result of their disability, totals $1.25 billion[417]. . . .

Over 21 million Americans suffer some hearing impairment. In 1988, 90.8 per 1000 people had hearing impairments and 7.5 per 1,000 were deaf in both ears.[410] An estimated 1 to 2 percent of infants and children have hearing impairment. Half of these cases are congenital or acquired during infancy.[415,418,419,420] Infants at greatest risk for hearing loss include those with low birth weight, congenital infection with rubella or other infections, malformations, trauma, perinatal asphyxia, prematurity, and hospitalization in the intensive care nursery.[415,419,421,422] Fluctuating hearing loss is common among children. At any given time, about 5 to 7 percent of children have a 25 dB hearing loss, usually a self-limited complication of otitis media with middle ear effusion.[423] Recurrent otitis media may result in serious long-term complications.[424,425]

The development of hearing loss between adolescence and age 50 can have diverse causes (e.g., Meniere's disease, otosclerosis, genetic conditions, head trauma, ototoxicity), but noise-induced hearing loss accounts for the major proportion of hearing impairment among people between the ages of 35 and 65. More than 5 million Americans are at increased risk for hearing impairment due to occupational exposure to hazardous noise levels (e.g., factory, maintenance, and farm workers).[426] Even by age 18, children have been exposed to sufficient noise—lawn mowing machines, amplified music, motorcycles, snow mobiles, firecrackers, cap guns, and rifle fire in ROTC programs—to affect their high frequency hearing significantly.[428,429]

* * *

Hearing impairment due to a number of conditions can be prevented or delayed in onset. Noise-induced hearing loss is often preventable. Some congenital hearing impairments and many of those acquired during infancy are also preventable. In children, hearing loss due to chronic otitis media and diseases like meningitis can be reduced through better primary care and the use of new vaccines, such as that for Hemophilus influenza (Hib). Even age-related hearing changes may not be related to structure deterioration as much as they reflect overexposure in industrialized societies to environmental noise and other ototoxic agents.

Early detection and intervention are critical in reducing functional limitation and disability due to hearing impairment. Early detection of hearing impairment in infants is particularly important (see Objectives 17.15 and 17.16). Older adults are also likely to benefit from evaluation (see Objective 17.17). Once detected, auditory thresholds in people with hearing impairment can be improved through electro-acoustic amplification with hearing aids and frequency modulation radio devices. Communication skills can be improved with auditory and speech and language training (known as aural rehabilitation). Other assistive listening, alerting, or caption decoder devices, like closed captioned television decoders, are available for improving communicative competence.

17.7 **Reduce significant visual impairment to a prevalence of no more than 30 per 1,000 people. (Baseline: Average of 34.5 per 1,000 during 1986-88)**

* * *

Note: Significant visual impairment is generally defined as a permanent reduction in visual acuity and/or field of vision which is not correctable with eyeglasses or contact lenses. Severe visual impairment is defined as inability to read ordinary newsprint even with corrective lenses. For this objective, self-reported blindness in one or both eyes and other self-reported visual impairments (i.e., any trouble seeing with one or both eyes even when wearing glasses or colorblindness) will be used as a proxy measure for significant visual impairment.

Baseline data source: National Health Interview Survey, CDC.

Vision is the most highly developed human sense, and its loss or impairment can have devastating effects on physical, emotional, and social well-being. Particularly in a modern technological society, vision is the most important source of information for coping with the intricacies of daily life. In a world where printed words and televised images convey knowledge, where transportation systems are mechanized and complex, and where a vast number of instruments and tools are required for the performance of many complicated tasks, good vision is of primary importance. According to a 1988 Gallup survey, blindness is the disability that Americans most fear.[430] Blindness ranked fourth after AIDS, cancer, and Alzheimer's disease as "the worst disease or ailment."

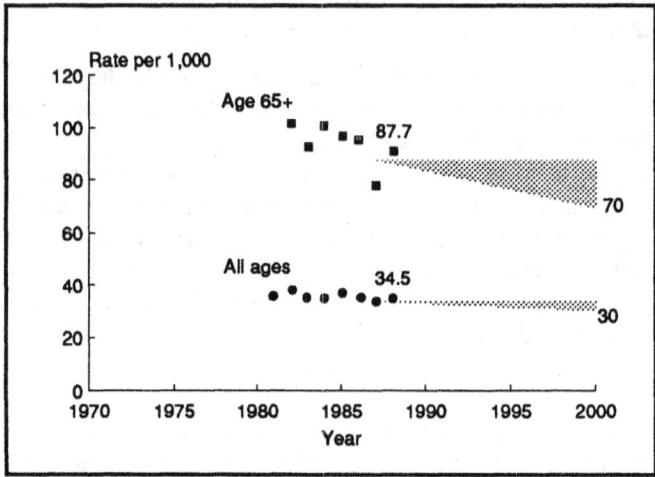

Fig. 17.7
Prevalence of visual impairment

Though seldom fatal, eye diseases and vision disorders cause suffering, disability, and loss of productivity for millions of people. In the United States, 8 to 10 million people suffer from visual impairment that cannot be corrected by eyeglasses or contact lenses.[410] Of these, 2 million people are so severely impaired that they cannot read ordinary newsprint. This includes approximately 800,000 who are legally blind, usually defined as having vision of 20/200 or less, even when wearing corrective lenses, or having a field of vision of 20 degrees or less. In addition, roughly 6 million people have low-vision, a visual acuity of 20/70 or worse, or visual field (peripheral vision) restriction that cannot be helped with standard eyeglasses or contact lenses. Added to the physical and emotional pain and hardship from visual disorders is a staggering economic burden. The National Eye Institute estimates that visual disorders and blindness cost the Nation more than $16 billion annually in direct medical care and indirect costs such as days lost from work.

In 1988, the prevalence of visual impairments was 35.7 per 1,000.[410] . . .

Diabetic retinopathy is the leading cause of new cases of blindness among people aged 20 through 44. . . . Early detection and laser photocoagulation treatment of diabetic retinopathy can prevent 60 percent of diabetes-related blindness or severe visual loss (see Objective 17.10).

Glaucoma, is a leading cause of blindness, affecting nearly 2 million Americans.[410] Of the various forms of glaucoma (e.g., congenital, open-angle, closed-angle, secondary), open-angle glaucoma is the most common (90 percent of cases) and insidious form. . . . In addition to age and race, other risk factors for glaucoma include diabetes mellitus, myopia, and a family history of glaucoma.[431,432] Early detection of glaucoma is essential to instituting treatment that will sharply reduce the risk of severe visual loss.

Cataract is an opacity in the eye's normally clear lens that interferes with vision. It is a common blinding eye condition, accounting for about 15 percent of blindness. At present, most cataract is believed to be an unavoidable and frequent accompaniment to advancing age, although there are types of cataract that may appear at any age due to diabetes or other metabolic disorders, or toxic environmental agents, such as steroids and other drugs, and radiation. . . .

An estimated 1.3 million people suffer from an eye injury each year. Approximately 1,000 per day or about 350,000 per year occur on the job. Over 100,000 of the injuries are permanently disabling. Yet, it is estimated that over 9 out of 10 injuries could have been prevented if appropriate eye safety practices and protective eyewear had been used.

In addition, 160,000 school-aged children suffer eye injuries and 100,000 product-related eye injuries occur in the home.

About 2 to 5 percent of American children suffer from amblyopia (lazy eye), anisometropia (unequal refractive error), and strabismus (ocular misalignment), and nearly 20 percent have simple refractive errors by age 16.[423,433,434,435] Amblyopia, anisometropia, and strabismus usually develop between infancy and ages 5 to 7.[423] As normal vision from birth is necessary for proper eye development, failure to treat amblyopia, anisometropia, and strabismus before school age may result in irreversible visual deficits, permanent amblyopia, loss of depth perception and binocularity, cosmetic defects, and educational and occupational restrictions.[433,435,436] Refractive errors such as myopia become common during school age. There is uncertainty whether uncorrected refractive errors cause diminished academic performance among schoolchildren.

Early detection and treatment of vision disorders in infants and young children improve the prospects for normal eye development (see Objective 17.15).... Finally, many optical devices are available to assist people with low-vision whose visual impairment cannot be corrected by glasses or contact lenses. These range from large-print books and extra-dark felt-tipped pens to magnifiers and telescopic lenses to sophisticated electronic reading systems and computer software that can enlarge print up to 60 times normal size.

17.8* **Reduce the prevalence of serious mental retardation in school-aged children to no more than 2 per 1,000 children. (Baseline: 2.7 per 1,000 children aged 10 in 1985-88)**

Note: Serious mental retardation is defined as an Intelligence Quotient (I.Q.) less than 50. This includes individuals defined by the American Association of Mental Retardation as profoundly retarded (I.Q. of 20 or less), severely retarded (I.Q. of 21-35), and moderately retarded (I.Q. of 36-50).

Baseline data source: Metropolitan Atlanta Developmental Disabilities Study, CDC.

More than 1,200,000 people in the noninstitutionalized population have mental retardation and 250,472 people with mental retardation lived in intermediate care facilities for the mentally retarded in 1986.[478] In 1983-85, the reported prevalence of mental retardation in the noninstitutionalized population was 4.7 per 1,000 people and mental retardation accounted for 2.9 percent of the activity limitation experienced.[411] Eighty-four percent of people with mental retardation had limitation in major activity, and 20 percent needed help in basic life activities.

In 1985-87, among school-aged children, the race-adjusted prevalence of mental retardation (I.Q. less than 70) was estimated to be 8.4 per 1,000 based on a study of 10-year-old children, the Metropolitan Atlanta Developmental Disabilities Study. The estimated rate of serious mental retardation (I.Q. less than 50) was 2.7 per 1,000 children.

A 25-percent reduction in the prevalence of serious mental retardation (I.Q. less than 50) among school-aged children is attainable with current technology. There are two major approaches. The first reduces the proportion of children with I.Q.s under 50 among children with disorders known to be associated with serious mental retardation. For example, the proportion of children with Down Syndrome with I.Q.s greater than 50 has increased in recent years presumably because of family-centered early intervention. Similarly, mental retardation has been prevented in children with phenylketonuria and hypothyroidism through screening and treatment programs (see Objective 14.15 in *Maternal and Infant Health*).

The second approach reduces the incidence of clinical disorders that are associated with mental retardation. There are important opportunities to reduce the incidence of the following five clinical disorders which account for more than half of serious mental retardation: fetal alcohol syndrome, fragile X syndrome, Down Syndrome, traumatic brain injury, and psychosocial disadvantage.

Mental retardation is associated with maternal use of alcohol in early pregnancy, especially heavy use. In a study of middle class pregnancies, infants born to mothers who reported using 2 or more drinks a day had, on average, a 7 point decrement in I.Q. at age 7 years.[437] Early intrauterine alcohol exposure is also associated with fetal alcohol syndrome (FAS). The prevalence of FAS is about 1.5 per 1,000 live births and about one-third of children with this disorder have mental retardation with I.Q. less than 70. Preventive interventions to reduce the prevalence of serious mental retardation associated with maternal heavy alcohol use include: (1) health education to increase awareness of the hazard of maternal alcohol use, (2) identification and treatment of alcohol abuse or addiction prior to conception or in early pregnancy, (3) early educational intervention for children with FAS, and (4) intervention by the courts to take custody of children. (See Objectives 14.4 and 14.10 in *Maternal and Infant Health* and Objective 4.19 in *Alcohol and Other Drugs*.)

The birth incidence of fragile X syndrome among males is estimated to be between 0.5 and 1 per 1,000 live births. More widespread use of diagnostic studies to identify families in which fragile X syndrome occurs can reduce this incidence.

The maternal age distribution of births is a very powerful predictor of Down Syndrome births. The birth incidence of Down Syndrome was over 2 per 1,000 live births in the 1920s and is now about 1 per 1,000. This 50-percent reduction in Down Syndrome rates occurred because the proportion of live births to women aged 35 and older decreased from over 15 percent to 5 percent during this interval. Continuation of the decreasing trend in Down Syndrome births is expected in the next decade as a result of a further reduction in the proportion of births to older women as the baby boomers born in the 1950s move beyond their childbearing years.

Infants with very low birth weight have a higher than average risk of having mental retardation. Interventions that reduce the proportion of infants with birth weights less than 1,500 grams will also contribute to the prevention of serious mental retardation (see Objective 14.5 in *Maternal and Infant Health*).

There is great potential for reducing mental retardation due to psychosocial deprivation. The intellectual enrichment provided by high quality preschool programs is thought an essential component of early educational interventions that reduce the risk of mental retardation among children born in families with psychosocial deprivation (see Objective 8.3 in *Educational and Community-Based Programs*).

Mental retardation in children due to traumatic brain injury can be reduced by measures to reduce motor vehicle, bicycle, and other injuries. The average annual incidence of traumatic brain injury is 2.3 per 1,000 children.[438] Given age-specific incidences, a child has a 40 per 1,000 risk of sustaining traumatic brain injury over the course of childhood and adolescence. Although the majority of these children do not have mental retardation, prevention of underlying injuries can help to reduce the prevalence of mental retardation (see Objectives 9.9, 9.12, 9.13, and 9.14 in *Unintentional Injuries*).

As the number of children with HIV infection grows, the virus is expected to become the leading infectious cause of mental retardation and developmental disability in children. The prevalence of central nervous system dysfunction in children with HIV infection ranges from 78 to 93 percent.[439] Neurologic effects include: global developmental delay, encephalopathy, acquired microcephaly, cognitive disorders, loss of previously achieved milestones, spasticity, motor function abnormalities, and sensory impairment.[440,441] Intervention programs for women who are intravenous drug users or the sexual partners of in-

17. Diabetes and Chronic Disabling Conditions

travenous drug users can help to slow and eventually reverse the increasing incidence of HIV infection among infants (see Objectives 18.2, 18.5, and 18.13 in *HIV Infection*).

Reducing the incidence and ultimately the prevalence of serious mental retardation will require increased education of health professionals regarding genetic and environmental contributions to birth defects and mental retardation. In order for many interventions to be effective, they must be applied prior to conception, a time at which adult medical specialists, such as family physicians and internists, are the principle care providers. Primary providers of obstetric services also need to become better informed about the importance of comprehensive preconception and prenatal risk assessment and counseling services. Couples identified to be at increased risk should be referred to genetic health care specialists (e.g., clinical/medical geneticists, clinical nurse specialists in genetics, and genetic counselors, teratogen information services or high risk obstetric services). Increased education of the public about these issues will be necessary to reduce the number of individuals exposed to avoidable hazards during pregnancies.

*This objective also appears as Objective 11.2 in *Environmental Health*.

Diabetes

* * *

17.10 **Reduce the most severe complications of diabetes as follows:**

Complications Among People With Diabetes	*1988 Baseline*	*2000 Target*
* * *		
Perinatal mortality[‡]	5%	2%
Major congenital malformations[‡]	8%	4%

* * *

[‡]*Among infants of women with established diabetes*

* * *

Baseline data sources: ... For perinatal mortality and congenital malformations, clinical series and selected States' data.

Individuals with diabetes face not only a shortened life span but also the probability of multiple acute and chronic complications, including chronic progressive renal failure, blindness, and lower extremity amputations. In 1987, diabetes accounted for approximately 10,000 new cases of end-stage renal disease (ESRD) or progressive chronic kidney failure in the United States. ...

Diabetic retinopathy is the most common eye complication of diabetes and is related to the duration and type of diabetes. An estimated 40 percent of those having Type I diabetes for less than 10 years, and 95 percent of those with the disease for more than 15 years, develop retinopathy. For those with Type II diabetes, the equivalent prevalences are 25 percent and 50 percent, respectively. ...

* * *

Women with diabetes have increased pregnancy complications and their babies are more likely to die at birth than women without diabetes. Infants born to women with diabetes have a threefold higher frequency of birth defects and a fivefold increase in other complications requiring intensive medical care in the early days of life. Whereas the rate of major congenital malformations for all women is about 2.5 percent, the rate among women with established diabetes is 8 percent. Strict glucose control before conception and throughout gestation coupled with high risk pregnancy management can be effective in reducing adverse outcomes among offspring of women with diabetes to about the level of the overall population. Therefore, reproductive-age women with established diabetes should receive prepregnancy counseling and should strive to strictly control their blood glucose prior to and after conception. Pregnant diabetic women also should be under the care of specialists and should deliver in hospitals that are equipped to take care of high-risk newborns. If 75 percent of women with established diabetes receive effective care, the rate of major congenital malformations should decrease to 4 percent.

17.11 **Reduce diabetes to an incidence of no more than 2.5 per 1,000 people and a prevalence of no more than 25 per 1,000 people. (Baselines: 2.9 per 1,000 in 1987; 28 per 1,000 in 1987)**

* * *

Baseline data sources: For total population incidence and prevalence, the National Health Interview Survey, CDC; for American Indians, Indian Health Service; for Hispanics, Hispanic Health and Nutrition Examination Survey, CDC; for blacks, National Health Interview Survey, CDC.

Approximately 7 million people in the United States have been diagnosed with diabetes, and an additional 5 million may unknowingly have the disease. Each year more than 650,000 new cases of diabetes are identified . . . .

* * *

Risk Reduction Objectives

17.12* **Reduce overweight to a prevalence of no more than 20 percent among people aged 20 and older and no more than 15 percent among adolescents aged 12 through 19. (Baseline: 26 percent for people aged 20 through 74 in 1976-80, 24 percent for men and 27 percent for women; 15 percent for adolescents aged 12 through 19 in 1976-80)**

* * *

*For commentary, see Objective 2.3 in *Nutrition*. This objective also appears as Objective 1.2 in *Physical Activity and Fitness* and as Objective 15.10 in *Heart Disease and Stroke*.

17.13* **Increase to at least 30 percent the proportion of people aged 6 and older who engage regularly, preferably daily, in light to moderate physical activity for at least 30 minutes per day. (Baseline: 22 percent of people aged 18 and older were active for at least 30 minutes 5 or more times per week and 12 percent were active 7 or more times per week in 1985)**

Note: Light to moderate physical activity requires sustained, rhythmic muscular movements, is at least equivalent to sustained walking, and is performed at less than 60 percent of maximum heart rate for age. Maximum heart rate equals roughly 220 beats per minute minus age. Examples may include walking, swimming, cycling, dancing, gardening and yardwork, various domestic and occupational activities, and games and other childhood pursuits.

Baseline data source: Behavioral Risk Factor Surveillance System, CDC.

*For commentary, see Objective 1.3 in *Physical Activity and Fitness*. This objective also appears as Objective 15.11 in *Heart Disease and Stroke*.

17. Diabetes and Chronic Disabling Conditions

Services and Protection Objectives

17.14 Increase to at least 40 percent the proportion of people with chronic and disabling conditions who receive formal patient education including information about community and self-help resources as an integral part of the management of their condition. (Baseline data available in 1991)

Type-Specific Targets

Patient Education	1983-84 Baseline	2000 Target
17.14a People with diabetes	32% (classes) 68% (counseling)	75%
17.14b People with asthma	—	50%

Baseline data source: For people with diabetes, Halpern 1989.

Patient education programs for people with diabetes, asthma, heart disease, impaired mobility and other chronic and disabling conditions can help to improve the efficiency and effectiveness of care, and reduce subsequent morbidity, and disability. To be effective, patient education should be provided in a manner that meets individual needs, fosters improved self-management, and facilitates prompt referral, followup, and coordination of care. Self-help and mutual aid groups, in particular, are an important source of information and social support for people with chronic conditions and their families.

For people with diabetes, studies have demonstrated that blood glucose levels can be reduced through combined patient and professional education.[442] Several studies have demonstrated reductions in morbidity after patient education.[443,444] At present, patient education is generally considered an integral aspect of patient management and a mainstay of patient self-care. It is so widely accepted as standard diabetes management that a rigorous study design that denies education to a control group would be unethical. Education programs should target specific complication prevention with a combined patient and professional education approach.

In asthma, patient education also plays a crucial role in alleviating morbidity and postponing mortality. Patient education programs for asthma have been found to be effective in developing self-management skills and reducing the number of asthma attacks, emergency room visits, hospitalizations, and days lost from work or school.[445] The National Asthma Education Program's asthma management guidelines emphasize the importance of active patient participation in the management of asthma. An informed patient who takes an active role in treatment is more likely to take preventive measures, take medications properly, recognize the signs of an attack, control an attack once it has begun, and have a crisis plan for emergencies.

Although national baseline data for this objective are unavailable, limited data are available for specific chronic conditions. A household survey in Michigan found that 68 percent of respondents with diabetes had received instruction or special counseling in diabetes and 32 percent had received instruction in a formal class.[440]

17.15 Increase to at least 80 percent the proportion of providers of primary care for children who routinely refer or screen infants and children for impairments of vision, hearing, speech and language, and assess other developmental milestones as part of well-child care. (Baseline data available in 1992)

Providers of primary care for children occupy a pivotal position regarding early identification of developmental problems.[447] If such problems can be identified early, children are more likely to make developmental progress.[448] Since one-third of all scheduled pediatric visits are for well-child care, the primary care setting is an ideal place for such screening to occur.[427] The major objectives of well-child care and regular developmental screening are: (1) prevention of disease, and (2) early detection and treatment of disease.

To be effective, developmental screening needs to: begin at an early age; be available to all children regardless of socioeconomic condition; and be conducted on a regular basis. Unfortunately, early and periodic screening of all children is not routinely occurring.[449] Although data are limited, fewer than 15 percent of all birth-to-5-year-old children receive regular screening for vision, hearing, language, and other developmental milestones. A national survey of 1,000 pediatricians revealed that 60 percent of birth to 5-year-old children receive no routine screening for vision even though such screening is very quick, simple, and inexpensive.[449] Another study demonstrated that primary care physicians identified less than 5 percent of children with speech and language disorders.[450] Finally, though mandated by law and paid for by Title XIX funds, only 40 percent of children eligible for Early Periodic Screening, Diagnosis, and Treatment (EPSDT) program services receive any level of screening.[451,452]

Normal vision from birth through ages 5 to 7 is necessary for proper eye development, development of the visual system, and cognitive development. About 2 to 5 percent of American children suffer from amblyopia (lazy eye), strabismus (ocular misalignment), and anisometropia (difference between the two eyes in nearsightedness, farsightedness, and astigmatism).[423,433,434,435] These visual problems, when untreated, can cause irreversible visual deficits, permanent amblyopia, loss of depth perception and binocularity, cosmetic defects, and educational and occupational restrictions.[433,435,436] Detection and treatment of strabismus and amblyopia by age 1 to 2 can increase the likelihood of developing normal or near-normal binocular vision and may improve fine motor skills.[434,435] Interventions for amblyopia and strabismus are considerably less effective if initiated after age 5, and such a delay increases the risk of irreversible amblyopia, ocular misalignment, and other visual deficits.[423,433] Clinical screening tests can detect these disorders earlier than parents or teachers as only half of children with ocular misalignment have a cosmetically noticeable defect.[434,453] Recently the U.S. Preventive Services Task Force recommended testing for amblyopia and strabismus for all children once before entering school, preferably at age 3 or 4.[45]

An estimated 1 to 2 percent of infants and children have hearing impairment. Half of these cases are congenital or acquired during infancy.[415,418,419,420] Left uncorrected, hearing impairment during infancy and early childhood may interfere with the development of speech and language skills (see Objective 17.15). Although the detrimental effect of hearing loss on language development occurs before age 3, the abnormality often is not detected until ages 2 to 6.[416,419,420,421] Therefore, screening tests have been recommended during infancy, preferably during the neonatal period, especially for high risk newborns. Most experts recommend screening infants beginning at birth. The U.S. Preventive Services Task Force recently recommended screening for hearing impairment on all high-risk neonates.[45] The American Speech-Language-Hearing Association (ASHA) recommends electrophysiologic testing between birth and 6 months of age (preferably before hospital discharge) of all infants meeting selected risk criteria.[418] A joint policy statement by ASHA, the American Academy of Otolaryngology, Head and Neck Surgery, the American Academy of Pediatrics, and the American Nurses Association is currently being developed.

Nearly 6 million children under age 18 have some form of speech or language disorder[454] and an estimated 8.5 percent of children aged 0 through 3 years have significant language delays.[455,456] Early treatment of speech and language problems can help some children improve their communication skills and avoid or reduce later language and academic problems.[454] In addition, communication disorders may be the earliest and most easily recognized symptom of other disabilities (e.g., mental retardation, cleft palate, cerebral palsy, emotional disturbances, autism, learning disabilities, attention-deficit disorders).[455,457,458,459]

In addition to screening children for impaired vision and communication disorders, routine developmental assessment of all children is an essential part of health maintenance. For children with developmental delays, the effectiveness of early intervention is well documented. Mental retardation due to psychosocial deprivation is especially amenable to intervention (see Objective 17.8). Early intervention is also effective for children with organic mental retardation, including Down syndrome, and has been shown to increase cognitive, social, and communication skills. Young children with cerebral palsy, hearing and visual impairment, and emotional disturbances also benefit from early training and habilitation.

17.16 Reduce the average age at which children with significant hearing impairment are identified to no more than 12 months. (Baseline: Estimated as 24 to 30 months in 1988)

Baseline data source: Commission on Education of the Deaf.

The future of a child born with a significant hearing impairment depends to a very large degree on early identification (i.e., audiological diagnosis before 12 months of age) followed by immediate and appropriate intervention. If hearing impaired children are not identified early, it is difficult, if not impossible, for many of them to acquire the fundamental language, social, and cognitive skills that provide the foundation for later schooling and success in society.[417,420,460,461] When early identification and intervention occurs, hearing impaired children make dramatic progress, are more successful in school, and become more productive members of society. The earlier intervention and habilitation begins, the more dramatic the benefits.[462,463]

Unfortunately, the average age at which children with significant hearing impairment (i.e., moderate to profound bilateral hearing loss) are identified in the United States is somewhere between 24 and 30 months of age.[464,465,466,467,468,469,470] This contrasts sharply with other countries such as Israel and Great Britain where the average age of identification is 7 months of age.[464] Factors which contribute to failure to identify children earlier in the United States include lack of parental awareness of the indicators of hearing loss in very young children, the "wait-and-see" attitude exhibited by many physicians when parents express concern about possible hearing impairments,[466] and the fact that only a handful of States have implemented screening programs for high-risk children.[471,472] Existing knowledge and technology provide the tools to address these obstacles and thereby reduce the average age at which hearing impaired children are identified.

* * *

17.20 Increase to 50 the number of States that have service systems for children with or at risk of chronic and disabling conditions, as required by Public Law 101-239. (Baseline data available in 1991)

Note: Children with or at risk of chronic and disabling conditions, often referred to as children with special health care needs, include children with psychosocial as well as physical problems. This population encompasses children with a wide variety of actual or potential disabling conditions, including children with or at risk for cerebral palsy, mental retardation, sensory deprivation, developmental disabilities, spina bifida, hemophilia, other genetic disorders, and health-related educational and behavioral problems. Service systems for such children are organized networks of comprehensive, community-based, coordinated, and family-centered services.

The establishment of systems of services that reflect the principles of comprehensive, community-based, coordinated, family-centered care are essential for effectively fostering and facilitating activities to: (1) avoid the initial occurrence of chronic and disabling conditions among children, (2) reverse or slow the progress of chronic and disabling conditions among children, and (3) minimize the complications and impact of chronic disabling conditions among children.[473,474] The establishment of these service systems is also essential to strengthen the ability of families to care for and cope with children with actual or potential chronic and disabling conditions, and enables children with more serious conditions to be placed in home and community-based living arrangements rather than in institutional living arrangements.[475]

Children with potential or actual chronic and disabling conditions and their families often require a range of different types of services.[476] Health activities and services, for example, are one necessary component, and should include: (1) health education and health promotion activities for children and their families, (2) preventive and primary care that includes routine screening for impairments of vision, hearing, speech and language, and assessment of physical and psychosocial milestones, (3) specialized diagnostic and therapeutic services, and (4) habilitation and rehabilitation services. Early intervention services are another necessary component as are educational, vocational, and mental health services for children, and support for their families.

Service systems should, to the extent possible, provide services in or near the home communities of these children. Community-based services enhance the ability of families to care for children at home, thereby promoting a normal pattern of living.

Service systems should provide coordination to overcome gaps and duplications in services.[477] Multiple services from different providers affiliated with different agencies, institutions, and organizations should be delivered in a complementary and consistent manner, in a timely fashion, and in proper sequences. The current fragmentation makes it difficult for children and families to obtain needed services.

Service systems should be family-centered in order to support and assist families in their natural and pivotal role as primary caretakers by involving families and professionals as partners in the care of children. Family-centered services recognize the importance of the family in the child's life and the fact that the family is constant in the child's life, whereas those providing health and other services are transitory.

Finally, service systems should include a continuum of services, starting with services for pregnant women and adolescents aimed at improving pregnancy outcomes and reducing the number of children with or at risk for chronic and disabling conditions. Strong linkages should be created between these systems and maternal health programs and services. Particular attention should be focused on programs and services for pregnant women and adolescents at high risk for physical or psychosocial problems. Models exist for providing effective preventive intervention and support services for this population.

The concept of service systems is reflected in recent Federal legislation. The Title V Maternal and Child Health Services Block Grant legislation of 1989 mandates State Programs for Children with Special Health Care Needs to promote the building of such service systems, and part H of the Education of the Handicapped Act (P.L. 99-457) establishes a discretionary program to build statewide systems for comprehensive, community-based, coordinated, family-centered services for infants and toddlers with, or at risk of, chronic and disabling conditions.

* * *

Research Needs

Disabilities

- The epidemiology of disabilities—the distribution of disabilities within the population, especially groups with disproportionately high or low prevalence, and risk factors for limitations in human activity (e.g., disability).
- Expanded basic biomedical and social science research into causes, and methods of intervention, of disabilities.
- Research on assistive technology.
- The role that Independent Living Centers, parent support groups, and other advocacy groups can play in the prevention of secondary conditions in people with existing disabilities.

Genetic Services

- Consensus standards to assure the quality of genetic services that will be made available as the number of chromosomal, biochemical, and molecular markers for genetic disorders increases.
- Thorough consideration of the ethical issues presented by the increasing availability of screening tools for genetic conditions.

Diabetes

- Basic and clinical research to better understand the etiology and pathogenesis of diabetes and its complications.
- Research to develop optimal capabilities for the diagnosis, treatment, cure, and prevention of diabetes and its complications.

Vision

* * *

- Research to improve the prevention, diagnosis, and treatment of retinal diseases, corneal disease, glaucoma, strabismus, and amblyopia.
- Research to develop new low vision devices to improve the vision of those visually impaired.

Hearing

* * *

- Research to speed the development of "voice in: text-out" and other computer technology as well as alternative assistive devices such as those for tactile recognition of speech.
- Research on wearable, signal processing and/or implantable devices for people with hearing impairments, including devices for those whom the most sophisticated amplification devices are not currently effective.

* * *

Healthy Children 2000

Related Objectives From Other Priority Areas

* * *

Baseline Data Source References

Behavioral Risk Factor Surveillance System, Centers for Disease Control, Public Health Service, U.S. Department of Health and Human Services, Atlanta, GA.

Halpern, M. The Impact of Diabetes Education in Michigan. *Diabetes* 38(2):151A, 1989.

Metropolitan Atlanta Developmental Disabilities Study, Center for Environmental Health and Injury Control, Centers for Disease Control, Public Health Service, U.S. Department of Health and Human Services, Atlanta, GA.

National Health Interview Survey, National Center for Health Statistics, Centers for Disease Control, Public Health Service, U.S. Department of Health and Human Services, Hyattsville, MD.

HIV Infection

Contents

18

18.1	AIDS
18.2	HIV infection
18.3	Adolescent postponent of sexual intercourse
18.4	Condom use
18.5	IV-drug abusers in treatment
18.6	IV-drug abusers using uncontaminated drug paraphernalia
18.7	Transfusion-transmitted HIV infection

* * *

18.9	Clinician counseling to prevent HIV and other sexually transmitted diseases
18.10	HIV education in schools
18.11	HIV education in colleges and universities

* * *

18.13	Clinic services for HIV and other sexually transmitted diseases

* * *

	[Research Needs]

18. HIV Infection

***

Health Status Objectives

18.1 Confine annual incidence of diagnosed AIDS cases to no more than 98,000 cases. (Baseline: An estimated 44,000 to 50,000 diagnosed cases in 1989)

Special Population Targets

Diagnosed AIDS Cases	1989 Baseline	2000 Target
***		
18.1b Blacks	14,000-15,000	37,000
18.1c Hispanics	7,000-8,000	18,000

Note: *Targets for this objective are equal to upper bound estimates of the incidence of diagnosed AIDS cases projected for 1993.*
Baseline data source: Center for Infectious Diseases, CDC.

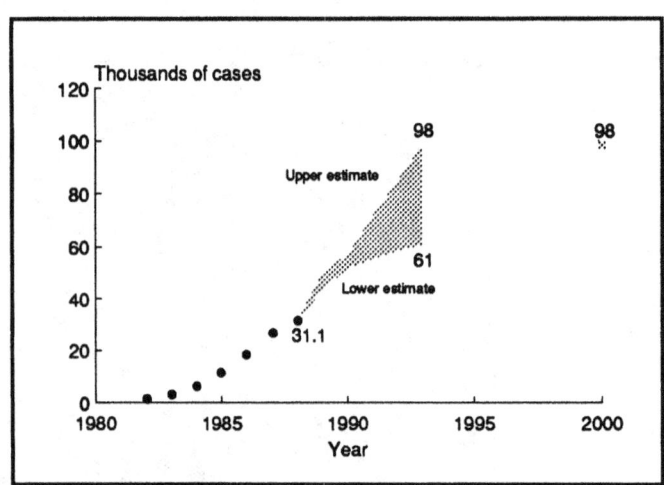

Fig. 18.1

Incidence of AIDS cases

The most important measure of progress in controlling the AIDS epidemic is the annual incidence of HIV infection. However, measuring reductions in the incidence of HIV infection would require that the same population be tested in a base period and tested again some time later to measure change. In comparison, the incidence of diagnosed AIDS cases is readily available and easy to track over time. AIDS diagnosis must be reported in all 50 States, the District of Columbia, and the U.S. Territories. A uniform case definition and case report form are used in each of these jurisdictions to report AIDS diagnosis.

Since the progression of HIV infection to AIDS is as high as 50 percent among untreated HIV-infected adults monitored for 10 years, the incidence of AIDS cases is a meaningful proxy for measuring progress in reducing the incidence of HIV infection. Various factors (e.g., age, duration of infection) that influence progression of the disease from asymptomatic HIV infection to AIDS have been recognized but require further study.

Continued progress in drug development and improvements in therapies to control the expression of HIV infection will improve ability to postpone illnesses associated with the development of AIDS. As a result, the number of HIV-infected people seeking chemoprophylaxis will grow during this decade. If chemoprophylaxis is successful, fewer people with HIV will develop AIDS; such progress will necessarily distort the measure used by this objective (incidence of AIDS cases).

The existence of medical interventions that can postpone onset of AIDS may encourage people whose behaviors put them at risk for HIV infection to seek HIV testing, creating new public health opportunities for counseling to prevent further spread and for partner notification. Currently, many people infected with HIV do not know they are infected and do not receive the counseling they need to avoid infecting others.

Although the year of peak annual incidence of AIDS cannot be predicted, prevention activities, including counseling to prevent further transmission and medical interventions to slow progression of HIV infection to AIDS, begun in the 1980s should show results in the 1990s. This objective sets as its target holding AIDS incidence to no more than the 1993 level. Achieving this target will require the concerted efforts of primary and secondary school teachers, health care providers, Federal, State, and local governments, community groups, youth-serving agencies, employers, and colleges and universities. Each has an important role to play in preventing further transmission of HIV.

18.2 Confine the prevalence of HIV infection to no more than 800 per 100,000 people. (Baseline: An estimated 400 per 100,000 in 1989)

Special Population Targets

Estimated Prevalence of HIV Infection (per 100,000)	1989 Baseline	2000 Target
* * *		
18.2b Intravenous drug abusers	30,000-40,000‡	40,000
18.2c Women giving birth to live-born infants	150	100
* * *		

‡*Per 100,000 intravenous drug abusers aged 15 through 24 in the New York city vicinity; in areas other than major metropolitan centers, infection rates in people entering selected drug treatment programs tested in unlinked surveys are often under 500 per 100,000*

Baseline data source: Center for Infectious Diseases, CDC.

Meaningful objectives to measure a change in the prevalence of HIV infection are challenging to formulate. Prevalence—the number of people with infections in a given population at a particular time—is usually expressed as a rate, such as percentage of the population infected or the number of infected people per 1,000 or 100,000 people in the population. Prevalence estimates require two pieces of information: the number of infected people and the total number of people within a given population. The true prevalence of HIV infection is difficult to estimate because it is hard to test an unbiased sample and the total size of the population group is rarely known. In addition, not only are newly infected people free of symptoms, the possibility of discrimination discourages people from participating in prevalence studies.

The Public Health Service has been able to document the magnitude of the HIV epidemic through examination of data on the prevalence of HIV infection among certain populations, using many separate surveys of childbearing women, young (aged 15 through 24) homosexual men visiting sexually transmitted disease (STD) clinics, and young (aged 15 through 24) intravenous drug abusers using drug abuse treatment facilities. These measures provide a rough indication of the prevalence of HIV infection; over time, they can describe trends among sentinel populations.

A useful proxy for measuring and tracking HIV prevalence is its prevalence among people whose behavior puts them at risk for infection. One such group is homosexual men who seek services at sexually transmitted disease clinics. Blood samples taken and analyzed in these clinics suggest that a substantial decline in the incidence of new infections in homosexual men has occurred. Recent data from the large San Francisco cohort showed almost no new infections in 1987. Considerable evidence points to reduced high-risk sexual behavior among white homosexual men, although data show some relapse to high-risk behavior in this group and continued risk-taking behavior among gay youth.[479]

Insight into the prevalence of HIV infection also may be gained through blood sampling in drug abuse treatment (mainly methadone maintenance) centers.[480] Prevalence rates as high as 7 percent of drug abusers sampled were found in one group in New York City in 1987.[481]

HIV infection among illicit drug abusers is likely to continue to increase because of continuing exchange of sex for drugs.[482] Effective programs may include comprehensive drug abuse treatment and outreach that includes information, education, and counseling to encourage entrance into drug abuse treatment programs, use of clean needles, testing for HIV infection, and the prevention of unwanted pregnancies. Programs should also target minority adult and adolescent women who are drug abusers or the sexual partners of drug abusers.

Newborn infants throughout the country are routinely screened for treatable metabolic disorders by blood samples collected shortly after birth. These samples can also be tested for the presence of HIV antibody that has been passively transferred from the mother, indicating that the mother is infected with HIV. It should be emphasized that HIV among women giving birth, not among their infants, is measured by this technique. Although reliable data on the prevalence of HIV among newborns is unavailable, an estimated 20 to 40 percent of the infants of infected mothers develop HIV infection.[483]

Most (70 percent) children with perinatally transmitted HIV come from families in which one or both parents are intravenous drug abusers. Data describing HIV infection among women giving birth to live infants (only live-born infants receive blood tests necessary to track this objective) can be used to target resources and assess the effectiveness of steps taken to prevent transmission of HIV to women of childbearing age and passively to their children. Perinatal transmission of HIV can be reduced by minimizing or eliminating risk of infection in young adults (especially women of childbearing age) and through programs that reduce drug abuse and unprotected sex among drug abusers and their partners.

Seroprevalence surveys have also been conducted on several college campuses. To avoid self-selection bias, seroprevalence was assessed through blind testing of blood specimens drawn for other purposes at college clinics. Preliminary results show only that there is HIV infection on college campuses (with a rate of approximately 200 per 100,000) and confirm that AIDS education and prevention should be targeted to this population.[484]

In the absence of national estimates of the prevalence and incidence of HIV infection based on probability samples, data from STD clinics, drug abuse treatment centers, and *ad hoc* surveys of at-risk populations will remain useful for targeting prevention resources and assessing the efficacy of prevention programs.

Risk Reduction Objectives

18.3* Reduce the proportion of adolescents who have engaged in sexual intercourse to no more than 15 percent by age 15 and no more than 40 percent by age 17. (Baseline: 27 percent of girls and 33 percent of boys by age 15; 50 percent of girls and 66 percent of boys by age 17; reported in 1988)

Baseline data sources: National Survey of Family Growth, CDC; National Survey of Adolescent Males.

*For commentary, see Objective 5.4 in *Family Planning*. This objective also appears as Objective 19.9 in *Sexually Transmitted Diseases*.

18.4* Increase to at least 50 percent the proportion of sexually active, unmarried people who used a condom at last sexual intercourse. (Baseline: 19 percent of sexually active, unmarried women aged 15 through 44 reported that their partners used a condom at last sexual intercourse in 1988)

Special Population Targets

Use of Condoms	1988 Baseline	2000 Target
18.4a Sexually active young women aged 15-19 (by their partners)	26%	60%
18.4b Sexually active young men aged 15-19	57%	75%
18.4c Intravenous drug abusers	—	60%

Note: Strategies to achieve this objective must be undertaken sensitively to avoid indirectly encouraging or condoning sexual activity among teens who are not yet sexually active.

Baseline data sources: National Survey of Family Growth, CDC; National Survey of Adolescent Males.

Abstinence from sexual intercourse, monogamous sexual relations with an uninfected partner, and avoidance of intravenous drug use are the most effective means of preventing HIV infection. Proper use of condoms, reducing the number of sexual partners, and abstinence from drug abuse decrease, but do not eliminate risk of HIV infection. Even with the proper use of condoms, high risk sexual behaviors, e.g., anal intercourse, should be avoided.

Although there is no absolute guarantee that using a condom will prevent people from getting sexually transmitted diseases, including HIV, risk can be greatly reduced if condoms are used properly. Failure of condoms to prevent the transmission of disease is more often caused by improper use than by product failure in the United States,[485] where condoms must adhere to quality control standards set by the Food and Drug Administration.

To be most effective in reducing the spread of HIV, condoms and instructions for their proper use should be made more widely available through health care providers who offer services to sexually active men and women, particularly in sexually transmitted disease clinics, family planning clinics, and drug abuse treatment centers. Counselors at these facilities should become more confident in counseling patients on infection prevention and should emphasize age-appropriate assertiveness skills. Instructions in correct condom use can be obtained from *Condoms and Sexually Transmitted Diseases . . . Especially AIDS*[486] or the National AIDS Hotline, 1-800-342-AIDS. More research is also needed to better understand why some people do not use condoms so that specific steps can be taken to increase their use.

At present, no national surveys accurately measure condom use for disease prevention among the total population. Existing studies are not sufficiently detailed to describe either the proportion of people who engage in high-risk behaviors and use condoms, or the proportion of high-risk sexual encounters in which condoms are being used. This objective uses the behavior of sexually active unmarried women as a proxy measure for the behavior of people who engage in high-risk sexual activity. Women aged 15 through 44 and adolescent males aged 15 through 19 are the only age groups for whom national data are gathered on condom use. For women aged 15 through 44, the data are limited to condom use for pregnancy prevention, not disease prevention.

*For additional commentary, see Objective 19.10 in *Sexually Transmitted Diseases*.

18.5 **Increase to at least 50 percent the estimated proportion of all intravenous drug abusers who are in drug abuse treatment programs. (Baseline: An estimated 11 percent of opiate abusers were in treatment in 1989)**

Baseline data source: National Institute on Drug Abuse, ADAMHA.

To prevent spread of HIV infection among intravenous drug abusers and their sexual partners, it is necessary to help drug abusers stop using illicit drugs. Comprehensive drug abuse treatment programs and risk reduction programs include information, education, and counseling to reduce risk, encourage testing, and prevent unintended pregnancies. Programs should target minority adults and adolescent women who are intravenous or nonintravenous drug abusers or the sexual partners of drug abusers. Because many drug abusers will not respond to treatment by stopping all drug use, the focus must also be on drug abuse prevention and abstinence from sharing drug paraphernalia.

Many children with perinatally transmitted AIDS come from families where one or both parents are intravenous drug abusers. Pediatric HIV infection is occurring disproportionately among blacks and Hispanics; 52 percent of pediatric AIDS patients are black, 25 percent are Hispanic.[487]

18.6 **Increase to at least 50 percent the estimated proportion of intravenous drug abusers not in treatment who use only uncontaminated drug paraphernalia ("works"). (Baseline: 25 to 35 percent of opiate abusers in 1989)**

Baseline data source: National Institute on Drug Abuse, ADAMHA.

As noted above, to prevent spread of HIV infection among intravenous drug abusers and their sexual partners, it is necessary to help drug abusers stop using illicit drugs. For those who cannot break their addiction, efforts are needed to reduce risk without condoning drug abuse. Some programs for drug abusers have succeeded in altering needle-sharing behavior and increasing the use of bleach to disinfect works.[481,488] These successes have been tempered, however, by numerous frustrations and barriers. For example, researchers have reported that even when drug abusers adopt safer drug use practices, they do not necessarily change high-risk sexual behavior. Therefore, public health approaches must include persistent efforts to counsel drug abusers about both high-risk drug use practices and high-risk sexual activities. Special efforts may be necessary to reach people who abuse illegal stimulants and depressants, as well as steroid abusers who share injection equipment.

18.7 **Reduce to no more than 1 per 250,000 units of blood and blood components the risk of transfusion-transmitted HIV infection. (Baseline: 1 per 40,000 to 150,000 units in 1989)**

Baseline data source: Center for Biologic Evaluation and Research, FDA.

18. HIV Infection

Efforts to prevent transfusion-associated HIV infection date from 1983, when voluntary self-exclusion of potential donors with high-risk behaviors was introduced. By mid-1985, tests to detect HIV antibodies were introduced nationwide by blood-collecting agencies. These advances have resulted in a blood supply that is among the safest in the world.

There are, however, recognized deficiencies in the ability of blood and plasma collecting facilities to educate donors about their own risk behaviors and to gain cooperation with voluntary self-deferral. Improvements in testing depend on scientific efforts to better define the time period between infection with HIV and the presence of antibodies and to narrow the interval between infection and detection of an indicator of infection. Thorough evaluation of the effectiveness of testing programs intended to reduce the chances of HIV infection are needed.

Other options for reducing transfusion-transmitted diseases include several alternatives to donor transfusion such as preoperative autologous blood donation, hemodilution, perioperative blood salvage, and use of pharmacologic agents, recombinant hematopoietic growth factors, recombinant coagulation factors, and red cell substitutes. These alternatives, if used effectively, would also help conserve the nation's blood supply. Physician education—for residents, medical students, surgeons, anesthesiologists, obstetricians, gynecologists, medical directors of blood centers, and members of hospital transfusion committees—is an integral part of promoting appropriate use of transfusion and transfusion alternatives.

The adequacy of the blood supply is also an important issue. The number of blood screening tests performed has risen in recent years, resulting not only in a greater measure of safety from transfusion-transmitted diseases, but also an increased number of deferred donors. Seasonal and geographic shortages continue to plague the blood supply. An estimated 4 to 6 percent of people have donated blood within the previous year, although more than half of the population has ever donated.[489] If a greater percentage of the population were current donors (donated within the previous year), and if more donors would give more frequently (more than once each year), the blood supply would be improved.

Services and Protection Objectives

* * *

18.9* Increase to at least 75 percent the proportion of primary care and mental health care providers who provide age-appropriate counseling on the prevention of HIV and other sexually transmitted diseases. (Baseline: 10 percent of physicians reported that they regularly assessed the sexual behaviors of their patients in 1987)

Special Population Target

Counseling on HIV and STD Prevention	1987 Baseline	2000 Target
18.9a Providers practicing in high incidence areas	—	90%

Note: Primary care providers include physicians, nurses, nurse practitioners, and physician assistants. Areas of high AIDS and sexually transmitted disease incidence are cities and States with incidence rates of AIDS cases, HIV seroprevalence, gonorrhea, or syphilis that are at least 25 percent above the national average.

Baseline data source: Lewis and Freeman 1987.

The primary purposes of counseling are to prevent further spread of HIV infection and, where possible, to slow progression of HIV to AIDS. HIV counseling can be used to (1) help uninfected individuals initiate and sustain behavioral changes that reduce their risk of infection, (2) help infected individuals adopt safe behaviors to avoid infecting others, (3) help spouses and sexual partners of infected people adopt safe behaviors, and (4) help infected people take better care of themselves.[489]

The U.S. Preventive Services Task Force[45] recommends that clinicians take a complete sexual and drug use history on all adolescent and adult patients. Sexually active patients should be advised that abstaining from sex or maintaining a mutually faithful monogamous relationship with a partner known to be uninfected with HIV or other sexually transmitted diseases are the most effective strategies for avoiding infection. Patients should also receive counseling about the indications and proper methods for using condoms and spermicides in sexual intercourse. Intravenous drug abusers should be encouraged to enroll in a drug abuse treatment program and warned against sharing drug injection equipment or using unsterilized needles and syringes.

This objective is particularly challenging. Available baseline data indicate that despite heavy media and national focus on HIV and AIDS, primary care providers are not, in general, taking a complete sexual and drug use history of their patients. Strong efforts should be made to modify primary care provider behavior, focusing programs on convincing providers that their efforts are often the key to modifying the risk behavior of their patients. The special population target is intended to focus particular attention on primary care providers in cities and States that have especially high rates of HIV infection and sexually transmitted diseases.

*This objective also appears as Objective 19.14 in *Sexually Transmitted Diseases*.

18.10 **Increase to at least 95 percent the proportion of schools that have age-appropriate HIV education curricula for students in 4th through 12th grade, preferably as part of quality school health education. (Baseline: 66 percent of school districts required HIV education but only 5 percent required HIV education in each year for 7th through 12th grade in 1989)**

Note: Strategies to achieve this objective must be undertaken sensitively to avoid indirectly encouraging or condoning sexual activity among teens who are not yet sexually active.
Baseline data source: General Accounting Office.

AIDS information and education programs have increased public knowledge and influenced attitudes about HIV and AIDS. However, some misinformation still persists at all levels of society. The first step toward reducing high-risk behaviors is for people to be able to use information about how HIV is transmitted to assess their own risk of becoming infected. Only when people know that they are at risk will they change their behavior.

Although intensive education has reduced high-risk sexual and drug abuse behaviors among some people, there is an urgent need to continue this trend and to ensure that low-risk behaviors are sustained. The public is generally aware of the linkage between intravenous drug abuse and HIV infection and of the risk for the spread of HIV infection from intravenous drug abusers to their sexual partners and children. Less well known is the risk of HIV infection among crack cocaine abusers, caused in part by the practice of exchanging sex for crack cocaine.

It is important to maintain and expand awareness for several reasons. First, educating children in school is a means of reaching the family members and sexual partners of intravenous drug abusers and crack cocaine abusers who are often difficult to contact through more focused outreach. Second, sexually active people should consider the possible drug-using practices of their current and potential sexual partners.

As of January 1990, only 29 States had policies regarding HIV/AIDS education; most of those States favored beginning such education before children reach the age of puberty, usually by 6th grade.[45] Ideally, HIV education would reach children before they develop patterns of high-risk sexual activity and drug abuse. School- and college- age youth, especially those in areas of high HIV incidence, should be a primary target of prevention education. To be effective, such training must be direct and unambiguous. In addition to information about transmission, HIV curricula should include training in the social and personal skills students need to resist peer pressure to participate in unhealthy sexual activity and drug abuse. For example, an effective curriculum might include the components recommended in the Centers for Disease Control's *Guidelines for Effective School Health Education to Prevent the Spread of AIDS*.[490] Special efforts will be needed to reach students who have special education needs. Optimally, HIV education should be provided as part of quality school health education. For a definition of quality school health education, see *Educational and Community-Based Programs*.

18.11 Provide HIV education for students and staff in at least 90 percent of colleges and universities. (Baseline data available in 1995)

High rates of sexually transmitted disease among students using college and university student health centers suggest that students are not practicing safe sex. For example, 40 percent of women seeking pregnancy tests at the University of Maryland student health center in 1987 tested positive for a sexually transmitted disease other than HIV.[484]

In a campus environment, many students encounter new independence, self-determination, and strong peer pressure to adopt certain behaviors. Experimentation with sex, alcohol, and drug use puts these students at risk for HIV infection. Further, students may underestimate their risk of acquiring HIV infection. Risk is heightened by beliefs by young adults that they are invincible and impervious to infection.

Colleges and universities can help prevent the spread of HIV infection by assuring that their students and staff are educated about how HIV is and is not transmitted, how to prevent transmission, and how to assess their own risk of infection accurately. In a campus community, students and faculty interact in many ways, allowing a well informed staff many opportunities to educate their students about HIV infection.

* * *

18.13* Increase to at least 50 percent the proportion of family planning clinics, maternal and child health clinics, sexually transmitted disease clinics, tuberculosis clinics, drug treatment centers, and primary care clinics that screen, diagnose, treat, counsel, and provide (or refer for) partner notification services for HIV infection and bacterial sexually transmitted diseases (gonorrhea, syphilis, and chlamydia). (Baseline: 40 percent of family planning clinics for bacterial sexually transmitted diseases in 1989)

Baseline data source: State Family Planning Directors.

People with tuberculosis have higher rates of HIV infection; rates are also higher among people with sexually transmitted diseases such as gonorrhea, syphilis, and lymphogranuloma venereum than among people who do not have these conditions. In addition, neuropsychological symptoms are common among people with HIV infection. Clinics and facilities that treat HIV-correlated diseases have a unique opportunity to reach some populations who are at the highest risk for HIV infection, notably intravenous drug abusers and the partners of intravenous drug abusers. In addition, public health clinics and community health centers are the major health care access points for low-income women of childbearing age who may also be at high risk for HIV infection. All women of childbearing age with known high-risk behaviors should be routinely counseled and tested for HIV antibodies and be given contraceptive counseling as appropriate. Many groups who are at high risk are often unaware of the risk behaviors of their partners and frequently will not admit, or will underestimate, their own high-risk behaviors. Particular emphasis should be placed on training people to accurately assess their own risk of contracting HIV infection and transmitting the disease to others.

*For additional commentary, see Objective 19.11 in *Sexually Transmitted Diseases*. This objective also appears as Objective 5.11 in *Family Planning*.

* * *

Research Needs

In addition to the priorities of discovering a cure for AIDS and a vaccine against HIV infection, research is also needed on the social and behavioral aspects of sexual and drug use practices, especially as they differ among cultures in the United States, so that high-risk behaviors and related factors can be better understood. Such research is essential for developing effective methods for promoting safer sexual practices and abstinence from drug abuse. The most pressing needs include research on the following:

- The epidemiology of nonopiate drug abusers, both those who are intravenous polydrug or cocaine abusers and those whose use of nonintravenous drugs increases their risk for HIV infection (i.e., those exchanging sex for drugs).

- The factors leading to higher HIV prevalence among blacks and Hispanics than among whites.

- Effective means of modifying high-risk behaviors.

* * *

Baseline Data Source References

AIDS Surveillance System, Center for Infectious Diseases, Centers for Disease Control, Public Health Service, U.S. Department of Health and Human Services, Atlanta, GA.

American College Health Association Task Force on AIDS, American College Health Association, Alexandria, VA.

Food and Drug Administration, Public Health Service, U.S. Department of Health and Human Services, Rockville, MD.

General Accounting Office. *AIDS Education: Public School Programs Require More Student Information and Teacher Training*. Washington, DC: the Office, 1990.

Lewis, C.F., and Freeman, H.E. The sexual history taking and counseling practices of California primary care physicians. *Western Journal of Medicine* 147:165-167, 1987.

National AIDS Program Office, Public Health Service, U.S. Department of Health and Human Services, Washington, DC.

National Institute on Drug Abuse, Alcohol, Drug Abuse, and Mental Health Administration, Public Health Service, U.S. Department of Health and Human Services, Rockville, MD.

National Survey of Family Growth, National Center for Health Statistics, Centers for Disease Control, Public Health Service, U.S. Department of Health and Human Services, Hyattsville, MD.

Sexually Transmitted Diseases

Contents

19.1	Gonorrhea
19.2	Chlamydia
19.3	Syphilis
19.4	Congenital syphilis
19.5	Genital herpes and genital warts
19.6	Pelvic inflammatory disease
19.7	Hepatitis B
19.8	Repeat gonorrhea infection
19.9	Adolescent postponent of sexual intercourse
19.10	Condom use
19.11	Clinic services for HIV and other sexually transmitted diseases
19.12	Sexually transmitted disease education in schools
19.13	Correct management of sexually transmitted disease cases
19.14	Clinician counseling to prevent sexually transmitted diseases
19.15	Partner notification of exposure to sexually transmitted disease
	[Research Needs]

19

19. Sexually Transmitted Diseases

* * *

Health Status Objectives

19.1 Reduce gonorrhea to an incidence of no more than 225 cases per 100,000 people. (Baseline: 300 per 100,000 in 1989)

Special Population Targets

Gonorrhea Incidence (per 100,000)	1989 Baseline	2000 Target
19.1a Blacks	1,990	1,300
19.1b Adolescents aged 15-19	1,123	750
19.1c Women aged 15-44	501	290

Baseline data source: Gonorrhea Surveillance System, CDC.

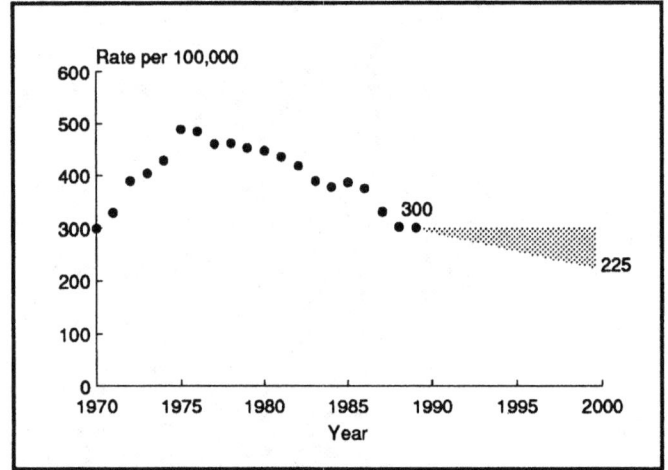

Fig. 19.1

Incidence of gonorrhea

Gonorrhea control efforts began in 1972 and have had remarkable success. Since 1981, cases of gonorrhea in males have fallen 29 percent and 24 percent in females. However, gonorrhea has not declined among racial and ethnic minorities and among teenagers. The benefit-cost ratio of gonorrhea screening and outreach efforts is estimated to be more than 2:1.[491] A major barrier to further gonorrhea reduction is the expected increase in antibiotic-resistant strains. The proportion of all gonorrhea organisms that are antibiotic-resistant grew from 0.8 percent in 1985 to 7.0 percent in 1989.[492]

Since gonorrhea continues to be the most frequently reported communicable disease in the United States, it is used as the key indicator of progress in reducing sexually transmitted diseases among populations that suffer from the highest disease rates. In the planning and implementation of sexually transmitted disease control programs, special emphasis should be given to the high-risk groups specifically targeted in the gonorrhea objective, namely, blacks, adolescents, and all women of childbearing age. No special population target has been included for Hispanics, since current gonorrhea rates are lower among Hispanics than among the total population (114 cases per 100,000 in 1989).

19.2 Reduce *Chlamydia trachomatis* infections, as measured by a decrease in the incidence of nongonococcal urethritis to no more than 170 cases per 100,000 people. (Baseline: 215 per 100,000 in 1988)

Baseline data source: National Disease and Therapeutic Index, CDC.

Chlamydia is the most common sexually transmitted bacterial pathogen in the United States, causing an estimated 4 million acute infections annually. Women and children bear an inordinate share of the burden of chlamydia infection, particularly in terms of its sequelae (acute PID, infant conjunctivitis, and infant pneumonia). Many people with uncomplicated chlamydia infection have no symptoms or signs of infection. Although chlamydia can be successfully treated with relatively inexpensive therapy, efforts to identify infected persons without symptoms have been hindered by the absence of inexpensive, widely available diagnostic tests. In addition, lack of compliance with the required 7-day treatment schedule is a major barrier to effective control.

Unlike other common sexually transmitted diseases such as gonorrhea and syphilis, no national surveillance system for chlamydia is fully functional.[493] Guidelines for chlamydia control in the United States were developed in 1985 and are being implemented.[494] Currently 42 States have at least 1 city or county sexually transmitted disease program offering comprehensive surveillance, diagnostic testing, and treatment services. Since 1985, the number of States that consider this infection a reportable disease has doubled, and the number of cases reported to the Centers for Disease Control has risen tenfold. The absence of nationwide surveillance for chlamydia has necessitated the use of nongonococcal urethritis as an indicator of progress in controlling chlamydia infections. As more States mandate reporting of chlamydia, and as use of available tests to diagnose infection becomes more widespread, it may be possible to track chlamydia itself rather than use nongonococcal urethritis as an indicator.

19.3 Reduce primary and secondary syphilis to an incidence of no more than 10 cases per 100,000 people. (Baseline: 18.1 per 100,000 in 1989)

Special Population Target

Primary and Secondary Syphilis Incidence (per 100,000)	1989 Baseline	2000 Target	Percent Decrease
19.3a Blacks	118	65	

Baseline data source: Syphilis Surveillance System, CDC.

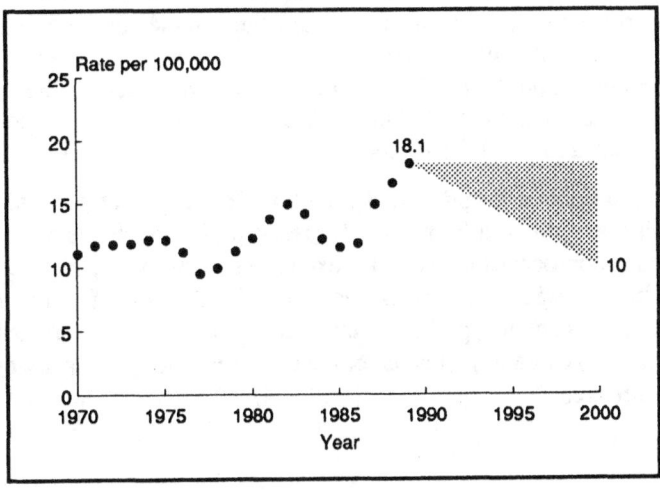

Fig. 19.3

Incidence of primary and secondary syphilis

Syphilis is the first sexually transmitted disease for which control measures were developed and tested. Since the initiation of Federal assistance for syphilis control in the 1940s, reported cases of all stages of syphilis declined from an all-time high of 575,600 in 1943 to fewer than 68,000 in 1985. In recent years, however, the number of syphilis cases has increased dramatically. Between 1986 and 1989, the number of reported cases of primary and secondary syphilis rose more than 55 percent, to the highest level in the United States since the early 1950s.

Decreases in reported syphilis noted through 1986 were caused, in part, by behavior changes among homosexual men in response to the HIV epidemic.[495] The recent increase may be due to the hard-to-reach crack cocaine users who are exchanging sex for drugs.[477] In addition, evidence increasingly confirms an association between genital ulcer disease (including infectious syphilis) and sexual HIV spread.[496] Thus, it is crucial that HIV prevention and syphilis control activities build upon and support each other.

Several supplementary approaches will help reverse the spiraling syphilis rates in the 1990s: (1) integrating syphilis control activities into community outreach efforts already underway with HIV resources; (2) training disciplines other than health professionals to recognize and appropriately refer syphilis cases; (3) concentrating syphilis control resources in the highest incidence areas; (4) expanding syphilis screening into facilities serving high-risk populations—e.g., drug treatment centers, correctional facilities, emergency rooms; and (5) applying prophylactic treatment in settings where epidemiologic indicators predict high levels of syphilis infection.

19.4 **Reduce congenital syphilis to an incidence of no more than 50 cases per 100,000 live births. (Baseline: 100 per 100,000 live births in 1989)**

Baseline data source: Syphilis Surveillance System, CDC.

Congenital syphilis causes fetal or perinatal death in 40 percent of the infants affected. Since 1970, the incidence of congenital syphilis has closely paralleled the incidence of primary and secondary syphilis in women. Reported cases of congenital syphilis among infants reached an all-time low of 3.1 cases per 100,000 live births in 1980, but since then have gradually increased. The rise in cases can be attributed to increases in heterosexual syphilis and improved reporting due to broader definitions. In 1989, more cases of congenital syphilis (925) were reported than in any of the previous 15 years; almost 1 of every 4,200 live-born infants in the United States had congenital syphilis.

The year 2000 congenital syphilis target takes into account the anticipated impact of the expanded case definition on the number of reported congenital syphilis cases.[497] Investigations have shown that previous surveillance underestimated the number of cases by four- to fivefold.[498] As such, the reported congenital syphilis rate of 21.4 per 100,000 live births in 1989 would be approximately 100 per 100,000 live births if adjusted for previous underreporting by use of the new definition. The objective targets a 50 percent reduction from the adjusted rate (50 per 100,000).

The Centers for Disease Control has published guidelines for the prevention and control of congenital syphilis that serve as a framework for reducing the incidence of this disease.[499] Recommended approaches include: (1) expanding syphilis screening of women of childbearing age in cities with high syphilis incidence; (2) developing community-based educational messages about syphilis and the need for prenatal care targeted to populations at risk; and (3) extending prenatal outreach services for pregnant women living in high-incidence areas.

19.5 Reduce genital herpes and genital warts, as measured by a reduction to 142,000 and 385,000, respectively, in the annual number of first-time consultations with a physician for the conditions. (Baseline: 167,000 and 451,000 in 1988)

Baseline data source: National Disease and Therapeutic Index, CDC.

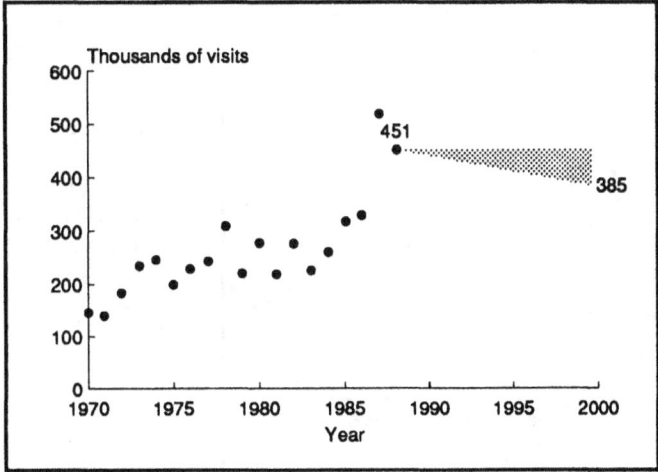

Fig. 19.5

Annual first-time physician consultations for genital warts

The estimated annual incidence of symptomatic genital herpes is 200,000 cases, with total prevalence estimates of genital herpes infection as high as 30 million cases.[500] These high levels are expected to continue, with recurrences among more people and increasingly serious complications for pregnant women and newborns. Control efforts for genital herpes are currently hampered because as many as three-fourths of genital herpes infections are transmitted by people who are unaware of their own infection and because no cure for the condition exists.[501] Progress is nevertheless expected in the development of antiviral agents capable of alleviating the disease.

Genital warts are a common sexually transmitted disease and account for approximately 5 percent of all sexually transmitted disease clinic visits. The warts are caused by human papillomavirus, which is strongly associated with cervical dysplasia and genital cancers. Genital human papillomavirus infections can also be passed to newborns who are delivered through infected birth canals. Many individuals infected with human papillomavirus are asymptomatic and thus transmit the virus unknowingly.[502] Because no culture method is available to diagnose human papillomavirus, diagnoses are made on largely clinical grounds. Genital human papillomavirus infections are difficult to treat and commonly recur. Increased research into diagnosis and treatment is essential for controlling human papillomavirus.

19.6 Reduce the incidence of pelvic inflammatory disease, as measured by a reduction in hospitalizations for pelvic inflammatory disease to no more than 250 per 100,000 women aged 15 through 44. (Baseline: 311 per 100,000 in 1988)

Baseline data source: National Hospital Discharge Survey, CDC.

Pelvic inflammatory disease is the most severe complication, with the greatest public health consequences, of lower genital tract infections such as gonorrhea and chlamydia in women. More than 1 million cases are diagnosed and treated each year, with a high percentage needing costly hospitalization. The cost of pelvic inflammatory disease and associated ectopic pregnancy and infertility alone exceeds $2.6 billion.[503]

The subclinical nature of PID results in unnecessary infertility among women whose condition goes unrecognized.[504] Specific diagnoses are difficult to make and expensive because they require laparoscopy. Effective prevention of this syndrome should be based on control of chlamydia and gonorrhea.

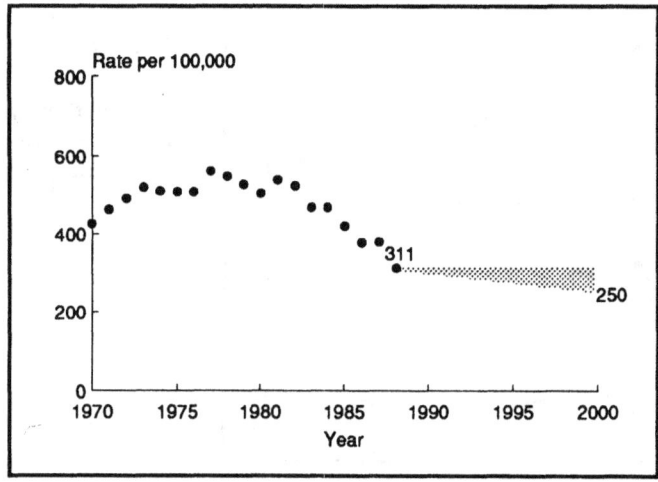

Fig. 19.6

Pelvic inflammatory disease hospitalization rate

The 1990 objective to reduce the incidence of PID to 560 cases per 100,000 women will probably not be met, although the 1990 target for gonococcal PID (60 per 100,000) will. The year 2000 objective is stated in terms of the hospitalization rate rather than total reported incidence, because data for hospitalization are more readily obtainable and more reliable than reported incidence.

19.7*   **Reduce sexually transmitted hepatitis B infection to no more than 30,500 cases. (Baseline: 58,300 cases in 1988)**

Baseline data source: Hepatitis Surveillance System, CDC.

Nationwide, the incidence of hepatitis B has increased steadily over the last decade despite the availability of a vaccine since 1982. Vaccination programs have focused primarily on three risk groups: health care workers exposed to blood; staff and resident patients of institutions for the developmentally disabled; and staff and patients in hemodialysis units. These groups, however, account for only 5 to 10 percent of acute hepatitis B cases. The people who account for most of the cases—intravenous drug abusers, sexual partners of infected heterosexuals, and homosexual men—are not being reached effectively by current vaccination programs.

Sexually transmitted hepatitis B has been decreasing among the homosexual population primarily because of changes in their sexual behavior to prevent HIV infection.[505] In contrast, the number of hepatitis B cases among heterosexuals has been increasing and parallels the recent increases in cases of primary and secondary syphilis among the heterosexual drug-abusing population.

Although hepatitis B is the only sexually transmitted disease for which an effective vaccine is available, cost and unfounded fear of HIV infection have limited its widespread acceptance. In addition, the ability to immunize high-risk groups is compromised by several factors: the failure of both health care providers and target populations to be aware of the specific groups at high risk of infection; difficulty in identifying members of

19. Sexually Transmitted Diseases

high-risk groups; problems in reaching these groups for delivery of vaccine; and the difficulties in dealing with transient at-risk populations.

Control of this virus will require active cooperation from agencies other than sexually transmitted disease clinics, such as drug treatment centers, adult immunization clinics, and private practitioners.

*This objective also appears as Objectives 20.3b and 20.3c in *Immunization and Infectious Diseases*.

19.8   **Reduce the rate of repeat gonorrhea infection to no more than 15 percent within the previous year. (Baseline: 20 percent in 1988)**

Note: As measured by a reduction in the proportion of gonorrhea patients who, within the previous year, were treated for a separate case of gonorrhea.
Baseline data source: STD Surveillance System, CDC.

As with other health problems, sexually transmitted diseases tend to cluster in certain core populations. In one longitudinal analysis, approximately 15 percent of infected individuals and their identified sexual partners accounted for nearly 30 percent of all gonorrhea cases.[506] Therefore, patients who have had previous infections are an important target group for reducing overall sexually transmitted disease rates and making the most cost-effective use of resources.

New methods of helping patients prevent repeat infections are required and will probably include improved psychosocial history-taking by clinicians. Possible interventions include consideration of social, economic, and environmental factors; psychosocial coping skills; referrals to community social agencies for other identified problems; and assistance in developing adequate social support systems. Gonorrhea is used as an indicator of repeat infection rates because it is the number one reportable communicable disease and is sensitive to changes in high-risk sexual behaviors. However, no uniform national data system exists to track repeat infections.

Risk Reduction Objectives

19.9*   Reduce the proportion of adolescents who have engaged in sexual intercourse to no more than 15 percent by age 15 and no more than 40 percent by age 17. (Baseline: 27 percent of girls and 33 percent of boys by age 15; 50 percent of girls and 66 percent of boys by age 17; reported in 1988)

Baseline data sources: National Survey of Family Growth; National Survey of Adolescent Males.
*For commentary, see Objective 5.4 in *Family Planning*. This objective also appears as Objective 18.3 in *HIV Infection*.

19.10* Increase to at least 50 percent the proportion of sexually active, unmarried people who used a condom at last sexual intercourse. (Baseline: 19 percent of sexually active, unmarried women aged 15 through 44 reported that their partners used a condom at last sexual intercourse in 1988)

Special Population Targets

Use of Condoms	1988 Baseline	2000 Target
19.10a Sexually active young women aged 15-19 (by their partners)	25%	60%
19.10b Sexually active young men aged 15-19	57%	75%
19.10c Intravenous drug abusers	—	60%

Note: Strategies to achieve this objective must be undertaken sensitively to avoid indirectly encouraging or condoning sexual activity among teens who are not yet sexually active.

Baseline data sources: National Survey of Family Growth, CDC; National Survey of Adolescent Males.

Abstinence or sexual intercourse with one mutually faithful uninfected partner are the only totally effective prevention strategies against sexually transmitted diseases. Proper use of condoms and reducing the number of sexual partners decrease, but do not eliminate, risk of sexually transmitted diseases. Even with the proper use of condoms, high risk sexual behaviors, e.g., anal intercourse, should be avoided. Research is needed to better understand resistance to effective condom use so that specific interventions can be implemented. Although reported condom use appears to be relatively high among sexually active adolescents, they are targeted because they are the age group at highest risk for sexually transmitted diseases, and because inculcating safer behaviors in this population will have long term positive implications for disease trends.

Failure of condoms to prevent disease is more often the fault of the user than of the product.[507] Condoms and instructions for their proper use should be made more widely available through health care providers who offer services to sexually active men and women, particularly in sexually transmitted disease clinics, family planning clinics, and drug treatment centers. These same facilities should become more assertive in counseling patients on sexually transmitted disease prevention. Instructions in correct condom use can be obtained from *Condoms and Sexually Transmitted Diseases . . . Especially AIDS*[481] or the National AIDS Hotline, 1-800-342-AIDS.

*For additional commentary, see Objective 18.4 in *HIV Infection*.

Services and Protection Objectives

19.11* Increase to at least 50 percent the proportion of family planning clinics, maternal and child health clinics, sexually transmitted disease clinics, tuberculosis clinics, drug treatment centers, and primary care clinics that screen, diagnose, treat, counsel, and provide (or refer for) partner notification services for HIV infection and bacterial sexually transmitted diseases (gonorrhea, syphilis, and chlamydia). (Baseline: 40 percent of family planning clinics for bacterial sexually transmitted diseases in 1989)

Baseline data source: State Family Planning Directors.

Expansion of comprehensive sexually transmitted disease services into other public health clinics serving high-risk patients is essential if the health status objectives for this priority area are to be achieved. Although screening for certain sexually transmitted infections (e.g., gonorrhea) is routine in some public health settings, the full range of clinical services (including partner notification) are often not available. Such expansion should also take place in the private sector. This is particularly important as sexually transmitted diseases become concentrated in hard-to-reach groups, such as intravenous drug abusers.

The objective includes only selected public facilities because they are more likely to have valid data to establish baselines and assess progress. However, other relevant public and private providers should also expand their sexually transmitted disease services in the coming decade.

*This objective also appears as Objective 5.11 in *Family Planning* and Objective 18.13 in *HIV Infection*.

19.12 Include instruction in sexually transmitted disease transmission prevention in the curricula of all middle and secondary schools, preferably as part of quality school health education. (Baseline: 95 percent of schools reported offering at least one class on sexually transmitted diseases as part of their standard curricula in 1988)

Note: Strategies to achieve this objective must be undertaken sensitively to avoid indirectly encouraging or condoning sexual activity among teens who are not yet sexually active.
Baseline data source: Alan Guttmacher Institute.

Awareness of the risks of sexual behavior and of sexually transmitted diseases is particularly crucial for adolescents. Through school-based education on family life and human sexuality, youth can be offered the knowledge and skills they need to reduce their risk of contracting sexually transmitted diseases. Because of emphasis deriving from the HIV epidemic, students are relatively well informed about prevention of HIV transmission, but are less knowledgeable about the symptoms of other sexually transmitted diseases. Programs should be modified to include sexually transmitted diseases as part of a total health education package. In addition, school curricula must build on the foundation of increased knowledge by including behaviorally based instruction (e.g., role playing) to develop skills in improving safer sexual behaviors. Optimally, sexually transmitted disease education should be provided as part of quality school health education. For a definition of quality school health education, see *Educational and Community-Based Programs*.

As messages about safer sexual behaviors have become more common, emphasis has also been placed on increasing the variety and specificity of these messages to reach different cultural and ethnic groups in more effective ways. HIV prevention messages should be expanded to include symptoms of other sexually transmitted diseases and services for diagnosing/treating them. The effect of these messages on adolescent behavior should be assessed so that the most successful messages can be more broadly distributed.

19.13 Increase to at least 90 percent the proportion of primary care providers treating patients with sexually transmitted diseases who correctly manage cases, as measured by their use of appropriate types and amounts of therapy. (Baseline: 70 percent in 1988)

Baseline data source: National Disease and Therapeutic Index, CDC.
Adequate clinical services are crucial for effectively controlling sexually transmitted diseases. Without effective treatment, opportunities for continued spread of infections are increased. Therefore, clinicians must be skilled in taking sexual histories, diagnostic procedures, and current treatment regimens. Although the proficiency of health care providers in sexually transmitted disease clinical management has improved in recent

years, it remains far short of the necessary quality and scope. For example, only 10 percent of primary care providers regularly assess the sexual behaviors of their patients.[508] In addition, a sizable proportion do not prescribe the combination of antibiotics required to treat polymicrobial PID.[509]

Selected sexually transmitted diseases will be used as indicators (i.e., gonorrhea and PID) in monitoring this objective, and the definition of appropriate therapy will be based on the sexually transmitted disease treatments recommended by the Centers for Disease Control.[510] Progress toward achieving this objective will reflect improvements in the knowledge and decision making skills of practitioners, as well as the effectiveness of medical and other allied health schools in improving sexually transmitted disease knowledge and clinical skills.

19.14* Increase to at least 75 percent the proportion of primary care and mental health care providers who provide age-appropriate counseling on the prevention of HIV and other sexually transmitted diseases. (Baseline: 10 percent of physicians reported that they regularly assessed the sexual behaviors of their patients in 1987)

Special Population Target

Counseling on HIV and STD Prevention	1987 Baseline	2000 Target
19.14a Providers practicing in high incidence areas	—	90%

Note: *Primary care providers include physicians, nurses, nurse practitioners, and physician assistants. Areas of high AIDS and sexually transmitted disease incidence are cities and States with incidence rates of AIDS cases, HIV seroprevalence, gonorrhea, or syphilis that are at least 25 percent above the national average.*

Baseline data source: Lewis and Freeman 1987.

According to the U.S. Preventive Services Task Force [45] clinicians should take a complete sexual and drug use history on all adolescent and adult patients. Sexually active patients should receive complete information on their risk for acquiring HIV or other sexually transmitted diseases. Patients should be advised against sexual activity with individuals whose infection status is uncertain. Patients who choose to have sexual intercourse with multiple partners or with people who may be infected, should be advised to use a condom at each encounter and to avoid anal intercourse. Women should be informed of the potential risks of HIV infection during pregnancy. People who abuse intravenous drugs should be encouraged to enroll in a drug treatment program, warned against sharing drug injection equipment and using unsterilized syringes and needles, and given sources for uncontaminated injection equipment or referred to community programs that have this information.

*For additional commentary, see Objective 18.9 in *HIV Infection*.

19.15 Increase to at least 50 percent the proportion of all patients with bacterial sexually transmitted diseases (gonorrhea, syphilis, and chlamydia) who are offered provider referral services. (Baseline: 20 percent of those treated in sexually transmitted disease clinics in 1988)

Note: *Provider referral (previously called contact tracing) is the process whereby health department personnel directly notify the sexual partners of infected individuals of their exposure to an infected individual.*

Baseline data source: STD Surveillance System, CDC.

Partner notification is a public health process for interrupting transmission of infectious diseases that has helped to find, treat, and prevent thousands of sexually transmitted disease cases annually.[511] The purpose of partner notification in sexually transmitted disease control is to identify people who should receive curative sexually transmitted disease treatment, and thus reduce transmission of infection within the community, and also to prevent further complications such as upper genital tract infections.

Previous temporal and geographic trends suggest that partner notification contributed to reducing the national prevalence of syphilis, and especially congenital syphilis.[511] Partner notification strategies have also been effective in helping to control focal outbreaks of infection due to antibiotic resistant gonorrhea and chancroid, and in targeting intervention activities for specific high-risk populations.[512]

Two types of partner notification are generally used by health departments: patient referral and provider referral. With patient referral, offered routinely to every person with a sexually transmitted disease, patients are encouraged and coached to inform their sex partners of exposure to infection; with provider referral (previously called contact tracing), health department personnel directly notify partners of their exposure to an infected individual. Advantages of provider referral include greater certainty that the sex partner(s) have been notified, delivery of risk-reduction messages during the process of notification, and identifying additional sex partners to be notified. However, because provider referral is labor intensive, it has not been possible, given current resources, to extend this prevention strategy to all persons with syphilis, gonorrhea, and chlamydia seen in sexually transmitted disease clinics.

* * *

Research Needs

Basic Science

- New technologies to detect asymptomatic sexually transmitted diseases. To be effective, new tests should be less expensive, easier to implement, and provide more timely information to the clinician and the patient than those currently available.

- Better antibacterial therapies. New research should focus on combating drug-resistant organisms and reducing difficulties in gaining patient compliance with regimens that require more than a single dose.

- Vaccines against sexually transmitted diseases other than hepatitis B and systems for administering the vaccines to high-risk adult populations. Convincing people to reduce high-risk behaviors is only part of the solution to the national sexually transmitted disease problem. Especially among those who are difficult to reach with risk-reduction messages (e.g., intravenous drug abusers), safe, effective vaccines hold tremendous potential for reducing the devastating effect of sexually transmitted diseases.

Behavioral Research

- Definition of the determinants of [adolescent and youth] sexual risk-taking behavior and development of appropriate behavioral interventions. Little is known about why people change (or fail to change) risk-taking behaviors. Without such basic knowledge, it is virtually impossible to design programs that are effective in helping people choose healthy behaviors.

- Understanding of the factors affecting use of preventive measures (condoms, chemical prophylaxis), so that such precautions will be more widely taken.

- Evaluation of counseling to promote safer sexual practices. The specific messages that promote sustained behavior modification for both individuals and communities need to be understood, and if effective, become more widely disseminated.

* * *

Baseline Data Source References

The Alan Guttmacher Institute. *Risk and Responsibility: Teaching Sex Education in America's Schools Today.* New York: the Institute, 1989.

Hepatitis Surveillance System, Center for Infectious Diseases, Centers for Disease Control, Public Health Service, U.S. Department of Health and Human Services, Atlanta, GA.

Gonorrhea Surveillance System, Center for Prevention Services, Centers for Disease Control, Public Health Service, U.S. Department of Health and Human Services, Atlanta, GA.

Lewis, C.F. and Freeman, H.E. The sexual history taking and counseling practices of California primary care physicians. *Western Journal of Medicine* 147:165-167, 1987.

National Disease and Therapeutic Index, Center for Prevention Services, Centers for Disease Control, Public Health Service, U.S. Department of Health and Human Services, Atlanta, GA.

National Hospital Discharge Survey, National Center for Health Statistics, Centers for Disease Control, Public Health Service, U.S. Department of Health and Human Services, Hyattsville, MD.

National Survey of Adolescent Males. In: Sonnenstein, F.L.; Pleck, J.H.; and Ku, L.C. Sexual activity, condom use, and AIDS awareness among adolescent males. *Family Planning Perspectives* 21(4): 152-158, 1989.

National Survey of Family Growth, National Center for Health Statistics, Centers for Disease Control, Public Health Service, U.S. Department of Health and Human Services, Hyattsville, MD.

STD Surveillance System, Center for Prevention Services, Centers for Disease Control, Public Health Service, U.S. Department of Health and Human Services, Atlanta, GA.

State Family Planning Association, Washington, DC.

Syphilis Surveillance System, Center for Prevention Services, Centers for Disease Control, Public Health Service, U.S. Department of Health and Human Services, Atlanta, GA.

Immunization and Infectious Diseases

20

Contents

20.1	Vaccine-preventable diseases

* * *

20.3	Viral hepatitis

* * *

20.7	Bacterial meningitis
20.8	Diarrhea among children in child care centers
20.9	Ear infections among children
20.10	Pneumonia-related illness
20.11	Immunizations
20.12	Rabies treatments
20.13	Immunization laws
20.14	Counseling about immunization by clinician
20.15	Financial barriers to immunization

* * *

20.17	Tuberculosis identification

* * *

[Research Needs]

20. Immunization and Infectious Diseases

* * *

Health Status Objectives

20.1 Reduce indigenous cases of vaccine-preventable diseases as follows:

Disease	1988 Baseline	2000 Target
Diphtheria among people aged 25 and younger	1	0
Tetanus among people aged 25 and younger	3	0
Polio (wild-type virus)	0	0
Measles	3,058	0
Rubella	225	0
Congenital Rubella Syndrome	6	0
Mumps	4,866	500
Pertussis	3,450	1,000

Baseline data source: Center for Prevention Services, CDC.

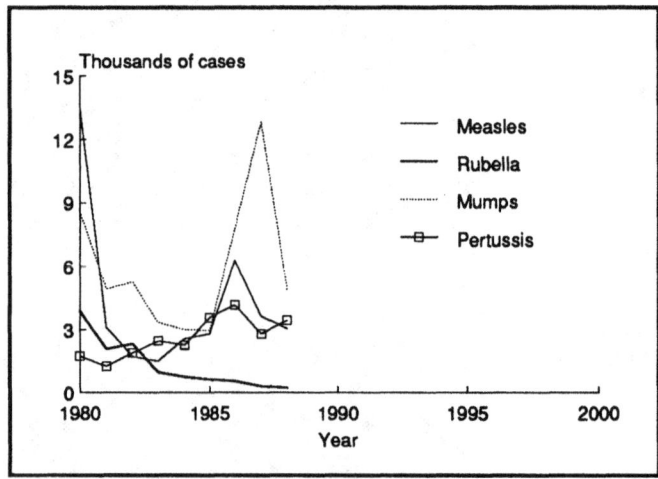

Fig. 20.1

Vaccine-preventable diseases

Diphtheria and Tetanus: With the availability of highly effective toxoids and school entry laws, no one attending school since the early 1980s should develop tetanus or diphtheria. The major barrier to the achievement of complete eradication of these diseases is failure to immunize as appropriate for their age all children, adolescents, and adults.

Polio (wild-type virus), Indigenous Measles, Rubella, and Congenital Rubella Syndrome: The World Health Organization has adopted a resolution for eradication of paralytic poliomyelitis from the world by the year 2000. No cases of indigenous polio caused by wild-type virus have been reported in the United States since 1979.[513]

Since 1978, the United States has had as a goal the elimination of indigenous measles; however, importations with limited spread will continue to occur, and approximately 500 cases of measles are expected each year, even after elimination of indigenous cases. Cases of measles decreased from 26,871 in 1978 to approximately 3,000 cases annually from 1981 through 1988. In 1989, there was a resurgence of measles with a provisional total of 16,236 cases reported.

Current illness can be divided into two major patterns—preschool outbreaks and school outbreaks.[514] The former are predominantly in unvaccinated children and require better immunization coverage at recommended ages. The latter occur primarily in vaccinated children and require more aggressive revaccination strategies during outbreak control efforts. Other requirements include continued high vaccine coverage at school entry, implementation of a two-dose schedule, identification and vaccination of at-risk groups, and use of every health care contact to provide all needed vaccines, including measles vaccine.[515] Because measles vaccine is usually administered with mumps and rubella vaccines (MMR) and because the latter diseases are less communicable than measles, high coverage with a two-dose MMR schedule should lead to elimination of rubella and congenital rubella syndrome and to marked decreases in mumps cases.

Mumps: Reported mumps cases decreased dramatically from 152,209 cases in 1968—the year after mumps vaccine licensure—to 2,982 cases in 1985. In 1986 and 1987, however, there were marked increases, peaking at 12,848 cases in 1987. Following the epidemic in 1987, mumps cases decreased to 4,866 in 1988 and a provisional total of 5,611 in 1989. These increases were due to cases occurring in unvaccinated children, predominantly in States without immunization requirements for mumps. Increased use of MMR, particularly in a two-dose schedule, should permit attainment of the target for reduction of mumps.[516] Currently, 11 States do not have mumps immunization requirements.

Pertussis: The majority of reported cases of pertussis occur in children up to age 5. The most significant morbidity and incidents of death occur in infants—predominantly in infants less than 6 months of age.[517] Pertussis vaccine, which is given with diphtheria and tetanus as DTP, is recommended in a four-dose primary schedule commencing at 6 to 8 weeks of age and ending with the fourth dose at 15 to 18 months of age. In addition, a booster dose is needed before school entry. Because at least three doses are considered necessary for protection against the disease, infants are not adequately protected against pertussis prior to 6 months of age.

Besides reducing illness and death in the age group most at risk for pertussis and its complications, increased vaccination against pertussis can reduce its overall transmission. High levels of age-appropriate vaccination of infants and young children need to be achieved, requiring the identification and vaccination of high-risk groups and the assurance that every health care encounter becomes an opportunity for vaccination. Efforts are continuing to develop a safer pertussis vaccine that is at least as effective as current whole-cell vaccines.[518] The availability of such a vaccine should lead to increased use of pertussis vaccine among the young. If usable in children and adults older than 6 years of age, the new vaccine may lead to decreased transmission of pertussis among older people and from older people to infants and young children.

The reduction of indigenous cases of vaccine-preventable diseases will require sensitive surveillance to detect and report cases as early as possible. It will also require broadening the definition of the at-risk population to include adults as well as children in some instances.

* * *

20.3* **Reduce viral hepatitis as follows:**

(Per 100,000)	1987 Baseline	2000 Target
Hepatitis B (HBV)	63.5	40
Hepatitis A	31	23
Hepatitis C	18.3	13.7

Special Population Targets for HBV

	HBV Cases	1987 Estimated Baseline	2000 Target
20.3a	Intravenous drug abusers	30,000	22,500
20.3b	Heterosexually active people	33,000	22,000
20.3c	Homosexual men	25,300	8,500
20.3d	Children of Asians/Pacific Islanders	8,900	1,800
20.3e	Occupationally exposed workers	6,200	1,250
20.3f	Infants	3,500	550 new carriers
20.3g	Alaska Natives	15	1

Baseline data source: Center for Infectious Diseases, CDC.

Hepatitis A continues to be an important disease, with 75,800 cases estimated annually. After a steady decrease from 1971 through 1983, disease rates are increasing, possibly related to increased transmission among drug abusers. Risk is also very high among American Indians, among whom cyclic epidemics occur every 5 to 10 years. Current control measures—namely immunoglobulin for case contacts—have historically had no impact on national disease rates. Candidate hepatitis A vaccines are undergoing clinical trials and may become available before the year 2000. If so, use of these vaccines in high-risk groups, such as American Indians and Alaska Natives, international travelers, and children attending child care centers, should begin to have an impact on disease incidence. Slow development of vaccines and difficulty in getting the vaccine to the target populations may impede efforts.

Incidence of hepatitis C (parenterally transmitted non-A non-B hepatitis) is more difficult to estimate, and until recently no effective control measures were available. Cloning and identification of one of the causative agents occurred in 1988, and a laboratory test to identify infected persons is now available. Such tests will permit universal screening of blood to prevent posttransfusion hepatitis, which accounted for about 20 percent of the disease through 1985, but for only 5 percent of the disease in 1986 and 1987. Diagnostic tests will also permit the epidemiology of this disease to be clearly defined and may allow evaluation of immunoglobulin prophylaxis and candidate vaccines.

Hepatitis B is primarily an infection of people in certain risk groups to whom available vaccines are now targeted. Risk is also very high among Alaska Natives, Pacific Islanders, Asians, and others who emigrate from areas of high hepatitis B endemicity. In 1987, the Centers for Disease Control (CDC) estimated the total number of hepatitis B virus infections to be 300,000 per year. Of these patients, 6 to 10 percent become carriers at risk of developing chronic liver disease and becoming infectious to others. Wider use of vaccine is recommended for infants and children in high-risk populations.

The incidence of hepatitis B cases continued to increase through 1985 despite availability of effective vaccines. By 1987, rates had decreased slightly—probably due to changing sexual behavior.

Licensure of new vaccines should decrease the cost of vaccine, which should stimulate much wider use by the year 2000. Disease incidence should be decreased by 80 to 90

20. Immunization and Infectious Diseases

percent among infants of hepatitis B-carrier mothers and among occupationally exposed workers (defined as those whose occupations cause them to be exposed on average one or more times per month) because of universal prenatal hepatitis B surface antigen (HBsAg) screening of mothers and implementation of industrywide standards for vaccination of occupationally exposed workers. Incidence in homosexual men should continue to decrease because of changes in sexual behavior and wider vaccine use. Decreases among drug abusers will be difficult to achieve unless drug use can be discouraged through behavior modification, users can be motivated to receive the vaccine, and programs can be established to deliver vaccine to these individuals. Achieving a 37-percent overall disease reduction will also depend on preventing disease transmission through heterosexual contact, which accounts for 21 percent of cases, and will require aggressive programs to deliver vaccine in sexually transmitted disease clinics, high schools, and colleges. When less costly vaccines become available, programs for universal vaccination of children or adolescents must be strongly considered as the best approach for long-term control of this disease.

* Special Population targets 20.3b, and 20.3c also appear as Objective 19.7 in *Sexually Transmitted Diseases*.

* * *

20.7 **Reduce bacterial meningitis to no more than 4.7 cases per 100,000 people. (Baseline: 6.3 per 100,000 in 1986)**

Special Population Target

Bacterial Meningitis Cases (per 100,000)	*1987 Baseline*	*2000 Target*
20.7a Alaska Natives	33	8

Baseline data source: Center for Infectious Diseases, CDC.

Bacterial meningitis is a major cause of death and neurologic impairment in children. A recent analysis of *Haemophilus influenzae* type b (Hib) disease, the most important cause of meningitis in children, estimated costs of approximately $2 billion per year in the United States. Reducing the rate of bacterial meningitis would both decrease childhood deaths and reduce the number of children with permanent neurologic damage, including deafness.

The projected reduction in Hib disease assumes that the newly developed vaccine will be licensed for use in infants, will be used by at least 75 percent of the eligible population, and will be at least 65 percent effective. Baseline data for Hib immunization levels are not currently available. The vaccination program will be promoted through public and medical educational materials and implemented through currently administered vaccination programs. Extending such programs to cover child day care can be an important step in this effort.

Group B streptococcal disease is the leading cause of meningitis in neonates. Reduction assumes peripartum chemoprophylaxis, hyperimmune globulin, and vaccines will prove effective in prevention of disease and will be used by the medical community.

20.8 **Reduce infectious diarrhea by at least 25 percent among children in licensed child care centers and children in programs that provide an Individualized Education Program (IEP) or Individualized Health Plan (IHP). (Baseline data available in 1992)**

Children in licensed child care centers have three to four times as much diarrheal disease as do those not in child care. Similar rates are reported among children with disabilities enrolled in special early childhood IEP and IHP programs administered by public school systems. Reducing this risk would improve the health of children attending day care and reduce the absenteeism costs to parents and employers in caring for sick children.

Keys to achieving this objective are the development of the following: (1) effective control programs based on findings from current studies to identify factors associated with infectious disease in child care centers, (2) adequate surveillance for child care-related disease, (3) identification of cost-effective prevention and control strategies, and (4) vaccines for specific agents, such as rotavirus. Attaining this objective will require the involvement of CDC, State and local health departments, regulatory agencies, universities and nongovernmental organizations, as well as the child care and early childhood education professionals who will be principally responsible for carrying out infection control measures in their programs.[519]

20.9 Reduce acute middle ear infections among children aged 4 and younger, as measured by days of restricted activity or school absenteeism, to no more than 105 days per 100 children. (Baseline: 131 days per 100 children in 1987)

Baseline data source: National Health Interview Survey, CDC.

Acute middle ear infections (otitis media) are a common cause of illness in young children and result in frequent use of antibiotics. Children with recurrent infections may develop hearing deficits and poor school performance and often require surgical procedures to improve middle ear drainage. *Streptococcus pneumoniae* is the most common etiologic agent. However, prevention through use of the currently available pneumococcal vaccine is not possible because the most frequent pneumococcal capsular types causing disease are very poor immunogens in children less than 2 years old, the group at highest risk for recurrent ear infections. A more immunogenic pneumococcal vaccine is currently being developed and is expected to be available for use before the year 2000. Immunization of children who have had an acute ear infection may decrease the number of episodes of recurrent disease. Federal, State, and local health departments and physicians with primary care responsibilities for children should promote the use of the new vaccine when it becomes available.

20.10 Reduce pneumonia-related days of restricted activity as follows:

	1987 Baseline	*2000 Target*
* * *		
Children aged 4 and younger (per 100 children)	27 days	24 days

Baseline data source: National Health Interview Survey, CDC

Pneumonia and other lower respiratory infections are a major cause of illness in the United States, primarily in older adults and the very young.... Respiratory syncytial virus, influenza virus, and parainfluenza virus type 3 are the most common causes of the most common illness in young children.... Vaccines are not available for respiratory syncytial virus and parainfluenza virus type 3, but candidate vaccines are being developed.

Achieving these objectives is contingent on ... the availability of new vaccines, better diagnostic methods, and earlier treatment.... Federal and private research funding agencies and vaccine manufacturers should be encouraged to expand programs for development and testing of vaccines for respiratory syncytial virus and parainfluenza type 3. The use of safe, effective vaccines may also decrease days of restricted activity in children under 5 years old. Federal, State, and local health departments, organizations of health professionals, and primary care physicians should all help in the promotion and delivery of vaccines to persons recommended for immunization. Third-party payers of health care can also do more to promote recommended immunizations.

Risk Reduction Objectives

20.11 Increase immunization levels as follows:

Basic immunization series among children under age 2: at least 90 percent. (Baseline: 70-80 percent estimated in 1989)

Basic immunization series among children in licensed child care facilities and kindergarten through post-secondary education institutions: at least 95 percent. (Baseline: For licensed child care, 94 percent; 97 percent for children entering school for the 1987-1988 school year; and for post-secondary institutions, baseline data available in 1992)

* * *

Hepatitis B immunization among high-risk populations, including infants of surface antigen-positive mothers to at least 90 percent; occupationally exposed workers to at least 90 percent; IV-drug users in drug treatment programs to at least 50 percent; and homosexual men to at least 50 percent. (Baseline data available in 1992)

Baseline data source: Center for Prevention Services and Center for Infectious Diseases, CDC.

One of the goals of the National Childhood Immunization Initiative, begun in 1978, is to establish a system for effective delivery of vaccines to the preschool population, i.e., adequately immunizing at least 90 percent of all children by 2 years of age. Although an effective national assessment of the preschool population has not been developed, the immunization level is believed to be approximately 70 to 80 percent, with certain pockets of the population having levels lower than 50 percent. Special efforts need to be targeted to minority populations, particularly blacks and Hispanics, since these groups appear to have substantially lower immunization levels than the general population.

A second goal of the initiative is to immunize at least 95 percent of the school children in the United States. Each State has enacted laws and/or regulations that specifically address the issue of immunization requirements to attend school, whether public or private. Similar laws and/or regulations pertaining to licensed day care facilities are in place or being drafted.

Approximately 40,000 persons die each year from complications associated with pneumococcal disease. Sequelae of influenza result in an additional 20,000 deaths. Obstacles include vaccine costs and lack of provider knowledge and motivation.[520] The provision of vaccine against pneumococcal pneumonia and influenza disease in institutions for the chronically ill and frail elderly is not legally mandated.... Reimbursement alone will not raise coverage levels. It will be necessary to have a concerted information and educational campaign directed at the lay and professional public to increase awareness of the need for influenza and pneumococcal vaccines.

Lifetime risk for hepatitis B disease varies from almost 100 percent in high-risk groups to 3 to 5 percent for the general population, yet only about 30 percent of people in high-risk groups have been immunized. To meet this objective, all pregnant women should be screened for hepatitis B surface antigen.[521] A delivery system needs to be established to ensure that all infants born to infected mothers begin their hepatitis B vaccine series at birth with followup to ensure that they complete the series according to the recommended schedule. Special attention should be given to Alaska Natives and Pacific Islanders, Southeast Asians, and women who migrate from areas of high endemicity....

20.12 Reduce postexposure rabies treatments to no more than 9,000 per year. (Baseline: 18,000 estimated treatments in 1987)

Baseline data source: Center for Infectious Diseases, CDC.

Each year approximately 18,000 people in the United States are vaccinated against rabies after being exposed to rabid or potentially rabid animals. Postexposure treatment includes a series of five vaccinations with rabies vaccine and one dose of rabies immunoglobulin administered concurrently with the first dose of vaccine. This treatment is expensive, with the cost of the biologicals alone ranging from $500 to $700. Since the decision to treat an exposed person is primarily based on the local presence of animal rabies, the number of people receiving postexposure treatment can be reduced by educating physicians and public health consultants about when postexposure rabies treatment is indicated.

Various domestic and wild animals can be immunized against rabies by ingesting baits containing recombinant DNA-derived rabies vaccines. Large-scale administration of such vaccines to targeted animal species could eradicate rabies in certain animal populations, for example, raccoons, skunks, and foxes, thereby further reducing the necessity for many postexposure treatments. In 1987, these three species represented 73 percent of the total number of rabid animals in the United States. Additional efficacy and safety testing of candidate vaccines will be necessary before large-scale immunization efforts can be undertaken.[522]

Services and Protection Objectives

20.13 Expand immunization laws for schools, preschools, and day care settings to all States for all antigens. (Baseline: 9 States and the District of Columbia in 1990)

Baseline data source: Center for Prevention Services, CDC.

Currently all 50 States and the District of Columbia have immunization laws or requirements for students in some or all grades from kindergarten through grade 12 and children attending licensed day care facilities (table 20.13). In general, the number of antigens required by day care and public school laws are quite similar. In recent years, there has been a marked increase in the number of States strengthening their existing immunization laws by adding new vaccine requirements and expanding coverage into the day care area.

Antigen	Day Care*	Some grades, including at least kindergarten - first grade	K-12th Grade
Measles	51	5	46
Mumps	41	20	20
Rubella	51	8	43
Polio	51	5	46
Diphtheria	51	5	46
Tetanus	40	5	43
Pertussis	46	42	NA
Haemophilus b	9	NA	NA

*Idaho is the only State without any day care regulation for immunization.

Fig. 20.13

Requirements of the 50 States and the District of Columbia

20.14 Increase to at least 90 percent the proportion of primary care providers who provide information and counseling about immunizations and offer immunizations as appropriate for their patients. (Baseline data available in 1992)

Currently, preschool children and adults in high-risk groups are underimmunized. Physicians, nurses, and other health care providers (including midwives) have a key role in influencing attitudes of patients regarding appropriate immunization. Shaping the attitudes and future practices of medical, nursing, and other health providers is critical to ensuring that appropriate immunizations are provided to their patients. Thousands of cases of illness and associated deaths can be prevented (especially in adults) with available vaccines. In the Rand Health Insurance Experiment, only 45 percent of infants received timely immunization against DTP and polio and only 4 percent of adults received a tetanus shot in the 3-year study period. Of particular importance is that free health care alone was not a sufficient incentive to ensure that participating patients received recommended levels of preventive services.[523]

Between 19 and 50 percent of primary care physicians offer tetanus immunization to patients.[524] . . .

Barriers to widespread administration of immunizations include patient reluctance to receive vaccines because of possible discomfort, potential side effects, or inconvenience and health care providers' failure to offer these primary preventive services to patients.

20.15 Improve the financing and delivery of immunizations for children and adults so that virtually no American has a financial barrier to receiving recommended immunizations. (Baseline: Financial coverage for immunizations was included in 45 percent of employment-based insurance plans with conventional insurance plans; 62 percent with Preferred Provider Organization plans; and 98 percent with Health Maintenance Organization plans in 1989; Medicaid covered basic immunizations for eligible children and Medicare covered pneumococcal immunization for eligible older adults in 1990)

Baseline data source: Health Insurance Association of America Survey 1989; Center for Prevention Services, CDC.

Immunization represents a partnership between the public and private sectors. The private sector is the source of immunizations for approximately 50 percent of children and almost all adults. Estimates of series completion among children by 2 years of age range from 50 percent to 82 percent. Vaccine coverage among adults is worse. Only about 20 percent of the target population receive annual influenza vaccinations, and 10 percent of the target population is believed to be immunized against pneumococcal disease. Cost, a potential barrier to immunization in both the private and public sectors, has escalated substantially in recent years. In 1982, the cost of vaccines to fully immunize a child in the private sector was approximately $23.29. In 1988, the cost had risen to approximately $128.06, not including any added costs for office visits.

* * *

20.17 Increase to at least 90 percent the proportion of local health departments that have ongoing programs for actively identifying cases of tuberculosis and latent infection in populations at high risk for tuberculosis. (Baseline data available in 1991)

Note: Local health department refers to any local component of the public health system, defined as an administrative and service unit of local or State government concerned with health and carrying some responsibility for the health of a jurisdiction smaller than a State.

People at high risk for tuberculosis include recent contacts of infectious cases, foreign-born persons from high-prevalence areas, high-risk minority populations, the homeless, migrant workers, people in nursing homes and correctional institutions, and known or suspected HIV-infected persons. It is estimated that at least one-half of reported cases, and a higher proportion of people infected without current disease, fall into one or more of these high-risk populations. Therefore, targeting, screening, and prevention activities aimed at these populations could have a profound impact on reducing future tuberculosis illness and death.

* * *

Research Needs

Priorities for research to improve immunization and infectious disease control during the 1990s include the following:

- Development and introduction of new or improved vaccines including (acellular) pertussis, *H. influenzae* type b, tuberculosis, respiratory syncytial virus, malaria, rotavirus, measles, *S. pneumoniae*, Group B streptococcus, measles, and parainfluenza virus type 3.

- Clarification of the relationship between whole-cell pertussis vaccines and serious neurologic reactions and investigation of possible adverse effects of vaccines.

- Evaluation of the effectiveness of a two-dose measles vaccines schedule.

- Elucidation and evaluation of the optimal schedule for combined use of inactivated and live poliovirus vaccines.

- Development and evaluation of rapid, sensitive, and specific diagnostic tests for measles and tuberculosis, as well as emerging infectious diseases such as Lyme disease.

- Development of effective immunoadjuvants to improve the efficacy of currently available vaccines for children, . . . and the immunocompromised.

- Refinement of *Streptococcus pneumoniae* vaccine for use in infants and young children to prevent otitis media complications.

* * *

Data Source References

Center for Infectious Diseases, Centers for Disease Control, Public Health Service, U.S. Department of Health and Human Services, Atlanta, GA.

Center for Prevention Services, Centers for Disease Control, Public Health Service, U.S. Department of Health and Human Services, Atlanta, GA.

Health Insurance Association of America, Washington, DC.

National Health Interview Survey, National Center for Health Statistics, Centers for Disease Control, Public Health Service, U.S. Department of Health and Human Services, Hyattsville, MD.

Clinical Preventive Services

21

Contents

***

21.2 Receipt of recommended services

21.3 Access to primary care

21.4 Financial barriers to receipt of services

21.5 Clinical preventive services from publicly funded programs

21.6 Provision of recommended services by clinicians

21.7 Public health department assurance of access

21.8 Racial/ethnic minority representation in the health professions

[Research Needs]

21. Clinical Preventive Services

* * *

Risk Reduction Objective

21.2 Increase to at least 50 percent the proportion of people who have received, as a minimum within the appropriate interval, all of the screening and immunization services and at least one of the counseling services appropriate for their age and gender as recommended by the U.S. Preventive Services Task Force. (Baseline data available in 1991)

Special Population Targets

	Receipt of Recommended Services	Baseline	2000 Target
21.2a	Infants up to 24 months	—	90%
21.2b	Children aged 2-12	—	80%
21.2c	Adolescents aged 13-18	—	50%
21.2d	Adults aged 19-39	—	40%
21.2g	Low-income people	—	50%
21.2h	Blacks	—	50%
21.2i	Hispanics	—	50%
21.2j	Asians/Pacific Islanders	—	50%
21.2k	American Indians/Alaska Natives	—	70%
21.2l	People with disabilities	—	80%

The effectiveness of preventive services in reducing morbidity and premature mortality is well documented. Yet the full public health benefit to be derived from clinical preventive services remains to be achieved. Many clinical preventive services are underutilized. Few, if any, individuals receive all of the services that would benefit them. Furthermore, many of those most in need of clinical preventive services are least likely to receive them.

No reliable national estimates are available on the extent to which individuals receive complete or even minimal sets of essential preventive services. Only a few studies have examined the receipt of services either as sets or in series. For example, the Rand Health Insurance Study found that although 93 percent of newborns had received at least one well-child examination, only 44 percent had received three or more doses of diphtheria-pertussis-tetanus (DPT) vaccine and three or more doses of polio vaccine by age 18 months.[517] An ambulatory care quality assurance study also found well-child care inadequate in delivering complete sets of recommended preventive services.[525]

Analysis of data from the National Health Interview Survey revealed significant increases in the use of eight routine preventive services among adults and children between 1973 and 1982.[526] The study also found that low-income people, people with low levels of education, and people of Hispanic origin were among the least likely to have ever received all eight screening procedures.

* * *

Access to optimal preventive care for the indigent and minorities may be further compromised by the type of settings in which they seek care. Physicians who serve more than a 50-percent minority Medicaid patient population see more patients, spend less time with each patient, and tend to incorporate fewer preventive practices into their encounters with patients than do physicians who have more affluent, predominantly white patients.[527]

This objective seeks to increase the proportion of Americans who receive a minimum set of recommended clinical preventive services: the age-, gender-, and risk-appropriate services recommended by the U.S.Preventive Services Task Force.[45] However, for reasons of attainability and tracking, this objective specifically targets a subset of the services recommended by the U.S. Preventive Services Task Force: all of the age- and gender-appropriate screening and immunization services and at least one age- and gender-appropriate counseling service. The receipt of risk-appropriate services and the receipt of all recommended counseling services will not be tracked. Baseline data are unavailable even for this subset of recommended services, however. But baseline estimates are available for many of the individual services, and the baseline estimate for any age group can be no higher than the estimate for the least utilized service recommended for that age group. For most age groups, immunizations appear to be the least utilized service (e.g., a tetanus-diphtheria booster within the preceding 10 years for people aged 13-18, 19-39, 40-64, and 65 and older; a pneumococcal vaccine and annual influenza vaccine for people aged 65 and older). Thus, the baseline estimates for this objective are largely driven by immunization rates (see *Immunization and Infectious Diseases*), and the age group targets have been set accordingly. Although the baseline estimates for low-income and racial and ethnic minority groups are likely lower than that for the total population, the targets for racial and ethnic minorities have been set at least equivalent to the overall population target to eliminate any gap in the receipt of a minimum set of essential clinical preventive services. Higher targets were established for American Indians and Alaska Natives and people with disabilities because of the opportunities these groups have for interaction with the Indian Health Service and the health care system, respectively.

Services and Protection Objectives

21.3 **Increase to at least 95 percent the proportion of people who have a specific source of ongoing primary care for coordination of their preventive and episodic health care. (Baseline: Less than 82 percent in 1986, as 18 percent reported having no physician, clinic, or hospital as a regular source of care)**

Special Population Targets

Percentage With Source of Care		1986 Baseline	2000 Target
21.3a	Hispanics	70%	95%
21.3b	Blacks	80%	95%
21.3c	Low-income people	80%	95%

Baseline data source: The Robert Wood Johnson Foundation 1986.

Access to clinical preventive services depends in part on access to an ongoing source of primary care. Increasing access to primary care can help to increase access to clinical preventive services for many of those most in need of these services. Ideally, access should be to a well-organized system of primary care, staffed by well-trained primary care providers, with established and well-functioning networks into the community.

In 1986, 18 percent of Americans—43 million Americans overall—reported having no physician, clinic or hospital as a regular source of medical care.[528] Sixteen percent reported needing health care but having difficulty obtaining it. The uninsured were almost twice as likely to be without a regular source of care as the insured—31 percent and 16 percent, respectively. Twenty percent of the poor (family income below 150 percent of the poverty level) reported no regular source of care. Blacks were less likely to have a regular source of care than whites, 20 percent compared to 16 percent. Between 1982 and 1986, the percentage of Hispanics reporting no regular source of care tripled from 10 percent to 30 percent. Urban and rural dwellers experience approximately equal access to the health care system.[528]

Even among Americans with a regular source of care, many lack access to a well-organized system of competent primary care. Competent primary care focuses on the health needs of individuals and families; is the "first contact" health care in the view of the patient; provides at least 80 percent of necessary care; provides a comprehensive array of services, on site or through referral, including health promotion and disease prevention as well as curative services; and is accessible and acceptable to the patient population. Primary care is typically rendered by general practitioners, family practitioners, internists, pediatricians, obstetrician/gynecologists, and mid-level practitioners (e.g., physician assistants, nurse practitioners). The primary care provider coordinates services for the family and patient; accepts continuing responsibility for the patient regardless of the presence or the type of diseases; provides continuity of care, with linkages to secondary and tertiary care; attempts to integrate and coordinate all of the physical, psychological, and social aspects of patient care; and is responsible for the quality and potential effects of the services. This type of care emphasizes caring for the patient's general health needs as opposed to a more specialized or fragmented approach to medical care. The concepts of comprehensiveness of services, coordination of services, and continuity of care are essential.[529,530,531,532,533]

Studies have demonstrated that comprehensive public/private collaborative community efforts can reduce access barriers to primary care and increase use of preventive services.[534,535,536,537] Several recent studies with discrete populations of underserved or uninsured and underinsured individuals have demonstrated improved health outcomes and reductions in inappropriate use of emergency services following increased access to primary care.[538]

21.4 Improve financing and delivery of clinical preventive services so that virtually no American has a financial barrier to receiving, at a minimum, the screening, counseling, and immunization services recommended by the U.S. Preventive Services Task Force. (Baseline data available in 1992)

A primary and often-cited barrier to the utilization of clinical preventive services is financial. Financial barriers can be reduced in several ways. These approaches reflect the multiple sources of financing for clinical preventive services—out-of-pocket payments by individuals, direct provision of services by public health clinics and programs, sponsorship by employers at the worksite, delivery by primary care providers in the context of a managed care program, or reimbursement as part of a conventional health insurance package.

For many Americans, out-of-pocket payments are currently the major source of financing for clinical preventive services. Consumers and providers alike list cost as a barrier to greater use of these services. However, a number of preventive services can be efficiently incorporated into routine acute and chronic disease care by primary care providers at little or no increased cost to consumers. Furthermore, many preventive services can be offered at lower cost to individuals when services are efficiently organized, take advantage of economies of scale, and rely more on allied health professionals for delivery.... Relative increases in the median per capita income can also reduce the financial barriers associated with out-of-pocket payments for preventive services.

The direct provision of clinical preventive services by publicly funded programs is an important mechanism for overcoming financial barriers, especially for low-income populations (see Objective 21.5).

Private and public insurance coverage for clinical preventive services and managed care plans such as Health Maintenance Organizations (HMOs) and Preferred Provider Arrangements/Organizations (PPAs/PPOs) can also reduce financial barriers. General principles of economics suggest and a number of empirical studies confirm that people utilize preventive services more when the out-of-pocket cost is reduced through insurance coverage or managed care....

* * *

	Adult Physical Exams	Well-Baby Care	Preventive Diagnostic Tests
Conventional plan	27%	45%	61%
PPO	39%	62%	72%
HMO	97%	98%	98%
All plans*	41%	56%	69%
Estimated percentage of all Americans	26%	35%	43%

*Weighted average

Fig. 21.4 Percentage of people with employer-sponsored health insurance coverage for selected clinical preventive services

* * *

The recommendations of the U.S. Preventive Services Task Force[45] can provide scientifically sound guidance to health insurers and purchasers of group plans regarding which preventive services, at a minimum, to cover. Implementation of this objective could be facilitated by additional information about (1) the potential health benefits to be achieved among insured groups by providing these services, (2) the incremental costs and full range of benefits likely to result from coverage of these services, and (3) the relative cost-effectiveness of these services. Information about the effectiveness of a set of preventive services in achieving a given intervention outcome in relation to costs is important in making decisions about insurance and program coverage. Such analyses help public and private payers to compare and rank choices among services according to the magnitude of their short- and long-term effects relative to costs. Models to protect against overutilization of preventive services in the face of increased coverage could also facilitate implementation of this objective. Finally, educational efforts to increase consumer demand for clinical preventive services could help to reduce perceived barriers, increase consumer willingness to pay for these services relative to other goods and services, and increase their utilization.

21.5 **Assure that at least 90 percent of people for whom primary care services are provided directly by publicly funded programs are offered, at a minimum, the screening, counseling, and immunization services recommended by the U.S. Preventive Services Task Force. (Baseline data available in 1992)**

Note: Publicly funded programs that provide primary care services directly include federally funded programs such as the Maternal and Child Health Program, Community and Migrant Health Centers, and the Indian Health Service as well as primary care service settings funded by State and local governments. This objective does not include services covered indirectly through the Medicare and Medicaid programs.

Publicly funded providers of health care serve various high-risk groups and derive their funds from several sources. Federal support is provided to the Maternal and Child Health program, Community and Migrant Health Centers, the National Health Service Corps, [and] the Indian Health Service (IHS), . . . among others. State and local governments also provide funding for primary care service settings, which present an opportunity to provide preventive services.

The Maternal and Child Health Block Grant Program provides Federal and matching State funds to enable States to promote health; prevent death, disease, and disability; and ensure access to high-quality, comprehensive, and coordinated systems of care for mothers, children, and other family members, particularly those with low incomes or limited access to care. Children with special health care needs due to chronic or disabling conditions also are included. Most States use a mix of service delivery mechanisms to provide screening, counseling, and immunization services for these populations. Services may be provided through local health departments, community health centers, private physicians, school-based clinics, and State-administered clinics.

The federally supported Community and Migrant Health Center and Health Care for the Homeless programs both deliver preventive services as part of comprehensive primary care. Currently, several categories of preventive services must be offered to clients through the Community and Migrant Health Center program, and additional services are provided, as required, to meet the needs of specific individuals or populations. Specific preventive services have been initiated to target underserved women and their children, populations at risk for HIV infection, HIV-infected people, and intravenous drug users. Where the services are high technology and high cost and not within the purview of the center, the center cannot necessarily assure these services at low cost to the consumer.

IHS provides preventive services through clinical staff on reservations and through community health personnel, forming integrated health teams that work within the Indian community. Services provided in these settings include prenatal, postnatal, and well-baby care; family planning; dental health; nutrition; immunizations; environmental health activities; and health education. IHS has an integrated approach to preventive care that combines community health nursing, dental health, medical social work, environmental health, and health education.

These and other publicly funded providers of health care services, such as the numerous State- and county-funded community programs, offer a wide range of opportunities to expand the range of preventive services offered. The recommendations of the U.S. Preventive Services Task Force[45] can provide scientifically sound guidance to publicly funded providers of health care regarding which preventive services to offer, at a minimum, to their clients. Additional information about the potential public health benefits and the relative cost-effectiveness of these services could facilitate implementation of this objective.

21.6 **Increase to at least 50 percent the proportion of primary care providers who provide their patients with the screening, counseling, and immunization services recommended by the U.S. Preventive Services Task Force. (Baseline data available in 1992)**

Primary care providers are optimally positioned in the health care system to provide preventive services. The public views physicians in particular as credible sources of health information. . . .

Primary care providers include general practitioners, family physicians, internists, pediatricians, obstetrician-gynecologists, physician assistants, nurse practitioners, and nurses. Advice from other health professionals (e.g., tobacco cessation counseling by oral health care providers, nutrition counseling by qualified dietitians) reaches even more people and serves to reinforce important messages for many patients. An interdisciplinary team approach to the provision of clinical preventive services is optimal.

* * *

Reasons given by physicians for their failure to practice more prevention include lack of time (70 percent), inadequate reimbursement (60 percent), and "unclear recommendations" (58 percent).[539] Other barriers include a lack of familiarity with current recommendations; attitudinal barriers such as lack of confidence, unrealistic expectations, and mistaken beliefs about efficacy; and lack of basic behavioral science skills and training.[540] Some of these barriers can be overcome through appropriate professional preparation and continuing education. Several randomized controlled trials have shown that physician compliance with disease prevention and control regimens can be improved with office reminder systems.[93,541,542] Among the tools used in practice are chart reminders and flowsheets, cues on computerized patient records, patient-held minirecords, and various forms of performance feedback.[543] Effectiveness in increasing the use of preventive services can be further enhanced by appropriate client tracking systems.

21.7 **Increase to at least 90 percent the proportion of people who are served by a local health department that assesses and assures access to essential clinical preventive services. (Baseline data available in 1992)**

Note: Local health department refers to any local component of the public health system, defined as an administrative and service unit of local or State government concerned with health and carrying some responsibility for the health of a jurisdiction smaller than a State.

The Institute of Medicine (IOM) report *The Future of Public Health* acknowledged past public health successes but described in detail problems within the U.S public health system.[276] The AIDS epidemic, which threatens the health of millions of Americans, has also brought the inadequacies of our public health system into high visibility. That same system is in critical need of improvement if the Nation is to address not only AIDS, but the burden of chronic diseases in our aging population and injuries and violence to our young. Both the Presidential Commission on HIV Infection and the IOM report outline steps necessary to strengthen the public health system and call for a plan of action for improvements. The desired outcome is a public health system effectively performing the core functions of public health agencies, which the IOM report identifies for all levels of government as assessment, policy development, and assurance. Specifically, with respect to access to care and clinical preventive services, public health agencies should (1) regularly and systematically collect, assemble, analyze, and make available information on the extent to which their constituents have full access to primary care and clinical preventive services, and (2) exercise their responsibility to serve the public interest in the development of comprehensive public health policies to assure their constituents' access to primary care and delivery of essential clinical preventive services.

The current public health system is built around a system of governmental agencies—primarily Federal, State, and local health departments. Other critical participants in the system include clinical medicine, voluntary agencies, schools and universities, business and industry, professional associations, community organizations, and third-party payers. A governmental presence is needed at the local level to provide the leadership to assure that necessary services are provided. Consensus must be developed and institutionalized on the appropriate roles, attributes, and standards of effective performance of all parties within the public health system to fully realize the benefits of primary care and clinical preventive services.

The public health community has recognized these problems and has initiated three landmark actions that have helped focus opinion on the need for definition and consensus with respect to the public health and health care systems. In 1979, the publication of *Model Standards: A Guide for Community Preventive Health Services* advanced the concept of a governmental presence at the local level to assure the public's health.[544] In 1988, *The Future of Public Health* proposed the core functions of public health.[276] In 1989, the U.S. Preventive Services Task Force published the *Guide to Clinical Preventive Services*.[45]

In addition, the 1990 objectives played an important role by providing direction and focus to the efforts of the public health system. However, the objectives did not specifically address the inadequacies in the system itself that might adversely affect their achievement. A public health system effectively carrying out the core functions will assure that scarce public health resources are directed to address identified health problems of high priority. If achievement of the year 2000 national health objectives is to be a reality, there must be a public health system with the capacity to effectively carry out the necessary strategies. This cross-cutting objective will help to assure the existence, effectiveness, and appropriate distribution of that capacity.

21.8 **Increase the proportion of all degrees in the health professions and allied and associated health profession fields awarded to members of underrepresented racial and ethnic minority groups as follows:**

Degrees Awarded To:	1985-86 Baseline	2000 Target
Blacks	5%	8%
Hispanics	3%	6.4%
American Indians/Alaska Natives	0.3%	0.6%

Note: Underrepresented minorities are those groups consistently below parity in most health profession schools—blacks, Hispanics, and American Indians and Alaska Natives.

Baseline data source: Health Resources and Services Administration.

Minority and disadvantaged communities lag behind the U.S. population on virtually all health status indicators. Furthermore, among the poor, minorities, and the uninsured, access to medical care has been deteriorating.[528] Increasing the number of minority health professionals may offer a partial solution to this public health crisis. Several studies have shown that underrepresented minority health profession graduates are more likely to enter primary care specialties and to voluntarily practice in or near designated primary care health manpower shortage areas.[545,546,547,548] In one study, 75 percent of black physicians were practicing in or near shortage areas, 90 percent had patient loads that were at least 50-percent minority, two-thirds had 70-percent minority patient loads, and one-third had 90-percent minority loads. Similarly, of Chicanos graduated from California medical schools, 75 percent chose to practice in or near designated shortage areas. Analyses of the regional distribution patterns of minority physicians show that the distribution patterns for black and American Indian physicians in particular appear to be influenced by the location of substantial numbers of like minorities.[546] It is estimated that 60 to 80 percent of the underrepresented minority students trained in the health professions voluntarily practice in or close to designated shortage areas with overwhelmingly minority patient populations.[548]

According to the 1980 census, members of racial and ethnic minority groups accounted for about 20 percent of the U.S. population: blacks accounted for an estimated 11.5 percent, Hispanics 6.4 percent, Asians and Pacific Islanders 1.5 percent, and Native Americans and Alaska Natives 0.6 percent. In the year 2000, racial and ethnic minorities are expected to comprise a little more than 25 percent of the population, with blacks and Hispanics accounting for more than 13 and 9 percent, respectively.

Though comprising a sizeable portion of the population, some minorities are not well represented among health and allied and associated health personnel. It is estimated that, in 1987, blacks accounted for only about 3 percent of practicing allopathic and osteopathic physicians, 2 percent of dentists, 4 percent of registered nurses, 7 percent of therapists, and 2 percent of dental hygienists. Hispanics were estimated to comprise about 5 percent of practicing physicians, 3 percent of dentists, and 1 percent of registered nurses.[549]

Although fewer than 1 in 10 undergraduates were from a minority group in the late 1960s, minorities dramatically increased their numbers in colleges and universities during the 1970s and early 1980s. By the academic year 1984-85, more than 1 in 6 undergraduate students and more than 1 in 9 students in graduate-level first professional degree programs were minorities.[545] (First professional degree programs include dentistry, medicine, optometry, osteopathic medicine, pharmacy, podiatry, veterinary medicine, chiropractic, law, and theological professions.)

In academic year 1985-86, underrepresented minorities comprised 8.3 percent of the graduates from schools of public health, 9.1 percent of the graduates from schools of allopathic medicine, 3.7 percent of schools of osteopathic medicine, and 7.2 percent of the graduates from schools of dentistry. Underrepresented minorities totaled 8 percent of the graduates of registered nurse (RN) baccalaureate programs in 1984-1985. Of those graduating from schools of medicine, schools of osteopathic medicine, schools of dentistry, and RN baccalaureate programs, blacks comprised 5.1, 1.5, 4.0, and 5.3 percent, respectively. Hispanics constituted 3.7 percent of the graduates from schools of medicine, 1.4 percent of the graduates from schools of osteopathic medicine, 3.1 percent of the graduates from schools of dentistry, and 2.4 percent of the graduates from RN baccalaureate programs. Only 0.3, 0.8, and 0.2 percent of the graduates from schools of medicine, osteopathic medicine, and dentistry, respectively, were Native Americans.[545,547,550]

Total enrollment figures for 1986-87 place the enrollment for underrepresented minorities at 8.7 percent in schools of allopathic medicine, 5.1 percent in schools of osteopathic medicine, and 10.1 percent in schools of dentistry. Of those enrolled in schools of allopathic medicine, osteopathic medicine, and dentistry, blacks comprised 5.9, 1.8, and 5.5 percent, respectively. Hispanics accounted for 5.3 percent of the enrollment in schools of allopathic medicine, 2.7 percent of the enrollment in schools of osteopathic medicine, and 4.3 percent of the enrollment in schools of dentistry. Native Americans comprised 0.4 percent of the enrollment in schools of allopathic medicine, 0.6 percent of the enrollment in schools of osteopathic medicine, and 0.3 percent of the enrollment in schools of dentistry. The most recent enrollment figures for schools of public health are for 1987-88. At that time, underrepresented minorities constituted 13.9 percent of total enrollment, with blacks representing 6.2 percent; Hispanics, 6.7 percent; and Native Americans, 1.0 percent, respectively.

Despite considerable effort to increase the number of minorities in health professional and allied and associated health professional schools, the rate of increase in the number of minority entrants, enrollees, and graduates has been slowing since the mid-1970s. Although the absolute number of underrepresented minorities entering, enrolled in, and graduating from many of these schools has increased, the percentage of these minorities in the universe of entrants and graduates has changed very little. The targets set for the year 2000 present a significant challenge. Attaining this objective will require an expansion of the following activities: financial assistance for minority students to pursue health care degrees; mentor relationships; early recruitment, such as expansion of the Health Careers Opportunities Program; and increasing minority faculty and administrative staff in schools that train health care professionals.

* * *

Research Needs

Gaps in the scientific evidence identified in the U.S. Preventive Services Task Force's *Guide to Clinical Preventive Services* underscore the magnitude of the research agenda in preventive medicine. For many of the topics evaluated in the *Guide*, the Task Force found inadequate evidence to evaluate their effectiveness or to determine their optimal frequency of delivery. In many cases, the necessary studies had never been performed. In other instances, studies performed lacked reliability due to improper study design or systematic biases. Better quality research, not merely more research, to evaluate the effectiveness of clinical preventive services is warranted. High priority research needs [in child and adolescent health] include:

- The impact of clinical preventive services on quality of life, not just survival.
- The efficacy, effectiveness, optimal frequency, and efficiency (i.e., cost-effectiveness) of clinical preventive services.
- The utilization of clinical preventive services.
- The impact of incentives and different forms of reimbursement on the implementation of clinical preventive services in primary care.

Baseline Data Source References

Bureau of Health Professions, Health Resources and Services Administration, Public Health Service, U.S. Department of Health and Human Services, Rockville, MD.

The Robert Wood Johnson Foundation. *Access to Health Care in the United States: Results of a 1986 Survey.* Special Report Number Two/1987. Princeton, NJ: the Foundation, 1987.

References

[1] Caspersen, C.J.; Powell, K.E.; and Christenson, G.M. Physical activity, exercise and physical fitness: Definitions and distinctions for health-related research. *Public Health Reports* 101:126-131, 1986.

[2] Leon, A.S.; Connett, J.; Jacobs, D.R.; and Raurama, R. Leisure-time physical activity levels and risk of coronary heart disease and death: The multiple risk factor intervention trial. *Journal of the American Medical Association* 258:2388-2395, 1987.

[3] Sallis, J.F.; Haskell, W.L.; Fortmann, S.P.; Wood, P.D.; and Vranizan, K.M. Moderate-intensity physical activity and cardiovascular risk factors: The Stanford five-city project. *Preventive Medicine* 15:561-568, 1986.

[4] Leon, A.S. Effects of physical activity and fitness on health. In: National Center for Health Statistics. *Assessing Physical Fitness and Physical Activity in Population-Based Surveys.* DHHS Pub. No. (PHS)89-1253. Hyattsville, MD: U.S. Department of Health and Human Services, 1989.

[5] Pollock, M.L.; Gettman, L.R.; Milesis, C.A.; Bah, M.D.; Durstine, J.L.; and Johnson, R.B. Effects of frequency and duration of training on attrition and the incidence of injury. *Medicine and Science in Sports and Exercise* 9:31-36, 1977.

[6] American College of Sports Medicine. American College of Sports Medicine position stand: The recommended quantity and quality of exercise for developing and maintaining cardiorespiratory and muscular fitness in healthy adults. *Medicine and Science in Sports and Exercise* 22:265-274, 1989.

[7] American College of Sports Medicine. *Guidelines of Exercise Testing and Exercise Prescription.* Philadelphia, PA: Lea and Febiger, 1988.

[8] Blair, S.N.; Kohl, H.W.; Paffenbarger, R.S.; Clark, D.G.; Cooper, K.H.; and Gibbons, L.W. Physical fitness and all-cause mortality: A prospective study of healthy men and women. *Journal of the American Medical Association* 262:2395-2401, 1989.

[9] Paffenbarger, R.S.; Wing, A.L.; and Hyde, R.T. Physical activity as an index of heart attack risk in college alumni. *American Journal of Epidemiology* 108:161-175, 1978.

[10] Buskirk, E.R. and Hodgson, J.L. Age and aerobic power: The rate of change in men and women. *Federal Proceedings* 46:1824-1829, 1987.

[11] Caspersen, C.J.; Pollard, R.A.; and Pratt, S.O. Scoring physical activity data with special consideration for elderly populations. In: *Data for an Aging Population*, pp. 30-34. DHHS Pub. No. (PHS) 88-1214. Washington, DC: U.S. Department of Health and Human Services, 1987.

[12] Caspersen, C.J.; Christenson, G.M.; and Pollard, R.A. Status of the 1990 physical fitness and exercise objectives—Evidence from NHIS-1985. *Public Health Reports* 101:587-592, 1986.

[13] Gettman, L.R.; Ayres, J.J.; Pollock, M.L.; and Jackson, A. The effect of circuit weight training on strength, cardiorespiratory function, and body composition of adult men. *Medicine and Science in Sports and Exercise* 10:171-176, 1978.

[14] Wilmore, J.H.; Parr, R.B.; Girandola, R.N.; Ward, P.; Vodak, P.A.; Barstow, T.J.; Pipes, T.V.; Romero, G.T.; and Leslie, P. Physiological alterations consequent to circuit weight training. *Medicine and Science in Sports and Exercise* 10:79-84, 1987.

[15] Wilmore, J.H. *Training for Sport and Activity.* 2nd edition. Boston, MA: Allyn and Bacon, 1982.

[16] Cady, L.D.; Bischoff, D.P.; O'Connell, E.R.; Thomas, P.C.; and Allan, J.H. Strength and fitness and subsequent back injuries in firefighters. *Journal of Occupational Medicine* 21:269-272, 1979.

[17] Passmore, R. The regulation of body weight in man. *Proceedings of the Nutrition Society* 30:122-127, 1971.

[18] Wood, P.D.; Stefanick, M.L.; Dreon, D.M.; Frey-Hewitt, D.; Garay, B.C.; Williams, P.T.; Superko, H.R.; Fortman, S.P.; Albers, J.J.; Vranizan, K.M.; Ellsworth, N.M.; Terry, R.B.; and Haskell, W.L. Changes in plasma lipids and lipoproteins in overweight men during weight loss through dieting as compared with exercise. *New England Journal of Medicine* 319:1173-1179, 1988.

[19] Epstein, L.H. and Wing, R.R. Aerobic exercise and weight. *Addictive Behavior* 3:371-388, 1980.

[20] U.S. Department of Health and Human Services. National children and youth fitness study. *Journal of Physical Education, Recreation, and Dance* 56:44-90, 1985.

[21] U.S. Department of Health and Human Services. National children and youth fitness study II. *Journal of Physical Education, Recreation, and Dance* 58:50-96, 1987.

[22] Bennett, W.J. *First Lessons: A Report on Elementary Education in America.* Washington, DC: U.S. Department of Education, 1986.

[23] Siedentop, D. *Developing Teaching Skills in Physical Education.* Palo Alto, CA: Mayfield, 1983.

[24] Sullivan, K. Personal communication. National Center for Health Statistics, 1990.

[25] Public Health Service. *The Surgeon General's Report on Nutrition and Health.* DHHS (PHS) Pub. No. 88-50210. Washington, DC: U.S. Department of Health and Human Services, 1988.

[26] Life Sciences Research Office, Federation of American Societies for Experimental Biology. *Nutrition Monitoring in the United States-An Update Report on Nutrition Monitoring.* DHHS Pub. No. (PHS)89-1255. Washington, DC: U.S. Department of Agriculture and U.S. Department of Health and Human Services, September, 1989.

[27] Rowland, M.L. A nomogram for computing body mass index. *Dietetic Concepts* 16(2):5-12, 1989.

[28] Stewart, A.L.; Brook, R.H.; and Kane, R.L., eds. Measurement of overweight and obesity as reported in the literature. In :*Conceptualization and Measurement of Health Habits for Adults in the Health Insurance Study: Vol. II*, pp. 5-20. Santa Monica, CA: The Rand Corporation, 1980.

[29] National Heart, Lung, and Blood Institute. *The Report of the Expert Panel on Population Strategies for Blood Cholesterol Reduction.* National Cholesterol Education Program of the National Heart, Lung, and Blood Institute Washington, DC: U.S. Department of Health and Human Services, 1990.

[30] National Research Council. *Diet and Health: Implications for Reducing Chronic Disease Risk.* Washington, DC: National Academy Press, 1989.

[31] Levy, A.S., and Stephenson, M.G. "Nutrition Knowledge Levels: 1983-88," submitted for publication.

[32] National Research Council. *Recommended Dietary Allowances.* 10th Edition. Washington, DC: National Academy Press, 1989.

[33] Food and Drug Administration, Division of Consumer Studies, *Health and Diet Survey.* Unpublished data, 1988.

[34] Life Sciences Research Office, Federation of American Societies for Experimental Biology. *Assessment of the Iron Nutritional Status of the U.S. Population Based on Data Collected in the Second National Health and Nutrition Examination Survey, 1976-1980.* Bethesda, MD: the Federation, 1984.

[35] Centers for Disease Control. CDC criteria for anemia in children and child-bearing/aged women. *Morbidity and Mortality Weekly Report* 38(22):400, 1989.

[36] Yip, R.; Binkin, N.; Fleshood, L.; and Trowbridge, F. Declining prevalence of anemia among low-income children in the United States. *JAMA* 258(12):1619-1623, 1987.

[37] U.S. Department of Agriculture and U.S. Department of Health and Human Services. *Dietary Guidelines for Americans.* Washington, DC: the Departments, 1985.

[38] Harris, L. and Associates. "Health: You've Got To Be Taught: An Evaluation of Comprehensive Health Education in American Public Schools, Summary." A survey conducted for Metropolitan Life Foundation. New York: the Foundation, 1988.

[39] American School Health Association; Association for the Advancement of Health Education; and Society for Public Health Education, Inc. *The National Adolescent Student Health Survey.* Oakland, CA: the Third Party Publishing Company, 1989.

[40] National Center for Health Statistics. *Health, United States, 1989.* DHHS Pub. No. (PHS)90-1232. Washington, DC: U.S. Department of Health and Human Services, 1990.

[41] Caggiula, A.W.; Christakis, G.; Farrand, M.; Hulley, S.B.; Johnson, R.; Lasser, N.L.; Stamler, J.; and Widdowson, G. The multiple risk intervention trial (MRFIT). IV. Intervention on blood lipids. *Preventive Medicine* 10:443-475, 1987.

[42] National Center for Health Statistics. Health Promotion and Disease Prevention: United States, 1985, by Schoenborn, C.A. *Vital and Health Statistics.* Series 10, No. 163. DHHS Pub. No. (PHS)88-1591. Washington, D.C.: U.S. Department of Health and Human Services, 1988.

[43] American College of Physicians. Results of the American College of Physicians membership survey of prevention practices in adult medicine. *Annals of Internal Medicine*, in press.

[44] Lewis, C.E. Disease prevention and health promotion practices of primary care physicians in the United States. *American Journal of Preventive Medicine* 4(suppl.):9-16, 1988.

[45] U.S. Preventive Services Task Force. *Guide to Clinical Preventive Services: An Assessment of the Effectiveness of 169 Interventions.* Baltimore, MD: Williams and Wilkins, 1989.

[46] Jenkins, C.; McPhee, S.J.; Bonilla, N.T.H.; and Khiem, T.V. "Cancer Risks and Prevention Behaviors Among Vietnamese Refugees." Paper presented at annual meeting of the American Public Health Association, Boston, MA, November, 1988.

[47] Levine, B.L. "Cigarette Smoking Habits and Characteristics in the Laotian Refugee: A Perspective Pre-and Post-Resettlement." Paper presented at Refugee Health Conference, San Diego, CA, 1985.

[48] Rumbaut, R. *IHARP Study Data.* San Diego State University, 1986.

[49] Goldbaum, G.M.; Kendrick, J.S.; Hogelin; G.C.; Gentry, E.M.; and Behavioral Risk Factors Surveys Group. The relative impact of smoking and oral contraceptive use on women in the United States. *JAMA* 258:1339-1342, 1987.

[50] Office on Smoking and Health. *Reducing the Health Consequences of Smoking: 25 Years of Progress. A Report of the Surgeon General.* DHHS Pub. No. (CDC)89-8411. Washington, DC: U.S. Department of Health and Human Services, 1989.

[51] Pierce, J.P.; Fiore, M.C.; Novotny, T.E.; Hatziandreu, E.J.; and Davis, R.M. Trends in cigarette smoking in the United States: Projections to the year 2000. *JAMA* 261:61-65, 1989.

[52] National Center for Health Statistics. Smoking and other tobacco use: United States, 1987, by Schoenborn, C.A., and Boyd, G. *Vital and Health Statistics* Series 10, No. 169. DHHS Pub. No.(PHS)89-1597. Hyattsville, MD: U.S. Department of Health and Human Services, 1989.

[53] Prager, K.; Malin, H.; Spiegler, D.; VanNatta, P; and Placek P.J. Smoking and drinking behavior before and during pregnancy of married mothers of live born infants and still born infants. *Public Health Reports* 99:117-127, 1984.

[54] Kleinman, J.C.; and Kopstein, A. Smoking during pregnancy 1967-1980. *American Journal of Public Health* 77:823-825, 1987.

[55] Freedman, M.A.; Gay, G.A.; Brockert, J.E.; Potrzebowski, P.W; and Rothwell, C.J. The 1989 revisions of the U.S. standard certificates of live birth and death and the U.S. standard report of fetal death. *American Journal of Public Health* 78:168-172, 1988.

[56] Bachman, J.G.; Johnston, J.G.; and O'Malley, P.M. *Monitoring the Future: Questionnaire Responses from the Nation's High School Seniors.* Ann Arbor, Michigan: Institute for Social Research, University of Michigan, 1980,1981,1982,1984,1985,1986.

[57] Johnston, L.D. University of Michigan press release. Ann Arbor, MI: University of Michigan News Information Services, February 13, 1990.

[58] Johnston, L.D.; Bachman, J.G.; and O'Malley, P.M. *Monitoring the Future: Questionnaire Responses from the Nation's High School Seniors.* Ann Arbor, Michigan: Institute for Social Research, University of Michigan, 1980,1982,1984,1986.

[59] Bureau of the Census. *Educational attainment in the United States: March 1987 and 1986.* Current Population Report, Series P-20, No. 428. Washington, DC: U.S. Department of Commerce, 1988.

[60] Pirie, P.L.; Murray, D.M.; and Luepker, R.V. Smoking prevalence in a cohort of adolescents, including absentees, drop outs, and transfers. *American Journal of Public Health* 78:176-178, 1988.

[61] Kleinman, J.C.; and Madans, J.H. The effects of maternal smoking, physical stature, and educational attainment on the incidence of low birthweight. *American Journal of Epidemiology* 121(6):843-55, 1985.

[62] Office of Disease Prevention and Health Promotion. *National Survey of Worksite Health Promotion Activities: A Summary.* Washington, DC: U.S. Department of Health and Human Services, 1987.

[63] Kleinman, J.C.; Pierre, M.B.; Madans, J.H.; Land, J.H.; and Schramm, W.F. The effects of maternal smoking on infant and fetal mortality. *American Journal of Epidemiology* 127:274-288, 1988.

[64] Windsor, R.A., and Orleans, C.T. Guidelines and methodologic standards for smoking cessation intervention research among pregnant women: Improving the science and the art. *Health Education Quarterly* 13(Summer):131-161, 1986.

[65] Ershoff, D.H.; Mullen, P.D.; and Quinn, V.P. A randomized trial of a serialized self-help smoking cessation program for pregnant women in an HMO. *American Journal of Public Health* 79:182-187, 1989.

[66] Fiore, M.C.; Novotny, T.E.; Pierce, J.P.; Hatziandreu, E.J.; Patel, K.M.; and Davis R.M. Trends in cigarette smoking in the United States: The changing influence of race and gender. *Journal of the American Medical Association* 261:49-55, 1989.

[67] National Research Council, Committee on Passive Smoking. *Environmental Tobacco Smoke: Measuring Exposure and Assessing Health Effects.* Washington, DC: National Academy Press, 1986.

[68] Office on Smoking and Health. *The Health Consequences of Involuntary Smoking. A Report of the Surgeon General.* DHHS Pub. No. (CDC)87-8398. Washington, DC: U.S. Department of Health and Human Services, 1986.

[69] Greenberg, R.A.; Bauman, K.E.; Glover, L.H.; Strecher, V.J.; Kleinbaum, D.G.; Haley, N.J.; Stedman, H.C.; Fowler, M.G.; and Loda, F.A. Ecology of passive smoking by young infants. *Journal of Pediatrics* 114:774-780, 1989.

[70] Schwartz-Bickenbach, D.; Schulte-Hobein, B.; Abt, S.; Plum, C.; and Nau, H. Smoking and passive smoking during pregnancy and early infancy: Effects on birth weight, lactation period, and cotinine concentrations in mother's milk and infant's urine. *Toxicology Letters* 35:73-81, 1987.

[71] U.S. Environmental Protection Agency. *Environmental Tobacco Smoke: Indoor Air Facts No. 5.* Washington, DC: the Agency, 1989.

[72] Office on Smoking and Health. 1986 Adult Use of Tobacco Survey, unpublished data.

73. National Institute on Drug Abuse. *National Household Survey on Drug Abuse, 1988. Population Estimates.* DHHS Pub. No.(ADH)89-1636. Rockville, MD: U.S. Department of Health and Human Services, 1989.

74. Centers for Disease Control. Prevalence of oral lesions and smokeless tobacco use in Northern Plains Indians. *Morbidity and Mortality Weekly Report* 37:608-611, 1988.

75. Centers for Disease Control. School policies and programs on smoking and health—United States, 1988. *Morbidity and Mortality Weekly Report* 38(12):202-203, 1989.

76. National School Boards Association. *Smoke-Free Schools: A Progress Report.* Alexandria, VA: the Association, 1989.

77. Glynn, T.J. Essential elements of school-based smoking prevention programs. *Journal of School Health* 59:181-188, 1989.

78. Chen, M.S. Multidisciplinary indicators to measure the impact of P.L. 99-252 on decreasing smokeless tobacco use. (Data from the Centers for Disease Control funded project.) Columbus, OH: Ohio State University, 1988.

79. Centers for Disease Control. Cigarette Advertising—United States, 1988. *Morbidity and Mortality Weekly Report* 39:261-265, 1990.

80. Reid, D. Prevention of smoking among school children: Recommendations for policy development. *Health Education Journal* 44:3-12, 1985.

81. Warner, K.E. Smoking and health implications of a change in the federal excise tax. *Journal of the American Medical Association* 255:1028-1032, 1986b.

82. Davis, R.M. Current trends in tobacco advertising and marketing. *New England Journal of Medicine* 316:725-732, 1987.

83. Warner, K.E. *Selling Smoke: Cigarette Advertising and Public Health.* Washington, DC: American Public Health Association, 1986a.

84. American Medical Association. *Tobacco Use in America Conference: Final Report and Recommendations from the Health Community to the 101st Congress and the Bush Administration.* Chicago, IL: the Association, 1989.

85. McCarthy, W.J. Testimony at the hearings on advertising of tobacco products before the Subcommittee on Health and the Environment of the Committee on Energy and Commerce; House of Representatives, 99th Congress, 2nd Session. Serial No. 99-167, July 18, August 1, 1986.

86. Popper, E.T. Testimony at the hearings on advertising of tobacco products before the Subcommittee on Health and the Environment of the Committee on Energy and Commerce; House of Representatives, 99th Congress, 2nd Session, Serial No. 99-167, July 18, August 1, 1986.

87. Davis, R.M., and Jason, L.A. The distribution of free cigarette samples to minors. *American Journal of Preventive Medicine* 4:21-26, 1988.

88. Warner, K.E. Cigarette advertising and media coverage of smoking and health. *New England Journal of Medicine* 312:384-388, 1985.

89. American Cancer Society. *A Survey Concerning: Cigarette Smoking, Health Check-ups, Cancer Detection Tests. A Summary of the Findings.* Princeton, NJ: Gallup Organization, 1977.

90. Kottke, T.E.; Battista, R.N.; DeFriese, G.H.; and Brekke, M.L. Attributes of successful smoking cessation interventions in medical practice: A meta-analysis of 39 controlled trials. *JAMA* 259:2882-2889, 1988.

91. Russell, M.A.H.; Wilson, C.; Taylor, C.; and Baker, C.D. Effects of general practitioners' advice against smoking. *British Medical Journal* 287:1782-1785, 1983.

92. Glynn, T.J., and Manley, M.W. *How To Help Your Patients Stop Smoking: A National Cancer Institute Manual for Physicians.* Bethesda, MD: National Cancer Institute, U.S. Department of Health and Human Services, 1989.

93. Cohen, S.J.; Stookey, G.K.; Katz, B.P.; Drook, C.A.; and Smith, D.M. Encouraging primary care physicians to help smokers quit. *Annals of Internal Medicine* 110:648-652, 1989.

94. National Center for Health Services Research. *National Health Care Expenditures Study—Data Preview.* DHHS Pub. No. (PHS)83-3361. Hyattsville, MD: U.S. Department of Health and Human Services, 1983.

95. National Center for Health Statistics. Current Estimates from the National Health Interview Survey: United States, 1981. *Vital and Health Statistics* Series 10, No 141. DHHS Pub. No. (PHS)82-1569. Rockville, MD: U.S. Department of Health, Education, and Welfare, Oct. 1982.

96. Sobal, J.; Valente, C.M.; Muncie, H.L.; Levine, D.M.; and Deforge, B.R. Physicians' beliefs about the importance of 25 health promoting behaviors. *American Journal of Public Health* 75:1427-1428, 1985.

97. Wells, K.B.; Lewis, C.E.; Leake, B.; Schleiter, M.K.; and Brook, R.H. The practices of general and subspecialty internists in counseling about smoking and exercise. *American Journal of Public Health* 76:1009-1013, 1986.

98. Ginzel, K.H. The underemphasis on smoking in medical education. *New York State Journal of Medicine* 85:299-301, 1985.

99. Horton, J. Education programs on smoking prevention and smoking cessation for students and house staff in U.S. medical schools. *Cancer Detection and Prevention* 9:417-420, 1986.

[100] Wells, K.B.; Lewis, C.E.; Leake, B.; and Ware, J.E. Do physicians preach what they practice? A study of physicians' health habits and counseling practices. *JAMA* 252:2846-2848, 1984.

[101] Weschler, H.; Levine, S.; Idelson, R.K.; Rohmman, M.; and Taylor, J.O. The physician's role in health promotion. A survey of primary-care practitioners. *New England Journal of Medicine* 308:97-100, 1983.

[102] Davis, R.M. Uniting physicians against smoking: The need for a coordinated national strategy. *Journal of the American Medical Association* 259:2900-2901, 1988.

[103] Ockene, J.K. Physician-delivered interventions for smoking cessation: Strategies for increasing effectiveness. *Preventive Medicine* 16:723-737, 1987.

[104] Schuman, L.M. Progress and responsibilities of educators in smoking control. *Medical and Pediatric Oncology* 11:375-382, 1983.

[105] Public Health Service. *Health United States 1989 and Prevention Profile.* Washington, DC: U.S. Department of Health and Human Services, 1990.

[106] National Highway Traffic Administration. *Fatal Accident Reporting System, 1987.* Washington, DC: Department of Transportation, 1988.

[107] Public Health Service. *Surgeon General's Workshop on Drunk Driving - Proceedings.* Washington, DC: U.S. Department of Health and Human Services, 1989.

[108] Kandel, D.B. Reaching the hard-to-reach: Illicit drug use among high school absentees. *Addictive Diseases* 1:465-480, 1975.

[109] National Institute on Drug Abuse. *National Trends in Drug Use and Related Factors Among American High School Students and Young Adults, 1975-1986.* DHHS Pub. No. (ADM)87-1535. Washington, DC: U.S. Department of Health and Human Services, 1987.

[110] Jessor, R., and Jessor, S.L. Theory testing in longitudinal research on marijuana use. In: Kandel, D.B., ed. *Longitudinal Research on Drug Use.* Washington, DC: Hemisphere, 1978.

[111] Robins, L.N., and Przybeck, T.R. Age of onset of drug use as a factor in drug and other disorders. NIDA Research Monograph No. 56. In: Jones, C.L., and Battjes, R.J., eds. *Etiology of Drug Abuse: Implications for Prevention.* Washington, DC: U.S. Department of Health and Human Services, 1985.

[112] Holmberg, M.B. Longitudinal studies of drug abuse in a fifteen-year-old population. *ACTA Psychiatrica Scandinavia* 16:129-136, 1985.

[113] Kandel, D.B. Epidemiological and psychological perspectives on adolescent drug abuse. *Journal of American Academic Clinical Psychiatry* 21:328-347, 1982.

[114] Clayton, R.R., and Voss, H.L.. *Technical Review on Drug Abuse and Drop-outs, Report for National Institute on Drug Abuse,* 1982.

[115] Kandel, D.B. Stages in adolescent involvement in drug use. *Science* 190:912-914, 1975.

[116] Brooks, S.; Williams, G.; Stinson, F.; and Noble, J. *Surveillance Report #13: Apparent Per Capita Alcohol Consumption, National, State, and Regional Trends, 1977-1987.* Washington, DC: U.S. Department of Health and Human Services, 1989.

[117] National Institute on Alcohol Abuse and Alcoholism. *Sixth Special Report to the U.S. Congress on Alcohol and Health.* Washington, DC: U.S. Department of Health and Human Services, 1987.

[118] Bachman, J.G.; Johnston, L.D.; O'Malley, P.M.; and Humphrey, R.H. Explaining the recent decline in marijuana use: Differentiating effects of perceived risks, disapproval, and general lifestyle factors. *Journal of Health and Social Behavior* 29:92-112, 1988.

[119] National Institute on Drug Abuse. *Anabolic Steroid Use.* Washington, DC: U.S. Department of Health and Human Services, in press.

[120] Donovan, D.M. Driving while intoxicated: Different roads to and from the problem. *Criminal Justice and Behavior.* In press.

[121] Coate, D; and Grossman, M. Change in alcoholic beverage prices and legal drinking ages: Effects on youth alcohol use and motor vehicle mortality. *Alcohol Health and Research World* 12:22-26, 1987.

[122] Grossman, M.; Coate, D; and Arluck, G.M. Price sensitivity of alcoholic beverages in the United States: Youth alcohol consumption. In: Holder, H.D., ed. *Control Issues in Alcohol Abuse Prevention: Strategies for States and Communities.* Greenwich, CT: JAI Press, 1987.

[123] Coate, D.; and Grossman, M. Effects of alcoholic beverage prices and legal drinking ages on youth alcohol use. *Journal of Law and Economics.* 31:145-171, 1988.

[124] Cook, P. The effect of liquor taxes on drinking, cirrhosis and auto accidents. In: Moore, M.; and Gerstein, D., eds. *Alcohol and Public Policy: Beyond the Shadow of Prohibition.* Washington, DC: National Academy Press, 1981.

[125] Saffer, H.; and Grossman, M. Beer taxes, the legal drinking age, and youth motor vehicle fatalities. *Evaluation and Health Professions* 10:5-27, 1987.

[126] Phelps, C.E. Death and taxes. *Journal of Health Economics* 7:1-24, 1988.

[127] Manning, W.G.; Keller, E.B.; Newhouse, J.P.; Sloss, E.M.; and Wasserman, J. The taxes of sin: Do smokers and drinkers pay their way? *Journal of the American Medical Association* 26(11):1604-1609, 1989.

References

[128] Atkin, C.K. Alcoholic-beverage advertising: Its content and impact. In: *Control Issues in Alcohol Abuse Prevention: Strategies for States and Communities. Advances in Substance Abuse.* Suyppl. 1. Greenwich, CT: JAI Press, 1987.

[129] Hilton, M.E. Demographic characteristics and the frequency of heaving drinking as predictors of self-reported drinking problems. *British Journal of Addictions* 82:913-925, 1987.

[130] Douglass, R.L. Youth, alcohol and traffic accidents. In National Institute on Alcohol Abuse and Alcoholism. *Special Population Issues* Alcohol and Health Monography No. 4, DHHS Pub. No. (ADM)82-1193. Washington, DC: U.S. Department of Health and Human Services, 1982.

[131] Breed, W.; Wallack, L.; and Grube, J.W. Alcohol advertising in college newspapers: A seven year follow-up. Journal of American College Health, in press.

[132] Defoe, J.R.; and Breed, W. The problem of alcohol advertisements in college newspapers. *Journal of American College Health* 27:195-199, 1979.

[133] Rosen, M.A.; Logsdon, D.M.; Demak, M.M. Prevention and health promotion in primary care: baseline results on physicans from the INSURE project on life cycle preventive health services. *Preventive Medicine.* 13:535-548, 1984.

[134] Hayward, R.A.; Shapiro, M.F.; Corey, C.R.; and Freeman, H.E. "Who gets preventive care? Results from a new national survey." Presented at Concurrent Symposium A, SREPCIM Abstracts, April 1, 1987.

[135] National Center for Health Statistics. National Vital Statistics System. National Center for Health Statistics, Centers for Disease Control, Public Health Service, U.S. Department of Health and Human Services, Hyattsville, MD.

[136] Jones, E.F.; Forrest, J.D.; Goldman, N; Henshaw, S.; Lincoln, R.; Rosoff, J.I.; Westoff, C.F.; and Wulf, D. *Teenage Pregnancy in Industrialized Countries: A Study Sponsored by the Alan Guttmacher Institute* New Haven, CT: Yale University Press, 1986.

[137] Henshaw, S.K.; Kenney, A.M.; Somberg, D.; and Van Vort, J. *Teenage Pregnancy in the United States: The Scope of the Problem and State Responses.* New York: The Alan Guttmacher Institute, 1989.

[138] National Center for Health Statistics. Health aspects of pregnancy and childbearing. *Vital and Health Statistics* Series 23 No. 16. DHHS Pub.(PHS)881992-2316. Washington, DC: U.S. Department of Health and Human Services, 1986.

[139] National Research Council. *Risking the Future: Adolescent Sexuality, Pregnancy, and Childbearing.* Washington, DC: National Academy Press, 1987.

[140] Baldwin, W., and Cain, V. The children of teenage parents. *Family Planning Perspectives* 12(1):34-43, 1980.

[141] Furstenberg, F.F. Jr. *Unplanned Parenthood: The Social Consequences of Teenage Childbearing.* New York: Free Press, 1976.

[142] Marks, J.S., and Kreuter, M.W. Youth pregnancy: A community solution. *Journal of the American Medical Association* 257(24):3410, 1987.

[143] Hatcher, R.A.; Guest, F.; Stewart, F.; et al. *Contraceptive Technology, 1988-1989.* Atlanta, GA: Printed Matter, Inc., 1988.

[144] Trussell, J., and Kost, K. Contraceptive failure in the United States: a critical review of the literature. *Studies in Family Planning.* 18(5): Table 2, 1987.

[145] Gold, R.B. *Abortion and Women's Health: A Turning Point for America?* New York: The Alan Guttmacher Institute, 1990.

[146] Westoff, C.F. Contraceptive paths toward reduction of unintended pregnancy and abortion. *Family Planning Perspectives* 20(1):4-13, 1988.

[147] National Center for Health Statistics. *National Survey of Family Growth.* Hyattsville, MD: U.S. Department of Health and Human Services, 1988.

[148] Institute of Medicine, National Academy of Sciences. *Prenatal Care: Reaching Mothers, Reaching Infants.* Washington DC: National Academy Press, 1988.

[149] National Center for Health Statistics. Interval between births: United States, 1970-1977. *Vital and Health Statistics,* Series 21, No. 39, DHHS Pub.No. (PHS)81-1917. Washington, DC: U.S. Department of Health and Human Services, 1981 as cited by Institute of Medicine. Committee to Study the Prevention of Low Birthweight. *Preventing Low Birthweight.* Washington, DC: National Academy Press, 1985.

[150] Institute of Medicine, National Academy of Sciences, Committee to Study the Prevention of Low Birthweight. *Preventing Low Birthweight.* Washington DC: National Academy Press, 1985.

[151] Office of Technology Assessment, U.S. Congress. *Infertility: Medical and Social Choices.* Washington, DC: The Office, May, 1988.

[152] National Committee for Adoption. *Adoption Factbook: United States Data, Issues, Regulations, and Resources.* Washington, DC: the Committee, 1985.

[153] Henshaw, S.K., and Orr, M.T. The need and unmet need for infertility services in the United States. *Family Planning Perspectives* 19(4):180-183,186, 1987.

[154] Hirsch, M.B., and Mosher, W.D. Characteristics of infertile women in the United States and their use of infertility services. *Fertility and Sterility* 46(4):618-625, 1987.

[155] Family Impact Seminars. *The Crisis in Foster Care: New Directions for the 1990s.* January 19, 1990.

[156] Planned Parenthood Federation of America, Inc. *First Things First.* New York: the Federation, 1989.

[157] Hogan, D.P., and Kitagawa, E.M. "Family Factors in the Fertility of Black Adolescents." Paper presented at the annual meeting of the Population Association of America, 1983.

[158] Jessor, R.; Costa, F.; Jessor, S.L.; and Donovan, J.E. The time of first intercourse: A prospective study. *Journal of Personality and Social Psychology* 44:608-626, 1983.

[159] National Center for Health Statistics. Married and unmarried couples: United States, 1982. *Vital and Health Statistics*, Series 23, No. 15. DHHS Pub.No.(PHS)871991-2315. Washington, DC: U.S. Department of Health and Human Services, 1987.

[160] Zabin, L.S. The association between smoking and sexual behavior among teens in U.S. contraceptive clinics. *American Journal of Public Health* 74:261-263, 1984.

[161] Zabin, L.S.; Hardy J.B.; Smith E.A., et al. Substance use and its relation to sexual activity among inner-city adolescents. *Journal of Adolescent Health Care* 7:320-331, 1986.

[162] Billy, J.O.G.; Landale, N.S.; Grady, W.R.; and Zimmerle, D.D. *Final Report: Effects of Sexual Activity on Adolescent Social and Psychological Development.* Seattle, WA: Battelle Human Affairs Research Centers, 1986.

[163] Devaney, B.L., and Hubley, K.S. *The Determinants of Adolescent Pregnancy and Childbearing.* Final report to the National Institute of Child Health and Human Development. Washington, DC: Mathematica Policy Research, 1981.

[164] Jessor, S.L., and Jessor, R. Transition from virginity to nonvirginity among youth: A social-psychological study over time. *Developmental Psychology* 11(4):473-484, 1975.

[165] Moore, K.A.; Peterson, J.L.; and Furstenberg, F.F., Jr. "Starting Early: The Antecedents of Early, Premarital Intercourse." Revised draft of a paper presented at the annual meeting of the Population Association of America, Minneapolis, MN 1985.

[166] Moore, K.A.; Simms, M.C.; and Betsey, C.L. *Choice and Circumstance: Racial Differences in Adolescent Sexuality and Fertility.* New Brunswick, NJ: Transaction Books, 1986 as cited in *Risking the Future: Adolescent Sexuality, Pregnancy, and Childbearing.* National Research Council, 1987.

[167] Mott, F.L. "Early Fertility Behavior Among American Youth: Evidence From the 1982 National Longitudinal Surveys of Labor Force Behavior of Youth." Paper presented at the annual meeting of the American Public Health Association. 1983.

[168] Udry, J.R.; Bauman, K.E.; and Morris, N.M. Changes in premarital coital experience of recent decade-of-birth cohorts of urban American women. *Journal of Marriage and the Family* 37:783-87, 1975.

[169] Simon, W.; Berger, A.S.; and Gagnon, J.H. Beyond anxiety and fantasy: The coital experiences of college youth. *Journal of Youth and Adolescence* 1:203-222, 1972.

[170] Nathanson, C.A., and Becker, M.H. The influence of client-provider relationships on teenage women's subsequent use of contraception. *American Journal of Public Health* 75(1):33-37, 1985.

[171] Vincent, M.L.; Clearie, A.R.; and Schluchter, M.D. Reducing adolescent pregnancy through school and community-based education. *Journal of the American Medical Association* 257:3382-3386, 1987.

[172] Governor's Task Force on Teenage Pregnancy Prevention: Preventing Pregnancy in Utah. Salt Lake City, UT. 1988.

[173] Boyer, D. *Victimization: An Unexplored Factor in Adolescent Pregnancy.* Olympia, WA: 1989.

[174] General Mills, Inc. *Family Health in an Era of Stress.* Minneapolis, MN: General Mills, 1979.

[175] Zabin, L.S.; Kantner, J.F.; and Zelnik, M. The risk of adolescent pregnancy in the first months of intercourse. *Family Planning Perspectives* 11:215-222, 1979. As cited in *Risking the Future: Adolescent Sexuality, Pregnancy, and Childbearing.* Working Papers and Statistical Appendixes. Washington, DC: National Research Council, 1987.

[176] The Alan Guttmacher Institute. *Teenage Pregnancy: The Problem that Hasn't Gone Away.* New York: the Institute, 1981. As cited in The Adolescent Obstetric - Gynecologic Patient, an article in the American College of Obstetricians and Gynecologists Technical Bulletin. Number 94, 1986.

[177] Bachrach, C.A., and Mosher, W. Use of contraception in the United States, 1982. *Advance Data From Vital and Health Statistics*, No 102. Hyattsville, MD: U.S. Department of Health and Human Services, 1984.

[178] Clark, S.D., Jr.; Zabin, L.S.; and Hardy, J.B. Sex, contraception, and parenthood: Experience and attitudes among urban black young men. *Family Planning Perspectives* 16(4):77-82, 1984.

[179] Sophocles, A.M., Jr., and Brozovich, E.M. Birth control failure among patients with unwanted pregnancies: 1982-1984. *Journal of Family Practice* 22:45-48, 1986.

[180] Jones, E.F., and Forrest, J.D. Contraceptive failure in the United States: Revised estimates from the 1982 National Survey of Family Growth. *Family Planning Perspectives* 21(3): 1989.

[181] Mosher, W. Fertility and family planning in the United States: Insights from the National Survey of Family Growth. *Family Planning Perspectives* 20(5): 207-217, 1988.

[182] Harris, L. and Associates for Planned Parenthood. *American Teens Speak: Sex, Myth, T.V., and Birth Control,*" New York, 1986. As cited in *First Things First*. New York: Planned Parenthood Federation of America, Inc., 1989.

[183] Miller, B.C. and Olson, T.D. "AANC, delivery and results." A research report presented to the annual meeting of the Utah Council on Family Relations. March 1985.

[184] Dietz, P. Youth serving agencies as effective providers of sexuality education. *SIECUS Report* 18(2):16-20, 1990.

[185] The Alan Guttmacher Institute *Risk and responsibility: teaching sex education in America's schools today* New York: the Institute, 1988.

[186] Dawson, D.A. The effects of sex education on adolescent behavior. *Family Planning Perspectives* 18(4): 1986.

[187] Marsiglio, W., and Mott, F.L. The impact of sex education on sexual activity, contraceptive use, and premarital pregnancy among American teenagers. *Family Planning Perspectives* 18(4): 1986.

[188] Stout, J.W., and Rivara, F.P. Schools and sex education: Does it work? *Pediatrics* 83(3):375-379, 1989.

[189] Zelnik, M., and Kim, Y.J. Sex education and its association with teenage sexual activity, pregnancy, and contraceptive use. *Family Planning Perspectives* 14(3):117-126, 1982.

[190] Miller, B.C.; McCoy, J.K.; Olson, T.D.; and Wallace, C.M. "Background and contextual factors in relation to adolescent sexual attitudes and behavior." Unpublished paper, submitted for review, 1985.

[191] Klerman, G.L. Clinical epidemiology of suicide. *Journal of Clinical Psychiatry* 48:33-38, 1987.

[192] Boyd, J.H., and Moscicki, E.K.. Firearms and youth suicide. *American Journal of Public Health* 76:1240-1242, 1986.

[193] Moscicki, E.K., and Boyd, J.H. Epidemiologic trends in firearm suicides among adolescents. *Pediatrician* 12:52-62, 1985.

[194] Friedman, J.M.H.; Asnis, G.M.; Boeck, M.B.; DiFiore, J. Prevalence of specific suicidal behaviors in a high school sample. *American Journal of Psychiatry* 144:1203-1206, 1987.

[195] Lester, D., and Murrell, M.E. The preventive effect of strict gun control laws on suicide and homicide. *Suicide and Life-Threatening Behavior* 12:131-140, 1982.

[196] Worden, J.W. Methods as a risk factor in youth suicide. In: Davidson, L., and Linnoila, M., eds. *Report of the Secretary's Task Force on Youth Suicide. Vol. II. Risk Factors for Youth Suicide*. DHHS Pub.No.(ADM)89-1622. Rockville, MD: U.S. Department of Health and Human Services, 1989.

[197] Centers for Disease Control. *Youth Suicide in the United States, 1970-1980*. Atlanta, GA: Division of Injury Epidemiology and Control, 1986.

[198] Alcohol, Drug Abuse, and Mental Health Administration. *Report of the Secretary's Task Force on Youth Suicide*. Pub. No. (ADM)899-1621. Washington, DC: U.S. Department of Health and Human Services, 1989.

[199] Meehan, P.J., et al. "Suicide Attempts Among Young Adults." Paper presented at the 39th Annual Epidemic Intelligence Service Conference at Atlanta, GA, April, 1990.

[200] Rosen, D.H. The serious suicide attempt: five-year follow-up study of 886 patients. *Journal of the American Medical Association* 235:2105-2109, 1976.

[201] Office of Technology Assessment, U.S. Congress. *Children's Mental Health: Problems and Services—A Background Paper*. Washington, DC: U.S. Government Printing Office, 1986.

[202] Shaffers, D.; Phillips. I; Enzer, N.B.; Anthony, V.Q. (eds). *Prevention in Child and Adolescent Psychiatry: The Reduction of Risk for Mental Disorders*. Washington, DC: American Academy of Child and Adolescent Psychiatry, 1990.

[203] Bond, L.A.; Compas, B.E. (eds). *Primary Prevention and Promotion in the Schools*. Newbury Park, CA: Sage Publishing Company, 1989.

[204] Robbins, L.N. The adult development of the antisocial child. *Seminar in Psychiatry* 6:420-434, 1970.

[205] Zins. J.E.; Forman, S.G. (eds). Primary prevention: From theory to practice. In *School Psychology Review* 17:4 Special Issue, 1988.

[206] Robins, E.; Murphy, G.E.; Wilkinson, R.H., Jr.; et al. Some clinical considerations in the prevention of suicide based on a study of 134 successful suicides. *American Journal of Public Health*. 49:888-899, 1959.

[207] Ramey, C.T.; Yeates, K.O.; and Short, E.J. The plasticity of intellectual development: Insights from preventive intervention. *Child Development* 55:1913-1925, 1984.

[208] Roberts, M.C.; Peterson, L. *Prevention of Problems in Childhood*. New York: John Wiley and Sons, 1984.

[209] Teplin, L.A. Detecting disorder: The treatment of mental illness among jail detainees. *Journal of Consulting and Clinical Psychology*, in press.

[210] Regier, D.A., et al. The NIMH Depression Awareness, Recognition, and Treatment program: structure, aims, and scientific basis. *American Journal of Psychiatry* 145:1351-1357, 1988b.

[211] Louis Harris Associates, Inc.. *A Study of the Sources, Correlates and Manifestations of Perceived and Experienced Stress in the United States.* DHHS Contract No. 282-85-0063. Report submitted to the Office of Disease Prevention and Health Promotion, Department of Health and Human Services, 1985.

[212] Bluementhal, S.J. Suicide: a guide to risk factors, assessment, and treatment of suicidal patients. *Medical Clinics of North America.* 72:937-71, 1988.

[213] Katon, W. The epidemiology of depress in medical care. *International Journal of Psychiatry Medicine.* 17:93-112, 1987.

[214] Nathan, R. Effects of a stress management course on grades and health of first year medical students. *Journal of Medical Education* 62:514-517, 1987.

[215] Offord, D.R. Conduct disorder: Risk factors and prevention. In: Shaffer, D., et al., eds. *Prevention of Mental Disorders, Alcohol and Other Drug Use in Children and Adolescents.* Rockville, MD: U.S. Department of Health and Human Services, 1989.

[216] Centers for Disease Control. *Homicide Surveillance: High-Risk Racial and Ethnic Groups/ Blacks and Hispanics, 1970 to 1983.* Atlanta, GA: U.S. Department of Health and Human Services, 1986.

[217] Mercy, J.A., and Saltzman, L.E. Fatal violence among spouses in the United States, 1976-1985. *American Journal of Public Health* 79(5):595-599, 1989.

[218] Browne, A. Assault and homicide in the home: When battered women kill. In: Saks, M.J., and Saxe, L., eds. *Advances in Applied Social Psychology.* Vol. 3. Hillsdale, NJ: Lawrence Erlbaum Associates, 1987.

[219] Jason, J. Child homicide spectrum. *American Journal of Diseases of Children* 137:571-81, 1983.

[220] U.S. Department of Health and Human Services. *Report of the Secretary's Task Force on Black and Minority Health.* Washington, DC: the Department, 1985.

[221] Smith, J.C.; Mercy, J.A.; and Rosenberg, M.L. Suicide and homicide among hispanics in the southwest. *Public Health Reports* 101(3): 265-270, 1986.

[222] Goldstein, P.J. The drugs violence nexus: A tripartite conceptual framework. *Drug Issues* 15:493-506, 1985.

[223] Goldstein, P.J. Homicide Related to drug traffic. *Bulletin of the New York Academy of Medicine* 62:509-16, 1986.

[224] McBride, D.C. Drugs and violence, In: Inciardi, J.A., ed. *The Drugs-Crime Connection.* Beverly Hills, CA: Sage Publications, 1981.

[225] Committee on Trauma Research, Commission on Life Sciences, National Research Council; Institute of Medicine. *Injury in America: A Continuing Public Health Problem.* Washington, DC: National Academy Press, 1985.

[226] Baker, S.P.; Teret, S.P.; and Dietz, P.E. Firearms and the public health. *Journal of Public Health Policy* 1:224-29, 1980.

[227] Mercy, J.A., and Houk, V.N. Firearm injuries: A call for science. *New England Journal of Medicine* 319:1283-85, 1988.

[228] Wintemute, G.J. Firearms as a cause of death in the United States, 1920-1982. *Journal of Trauma* 27:532-6, 1987.

[229] Westat, Inc. *Study Findings: Study of National Incidence of Child Abuse and Neglect.* Washington, DC: U.S. Department of Health and Human Services, 1988.

[230] Straus, M.A.; Gelles, R.J.; and Steinmetz, S.K. *Behind Closed Doors: Violence in the American Family.* New York: Anchor Books, 1981.

[231] Stark, E., and Flitcraft, A. Violence among intimates: An epidemiologic review. In: Van Hassett, V.B.; et al., eds. *Handbook of Family Violence.* pp. 293-318. New York: Plenum, 1988.

[232] Stark, E., and Flitcraft, A. Medical therapy as repression: The case of battered women. *Health and Medicine* Summer/Fall:29-32, 1982.

[233] Straus, M.A. Violence and homicide antecedents. *Bulletin of the New York Academy of Medicine* 62:446-62, 1986.

[234] Stark, E.; et al. *Wife Abuse in the Medical Setting: An Introduction for Health Personnel.* Monograph No. 7. Washington, DC: U.S. Department of Health and Human Services, 1981.

[235] Stark, E., and Flitcraft, A. Women and children at risk: A feminist perspective on child abuse. *International Journal of Health Services* 18(1):97-118, 1988.

[236] Harlow, C.W. *Injuries from Crime.* Washington, DC: U.S. Department of Justice, 1989.

[237] Grahm, P.M., and Weingarden, S.I. "Targeting Teen-agers in a Spinal Cord Injury Violence Prevention Program" A presentation at the 14th Annual Scientific Meeting of the American Spinal Cord Injury Association, San Diego, 1988.

[238] Interagency Office of Prevention. *Injury Studies of Florida Populations/Head Injury and Spinal Cord Injury: An Epidemiologic Analysis.* Tallahassee, FL: U.S. Department of Health and Rehabilitative Services and U.S. Department of Labor, 1989.

[239] Kraus, J.F.; et al. Incidence of traumatic spinal cord lesions. *Journal of Chronic Diseases* 28:471-492, 1975.

[240] Arkansas Spinal Cord Commission, Annual Report, 1985. Little Rock, AR: the Commission, 1985.

[241] Makintubee, S. Personal communication. National Center for Health Statistics, 1989.

[242] Bureau of Justice Statistics. *Intimate Victims: A Study of Violence Among Friends and Relatives, a National Crime Survey Report.* Pub. No. SD-NCS-N-14, NCJ-62319. Washington, DC: U.S. Department of Justice, 1980.

[243] Bureau of Justice Statistics. *The Crime of Rape.* Pub. No. NCJ-96777. Washington, DC: U.S. Department of Justice, 1985.

[244] Kikuchi, J.J. Rhode Island develops successful intervention program for adolescents. *NCASA News.* Fall, 1988.

[245] O'Carroll, P.W., and Smith, J.A. Suicide and homicide. In: Wallace, H.M.; Ryan, G.; and Oglesby, A.C., eds. *Maternal and Child Health Practices.* pp. 583-597. Oakland, CA: Third Party Publishing, 1988.

[246] Prothrow-Stith, D. *Violence Prevention Curriculum for Adolescents.* Newton, MA: Education Development Center, 1987.

[247] Rivara, F.P. Traumatic deaths of children in the United States: Currently available prevention strategies. *Pediatrics* 75(3):456-62, 1985.

[248] Office of Juvenile Justice and Delinquency Prevention, Weapons in Schools. *OJJDP Juvenile Justice Bulletin.* Washington, DC: Department of Justice, 1989.

[249] Baker, S.P. Without guns, do people kill people? *American Journal of Public Health* 75(6):587-88, 1985.

[250] Sloan, J.H.; et al. Handgun regulations, crime, assaults and homicidal death: A tale of two cities. *New England Journal of Medicine* 319:1256-62, 1988.

[251] Shaffer, D. Strategies for prevention of youth suicide. *Public Health Reports* 102-611-13, 1987.

[252] Zimring, F.E. Is gun control likely to reduce violent killings? *University of Chicago Law Review* 35:721-37, 1968.

[253] Zimring, F.E. The medium is the message: Firearm calibre as a determinant of death from assault. *Journal of Legal Studies* 4(1):97-124, 1972.

[254] Bell, C.C.; et al. The need for victimization screening in a poor outpatient medical population. *Journal of the National Medical Association* 80(8):853-60, 1988.

[255] Klingbeil, K. "Comprehensive Model to Detect, Assess, and Treat Assaultive Violence in Hospital Settings." Background paper for the Secretary's Task Force on Black and Minority Health, U.S. Department of Health and Human Services, 1985.

[256] McLeer, S.V., and Anwar, R. A study of battered women in an emergency department. *American Journal of Public Health* 79(1):65-66, 1989.

[257] Klugman, R.D. Advances and retreats in the protection of children. *New England Journal of Medicine* 320(8):531-32, 1989.

[258] Widom, C.S. The cycle of violence. *Science* 244:160-166, 1989.

[259] Conner, M. "Treatment Programs for Abused Children." Working paper number 837, National Committee for Prevention of Child Abuse, 1987.

[260] Daro, D. *Confronting Child Abuse.* New York: The Free Press, 1988.

[261] Statistics provided from the 1987 Domestic Violence Statistical Survey conducted by the National Coalition Against Domestic Violence, P.O. Box 15127, Washington, DC 20003-0127.

[262] National Committee for Injury Prevention and Control. Injury prevention: Meeting the challenge. *Supplement to American Journal of Preventive Medicine,* 1989.

[263] Centers for Disease Control. The effectiveness of school health education. *Morbidity and Mortality Weekly Report* 35(38):593-95, 1986a.

[264] Daro, D.; Abrahams, N.; and Robson, K. "Reducing Child Abuse 20% by 1990: 1985-86 Baseline Data." Working paper number 843 of the National Center on Child Abuse Prevention Research, a program of the National Committee for Prevention of Child Abuse, May, 1988.

[265] DeJong, W. *Project DARE Evaluation Results.* Newton, MA: Education Development Center, 1986.

[266] McCarthy, W.J. The cognitive developmental model and other alternatives to the social deficit model of smoking onset. In: Bell, C.S., and Battjes, R., eds. *Prevention Research: Deterring Drug Abuse Among Children and Adolescents.* NIDA Research Monograph 63. Rockville, MD: U.S. Department of Health and Human Services, 1985.

[267] Moskowitz, J. Preventing adolescent drug substance abuse through drug education. In: Glynn, T.J.; et al., eds. *Preventing Adolescent Drug Abuse: Intervention Strategies.* Rockville, MD: U.S. Department of Health and Human Services, 1983.

[268] Selman, R.L., and Glidden, M. Negotiation strategies for youth. *School Safety* Fall:18-21, 1987.

[269] Guerra, G., and Slaby, R.G. Cognitive Mediators of Aggression in Adolescent Offenders: Intervention, in press.

[270] Daro, D. "Intervening with New Parents: An Effective Way to Prevent Child Abuse." Working paper number 839, National Committee for Prevention of Child Abuse, 1988.

[271] Education Commission of the States. Recommendations for school health education: A handbook for policy makers. Denver, CO: the Commission, 1981.

[272] National Professional School Health Education Organizations. Comprehensive school health education as defined by the national professional school health education organizations. *Journal of School Health* 57(6):312-315, 1984.

[273] World Health Organization. *Global Strategy for Health for All by the Year 2000*, Health for All Series (No. 3). Geneva: the Organization, 1981.

[274] Connell, D.; Turner, R.; and Mason, E. Summary of findings of the school health education evaluation: Health promotion effectiveness, implementation, and costs. *Journal of School Health* 55(8):316-321, 1985.

[275] World Health Organization. *Statistical Indices of Family Health* Report No. 589:17, 1976.

[276] Campbell, T.L. *Family's Impact on Health: A Critical Review and Annotated Bibliography.* ADAMHA and NIMH (joint report). Rockville, MD: U.S. Department of Health and Human Services, 1986.

[277] Institute of Medicine, National Academy of Sciences. *The Future of Public Health.* Washington, DC: National Academy Press, 1988.

[278] American Public Health Association. *Model Standards.* Washington, DC: the Association, 1979.

[279] National Highway Traffic Safety Administration. *The Economic Cost to Society of Motor Vehicle Accidents.* Technical Report DOT HS 809-195, p. 1. Washington, DC: Department of Transportation, 1987.

[280] National Highway Traffic Safety Administration. *Motorcycle Accident Cause Factors and Identification of Countermeasures.* Technical Report DOT HS 805-862. Washington, DC: Department of Transportation, 1981.

[281] National Highway Traffic Administration. *The Effectiveness of Motorcycle Helmets in Preventing Fatalities.* Technical Report DOT HS 807-416. Washington, DC: Department of Transportation, 1989.

[282] Preusser, D.F. and Lund, A.K. And keep on looking: A film to reduce pedestrian crashes among 9 to 12 year olds. *Journal of Safety Research* 19(Winter):177-85, 1988.

[283] Federal Highway Administration. "Speed Limit Enforcement Certification Data, 1987." U.S. Department of Transportation, unpublished data.

[284] Robertson, L.S. Future directions: Where do we go from here? Roadway modifications, in special section: 1987 conference on injury in America. *Public Health Reports* 102(6):671, 1987.

[285] Gallagher, S.S.; Fineson, K.; Guyer, B.; and Goodenough, S.S. The incidence of injuries among 87,000 Massachusetts children and adolescents. *American Journal of Public Health* 10:1340-7, 1984.

[286] Sacks, J.J.; Smith, J.D.; Kaplasn, K. M.; Lambert, D.A.; Sattin, R.W.; and Sikes, K. The epidemiology of injuries in Atlanta day-care centers. *Journal of the American Medical Association* 260:262-1641-5, 1989.

[287] Division of Injury Epidemiology and Control. Unintentional poisoning mortality: United States, 1980-1986. *Morbidity and Mortality Report* 38(10):153-157, 1989.

[288] Spiegel, C.N. and Lindaman, F.C. Children can't fly: A program to prevent childhood morbidity and morality from window falls. *American Journal of Public Health* 67:1143-7, 1977.

[289] Gulaid, J.A. and Sattin, R.W. Drowning in the United States, 1978-1984. In: CDC Surveillance Summaries, February 1988. *Morbidity and Mortality Report* 37(SS-1):27-33, 1988.

[290] Nixon, J.; Pearn, J.; Wilkey, I, et al. Fifteen years of child drowning: A 1967-1981 analysis of all fatal cases from the Brisbane drowning study, an 11 year study of consecutive near-drowning cases. *Accident Analysis and Prevention* 18:199-201, 1986.

[291] O'Carroll, P.W.; Alkon, E.; and Weiss, B. Drowning mortality in Los Angeles, 1976 to 1984. *Journal of the American Medical Association* 260:380-383, 1988.

[292] Micik, S. Drowning and near drowning in California. In: Brill, D.; Micik, S.; and Yuwiler, J., eds. *Childhood Drowning: Current Issues and Strategies for Prevention, Summary Report of Conference Proceedings held in Orange County, California.* Washington, DC: U.S. Consumer Product Safety Commission, 1987.

[293] Gulaid, J.A.; Sattin, R.W.; and Waxweiler, R.J. Deaths from residential fires, 1978-1984. In: CDC Surveillance Summaries, February 1988. *Morbidity and Mortality Report* 37(SS-1):39-45, 1988.

[294] U.S. Fire Administration. *Fire in the United States: Death, Injuries, Dollar Loss, and Incidents at the National, State, and Local Levels in 1983.* 6th ed. Washington, DC: Federal Emergency Management Agency, 1983.

[295] Litovitz, T.L.; Schmitz, B.F.; Matyunas, N.; et al. 1987 annual report of the American Association of Poison Control Centers national data collection system. *American Journal of Emergency Medicine* 6(5):479-544, 1988.

[296] Frankowski, R.F.; Annegers, J.F.; and Whitman, S. Epidemiologic and descriptive studies, part I: The descriptive epidemiology of head trauma in the United States. In: Becker, D.P. and Povlishock, J.T., eds. *Central Nervous System Trauma Status Report, 1983.* Bethesda, MD: Department of Health and Human Services, 1983. pp. 33-42.

[297] Kalsbeck, W.D. The national head and spinal cord injury survey: Major findings. *Journal of Neurosurgery* 53:S19-S31, 1980.

[298] Kraus, J.F.; Frant, D.C.; Riggins, R.S.; Richards, D.; and Borhani, N.O. Incidence of traumatic spinal cord lesions. *Journal of Chronic Diseases* 28:471-492, 1975.

[299] Kraus, J.F. Epidemiologic aspects of acute spinal cord injury: A review of incidence, prevalence, causes and outcome. In: Becker, D.P. and Porlishock, J.T., eds. *Central Nervous System Trauma Status Report - 1983.* Bethesda, MD: Department of Health and Human Services, 1983.

[300] Carter, R.E. Traumatic spinal cord injuries due to automobile accidents. *Southern Medical Journal* 70:709, 1977.

[301] Stover, S.L. and Fine, P.R., eds. *Spinal Cord Injury: The Facts and Figures.* Birmingham, AL: University of Alabama, 1986.

[302] Institute of Medicine. *National Agenda on Disability.* Washington, DC: National Academy of Sciences Press, in press.

[303] National Institute on Disability and Rehabilitation Research. NIDRR National Consensus Conference, 1989. Washington, DC: U.S. Department of Education, in press.

[304] Rice, D.P.; MacKenzie, E.J.; et al. *Cost of Injury in the United States: A Report to Congress, 1989.* San Francisco, CA: Institute for Health and Aging of the University of California-San Francisco and Injury Prevention Center, The Johns Hopkins University, 1989.

[305] National Highway Traffic Safety Administration. *A Report to the Congress on the Effect of Motorcycle Helmet Use Law Repeal: A Case for Helmet Use.* Washington, DC: Department of Transportation, 1980.

[306] Thompson, R.S.; Rivara, F.P.O.; and Thompson, D.C. A case-control study of the effectiveness of bicycle safety helmets. *New England Journal of Medicine* 320(21):1364-1366, 1989.

[307] National Center for Statistics and Analysis. *Occupant Protection Facts.* Washington, DC: Department of Transportation, 1989.

[308] National Center for Statistics and Analysis. *Facts About Motorcycle Crashes and Safety Helmet Use.* Washington, DC: Department of Transportation, 1989.

[309] Sosin, D.M.; Sacks, J.J.; and Holmgreen, P. Head injury-associated deaths from motorcycles, United States, 1979 to 1986. Submitted in 1990 to *Journal of the American Medical Association*.

[310] U.S. Department of Commerce. *Estimating the Effectiveness of the State of the Art Detectors and Automatic Sprinklers on Life Safety in Residential Occupancies.* Washington, DC: the Department, 1984. Pub. No. NB-SIR 842819.

[311] Johns Hopkins University Applied Physics Laboratory. *Assessment of the Potential Impact of Fire Protection Systems on Actual Fire Incidents.* Washington, DC: U.S. Fire Administration, 1980.

[312] Hall, J.R. A decade of detectors: Measuring the effect. *Fire Journal* 79:37-43, Sept. 1985.

[313] Thornberry, O.T.; et al. Health promotion data for the 1990 objectives: Estimates from the national health interview survey of health promotion and disease prevention: United States, 1985. *Advance Data From Vital Statistics* 126:Sept. 19, 1986.

[314] Cales, R.H.; et al. Preventable trauma deaths: a review of trauma care systems development. *Journal of the American Medical Association* 254:1059-1063, 1985.

[315] U.S. General Accounting Office. *States Assume Leadership in Providing Emergency Medical Services.* Pub. No. GAO/HRD-86-132. Washington, DC: the Office, 1986.

[316] Office of Technology Assessment. *Rural Emergency Medical Services-Special Report.* Pub. No. OTA-H-445. Washington, DC: U.S. Congress, 1989.

[317] National EMS Clearinghouse. *State EMS Office: Evaluation/Information Systems and Public Information/Education.* Lexington, KY: National Association of State EMS Directors and the Council of State Governments, 1988.

[318] Eastman, A.B.; Lewis, F.R.; Champion, H.R.; and Mattox, K.L. Regional trauma system design: Critical concepts. *American Journal of Surgery* 154:79-87, 1987.

[319] Maryland Institute for Emergency Medical Services Systems. *Annual Report 1984-1985.* Baltimore, MD: the Institute, 1987.

[320] West, J.G.; Williams, M.J.; Trunkey, D.D.; and Wolferth, C.C. Trauma systems: Current status—future challenges," *Journal of American Medical Association* 259:3597-3600, 1988.

[321] National Heart, Lung, and Blood Institute. *Infomemo* December 1989.

[322] Agency for Toxic Substances and Disease Registry *The Nature and Extent of Lead Poisoning in Children in the United States: A Report to Congress.* Washington, DC: U.S. Department of Health and Human Services, July 1988.

[323] Environmental Protection Agency. *Environmental Progress and Challenges: EPA's Update.* EPA-230-07-88-033 Washington, DC: U.S. Environmental Protection Agency, 1988.

[324] Committee on the Biological Effects of Ionizing Radiations: "Health Risks of Radon and Other Internally Deposited Alpha-Emitters." Biologic Effects of Ionizing Radiation IV. Washington, DC: National Academy Press, 1988.

[325] International Commission on Radiological Protection. *Lung Cancer Risk from Indoor Exposure to Radon Daughters.* ICRP 50. New York: Pergamon Press, 1986.

[326] National Center for Health Statistics. Blood Lead Levels for Persons ages 6 months to 74 years: United States, 1976-80. Data from the National Health and Nutrition Examination Survey. *Vital and Health Statistics*, Series 11, No. 233, DHHS Pub. No. DHHS(PHS)84-1683. Washington, DC: U.S. Department of Health Human Service, 1984.

[327] Center for Environmental Health and Injury Control, Centers for Disease Control, Public Health Service, Atlanta, GA. U.S Department of Health and Human Services, August, 1990.

[328] Kilbourne, E.M. "Heat Waves." *The Public Health Consequences of Disasters.* Centers for Disease Control, Public Health Service, Atlanta, GA: U.S. Department of Health and Human Services, 1989.

[329] Upton, A.C. Carcinogenic effects of low-level ionizing radiation. *Journal of the National Cancer Institute.* 82(6) March 21, 1990.

[330] National Institute of Dental Research. *Oral Health of United States Children. The National Survey of Dental Caries in U.S. School Children, 1986-1987.* DHHS Pub.No. (NIH) 89-2247. Bethesda, MD: U.S Department of Health and Human Services, 1989.

[331] Woolfolk, M.; Hamard, M.; and Bagramian, R.A. Oral health of children of migrant farm workers in northwest Michigan. *Journal of Public Health Dentistry* 44:101-105, 1984.

[332] Burt, B.A. Proceedings for the workshop: Cost effectiveness of caries prevention in dental public health. *Journal of Public Health Dentistry* 49(5), 1989.

[333] Centers for Disease Control. *Estimates of U.S. Population Served by Fluoridated Water Systems, 1985.* Atlanta, GA: U.S. Department of Health and Human Services, July 1986.

[334] Broderick, E.; Mabry, J.; Robertson, D.; and Thompson, J. Baby bottle tooth decay in Native American children. *Public Health Reports* 104:50-54, 1989.

[335] Kelly, M.; and Bruerd, B. The Prevalence of Nursing Bottle Decay Among Two Native American Populations *Journal of Public Health Dentistry* 47:94-97, 1987.

[336] National Center for Health Statistics. *Use of Dental Services and Dental Health United States, 1986.* DHHS Pub.No. (PHS) 88-1593. Hyattsville, MD: U.S. Department of Health and Human Services, 1988.

[337] Jansen, J.A.; Flanders, R.; and Aduss, M.K. "Strategy to Improve Identification and Reporting of Craniofacial Anomalies," American Public Health Association abstract for session #2073, October, 1989.

[338] Buehler, J.W.; Kleinman, J.C.; Hogue, C.J.R.; Strauss, L.T.; and Smith, J.C. Birthweight-specific infant mortality, United States, 1960 and 1980. *Public Health Reports* 102(2):151-161, 1987.

[339] Kessel, S.S.; Kleinman, J.C.; Koontz, A.M.; Hogue, C.J.R.; and Berendes, H.W. Racial differences in pregnancy outcomes. *Clinics in Perinatology* 14:745-54, 1988.

[340] WHO Collaborating Center in Perinatal Care and Health Service Research in Maternal and Child Care. Unintended pregnancy and infant mortality/morbidity. In: Amler, R.W., and Dull, H.B., eds. *Closing the Gap: The Burden of Unnecessary Illness.* New York: Oxford University Press, 1987.

[341] Hogue, C.J.R., and Yip, R. Preterm delivery: Can we lower the black infant's first hurdle? *Journal of the American Medical Association* 262:548-550, 1989.

[342] National Center for Health Statistics. *Health Aspects of Pregnancy and Childbirth: United States, 1982,* by Pamuk, E.R., and Mosher, W.D. Vital and Health Statistics. Series 23, No. 16, DHHS Pub. No. (PHS) 89-1992. Washington, DC: U.S. Department of Health and Human Services, 1988.

[343] Friede, A.; Rhodes, P.H.; Guyer, B.; Binkin, N.J.; Hannan, M.T.; and Hogue, C.J.R. The postponement of neonatal deaths into the postneonatal period: Evidence from Massachusetts. *American Journal of Epidemiology* 127:161-170, 1988.

[344] Kleinman, J.C. Underreporting of infant deaths: Then and now, (invited editorial). *American Journal of Public Health* 76(4):365-366, 1988.

[345] Pritchard, J.A., and Macdonald, P.C. *Williams Obstetrics.* 16th ed. New York: Appleton-Century-Crofts, 1980.

[346] National Center for Health Statistics. *Vital Statistics: Instructions for Classifying the Underlying Cause of Death, 1979.* Washington, DC: U.S. Department of Health and Human Services, 1978.

[347] Smith, J.C.; Hughes, J.M.; Pekow, P.S.; et al. An assessment of the incidence of maternal mortality in the United States. *American Journal of Public Health* 74(8):780-784, 1984.

[348] Rochat, R.W.; Koonin, L.M.; Atrash, H.K.; and Jewett, J.F. Maternal mortality in the United States: Report from the maternal mortality collaborative. *Obstetrics and Gynecology* 72(1):91-97, 1988.

[349] Rosett, H.L., and Weiner, L. *Alcohol and the Fetus: A Clinical Perspective*. New York: Oxford University Press, 1984.

[350] Streissguth, A.P.; Barr, H.M.; and Sampson, P.D. Effects on child IQ and hearing problems at age 7 and a half years. Clinical and Experimental Research, In Press.

[351] May, P.A.; Hynbaugh, K.J.; Aase, J.M.; and Samet, J.M. Epidemiology of fetal alcohol syndrome among American Indians of the southwest. *Social Biology* 30:374-387, 1983.

[352] Kessel, S.S.; Villar, J.; Berendes, H.W.; and Nugent, R.P. The changing pattern of low birthweight in the United States: 1970-1980. *Journal of the American Medical Association* 251:1978-1982, 1984.

[353] Kleinman, J.C., and Kessel, S.S. Racial differences in low birthweight: Trends and risk factors. *New England Journal of Medicine* 317:749-753, 1987.

[354] Kleinman, J.C., and Madans, J. The effects of maternal smoking, physical stature, and educational attainment on the incidence of low birthweight. *American Journal of Epidemiology* 121(6):843-855, 1985.

[355] MacGregor, S.N.; Keith, L.G.; Chasnoff, I.J.; Rosner, M.A.; Chisum, G.M.; Shaw, P.; and Minogue, J.P. Cocaine use during pregnancy: Adverse perinatal outcome. *American Journal of Obstetrics and Gynecology* 157:686-690, 1987.

[356] Stein, Z., and Kline, J. Smoking, alcohol and reproduction. *American Journal of Public Health* 73:1154-1156, 1983.

[357] Zuckerman, B.; Frank, D.A.; Hingson, R.; Amaro, H.; Levenson, S.M.; Kayne, H.; Parker, S.; Vinci, R.; Aboagye, K.; Fried, L.E.; Cabral, H.; Timperi, R.; and Bauchner, H. Effects of maternal marijuana and cocaine use on fetal growth. *New England Journal of Medicine*. 320:762-768, 1989.

[358] Chasnoff, I.J. Drug use in pregnancy: Parameters of risk. *The Pediatric Clinician of North America* 35(6):1403-1412, 1988.

[359] Office of Technology Assessment, U.S. Congress. *Neonatal Intensive Care for Low Birthweight Infants: Costs and Effectiveness*. OTA-HCS-38. Washington, DC: Office of Technology Assessment, December 1987.

[360] Institute of Medicine, National Academy of Sciences, Subcommittee on Nutritional Status and Weight Gain During Pregnancy. *Nutrition During Pregnancy*. Washington, DC: National Academy Press, 1990.

[361] Niswander, K.R., and Gordon M. *The women and their pregnancies: The collaborative study of the National Institute of Neurologic Disease and Stroke*. Philadelphia, PA: W.B. Saunder, 1972.

[362] Orstead, C.; Arrington, D.; Kamath, S.K.; Olson, R.; and Kohrs, M.B. Efficacy of prenatal nutrition counseling: Weight gain, infant birthweight, and cost-effectiveness. *Journal of the American Dietetic Association* 85(1):40-45, 1985.

[363] Taffel, S.M. *Maternal weight gain and the outcome of pregnancy*. Vital and Health Statistics, Series 21, No. 44, DHHS Pub No. (PHS) 86-1922. Washington, DC: U.S. Department of Health and Human Services, June 1986.

[364] Taffel, S.M. Cesarean section in America: Dramatic trends, 1970-1987. *Statistical Bulletin* Oct-Dec:2-11, 1989.

[365] Broe, S., and Khoo, S.K. How safe is cesarean section in current practice? A survey of mortality and serious morbidity. *Australian and New Zealand Journal of Obstetrics and Gynecology* 29(2):93-98, 1989.

[366] Petitti, D.B.; Cefalo, R.C.; Shapiro, S.; and Whally, P. In-hospital maternal mortality in the United States: Time trends and relation to method of delivery. *Obstetrics and Gynecology* 59(1):6-12, 1982.

[367] Rubin, G.L.; Peterson, H.B.; Rochat, R.W.; McCarthy, B.J.; and Terry, J.S. Maternal death after cesarean section in Georgia. *American Journal of Obstetrics and Gynecology* 139(6):681-685, 1981.

[368] Myers, S.A.; and Gleicher, N. A successful program to lower cesarean-section rates. *New England Journal of Medicine* 319(23):1511-1516, 1988.

[369] American College of Obstetricians and Gynecologists. Committee on obstetrics: Maternal and fetal medicine. Guidelines for vaginal delivery after a previous cesarean section. ACOG Committee 64:1-2, 1988.

[370] Goldman, A.S.; Garza, C.; Nichols, B.L.; and Goldblum, R.M. Immunologic factors in human milk during the first year of lactation. *Journal of Pediatrics* 100(4):563-567, 1982.

[371] Lawrence, R. *Breastfeeding: A Guide for the Medical Profession*. St. Louis, MO: C.V. Mosby, 1985.

[372] Martinez, G.A. "Ross Laboratories Mothers Survey: Sample Design and Methodology Trends in Infant Milk Feeding." Unpublished data from Ross Laboratories, Columbia, OH, 1989.

[373] Howard, J.; Beckwith, L.; Rodning, C.; and Kropenske, V. National Center for Clinical Infant Programs. The development of young children of substance abusing parents: Insights from seven years of intervention and research. *Zero to Three* IX(5):8-12, 1989.

[374] Keith, L.G.; McGregor, S.N.; and Sciarra, J.J. Drug abuse in pregnancy. In: Chasnoff, I.J, ed. *Drugs, Alcohol, Pregnancy and Parenting.* Bingham, MA: Kluwer Academic Publishers, 1988. pp. 17-44.

[375] Singh, S.; Torres, D.; and Forrest, J.D. The need for prenatal care in the United States: Evidence from the 1980 national natality survey. *Family Planning Perspectives.* 17:118-124, 1985.

[376] Alan Guttmacher Institute. *Blessed Events and the Bottom Line: The Financing of Maternity Care in the United States.* New York: the Institute, 1987.

[377] Public Health Service. Expert Panel on the Content of Prenatal Care. *Caring for Our Future: The Content of Prenatal Care.* Washington, DC: U.S. Department of Health and Human Services, 1989.

[378] Lammer, E.J.; Chen, D.T.; Hoar, R.M.; Agnish, N.D.; Benke, P.J.; et. al. Retinoic acid embryopathy. *New England Journal of Medicine* 313(14):837-841, 1985.

[379] American Society of Human Genetics. Policy statement for maternal serum alpha-fetoprotein screening programs and quality control for laboratories performing maternal serum and amniotic fluid alpha fetoprotein assays. *American Journal of Human Genetics* 40:75-82, 1987.

[380] Palomaki, G.E.; Knight, G.J.; Holman, M.S.; and Haddow, J.E. Maternal serum alpha-fetoprotein screening for fetal down syndrome in the United States: Results of a survey. *American Journal of Obstetrics and Gynecology* 162:317-321, 1990.

[381] American College of Obstetricians and Gynecologists, Department of Professional Liability. *DPL Alert: Professional Liability Implications of AFP Tests.* Washington, DC: the College, 1985.

[382] American College of Obstetricians and Gynecologists, Committee on Professional Standards. *Standards for Obstetric-Gynecological Services.* 7th ed. Washington, DC: the College, 1989.

[383] Cooke, S.A.; Schwartz, R.M.; and Gagnon, D.E. *The perinatal partnership: An approach to organizing care in the 1990s.* Providence, RI: National Perinatal Information Center, 1988.

[384] National Institutes of Health. *Consensus Development Conference Statement.* 6(9). Bethesda, MD: *U.S. Department of Health and Human Services*, 1987.

[385] Gaston, M.H.; Verter, J.I.; Woods, G.; Pegelow, C.; Kelleher, J.; et. al. Prophylaxis with oral penicillin in children with sickle cell anemia: A randomized trial. *New England Journal of Medicine* 324(25):1593-1599, 1986.

[386] American Academy of Pediatrics, Committee on Genetics. 1989 newborn screening fact sheets. *Pediatrics* 83(3):*449-464*, 1989.

[387] Council of Regional Networks for Genetic Services, Data and Evaluation Committee. "1988 Comprehensive Newborn Screening Report." Unpublished data.

[388] American Academy of Pediatrics, Committee on Psychosocial Aspects of Child and Family Health. *Guidelines for Health Supervision II.* Elgrove Village, IL: the Academy, 1988.

[389] American Cancer Society. *Cancer Facts and Figures—1989.* New York: the Society, 1990.

[390] National Cancer Institute and the National Center for Health Statistics. 1987 National Health Interview Survey, Cancer Control Supplement, unpublished data.

[391] International Agency for Research on Cancer Working Group on Evaluation of Cervical Cancer Screening Programs. Screening for squamous cervical cancer: Duration of low risk after negative results of cervical cytology and its implications for screening policies. *British Medical Journal* 293:659-664, 1986.

[392] National Cancer Institute. *1987 Annual Cancer Statistics Review.* DHHS Pub.No. (NIH)88-2789. Bethesda, MD: U.S. Department of Health and Human Services, 1988.

[393] Eddy, D.M.; Hasselblad, V.; McGiveny, W.; and Hendee W. The value of mammography screening in women under 50 years. *JAMA* 259:1512-1519, 1988.

[394] National Cancer Institute. *Cancer Statistics Review 1973-1986.* DHHS Pub. No. (NIH)89-2789. Bethesda, MD: U.S. Department of Health and Human Services, 1989.

[395] National Cancer Institute. *Cancer Rates and Risks.* DHHS Pub. No. (NIH)85-691. Bethesda, MD: U.S. Department of Health and Human Services, 1985.

[396] Pathak, M.A. Sunscreens and their use in the preventive treatment of sunlight-induced skin damage. *Journal of Dermatologic Surgery and Oncology* 13:739-750, 1987.

[397] Kligman, L.H.; Akin, F.J.; and Kligman, M. Suncreens prevent ultraviolet photocarcinogenesis. *Journal of the American Academy of Dermatology* 3:30-35, 1980.

[398] Wulf, H.C.; Poulsen, T.; Brodthagen, H.; and Hou-Jensen, K. Sunscreens for delay of ultraviolet induction of skin tumors. *Journal of the American Academy of Dermatology* 7:194-202, 1982.

399 American Academy of Dermatology and Opinion Research Corporation. *Public Awareness of the Effects of Sun on Skin. A Survey Conducted for the American Academy of Dermatology.* Princeton, NJ: Opinion Research Corporation, 1987.

400 Boyes, D.A.; Morrison, B.; Knox, E.G.; Draper, G.J.; and Miller, A.B. A cohort study of cervical cancer screening in British Columbia. *Clinic of Investigative Medicine* 5:1-29, 1982.

401 Choi, N.W.; Nelson, N.A.; and Abu-Zeid, H.A.H. Cervical cytology program and its effects on cervical cancer incidence and mortality by geographical areas in Manitoba. In: Nieburgs, H.E., ed. *Prevention and Detection of Cancer.* New York: Marcel Dekke, 1980. pp. 1891-1907.

402 Johannesson, G.; Geirsson, G.; and Day, N.E. The effect of mass screening in Iceland 1965-74 on the incidence and mortality of cervical carcinoma. *International Journal of Cancer* 21:418-425, 1978.

403 Johannesson, G.; Geirsson, G.; Day N.; Tulinius, H. Screening for cancer of the uterine cervix in Iceland 1965-1978. *Acta Obstetricia et Gynecologica Scandinavica* 61:199-203, 1982.

404 MacGregor, J.E.; Moss, S.M.; Parkin, D.M.; and Day, N.E. A case-control cancer on N.E. Scotland. *Tumori* 62:287-295, 1985.

405 Office of Technology Assessment, U.S. Congress. The costs and effectiveness of screening for cervical cancer in elderly women—background paper. Pub. No. OTA-BP-H-65. Washington, DC: U.S. Department of Congress, 1990.

406 Shy, K.; Chu, J.; Mandelson, M.; Greer, B.; and Figge, D. Papanicolaou smear screening interval and risk of cervical cancer. *Obstetrics and Gynecology* 74:838-843, 1989.

407 American Medical Association, Council on Scientific Affairs. Quality assurance in cervical cytology: The Papanicolaou smear. *Journal of the American Medical Association* 262:1672-1679, 1989.

408 Koss, L.G. The Papanicolaou test for cervical cancer detection: A triumph and a tragedy. *Journal of the American Medical Association* 261:737-743, 1989.

409 National Cancer Institute Workshop. The 1988 Bethesda System for reporting cervical/vaginal cytological diagnosis. *Journal of the American Medical Association* 262:931-934, 1989.

410 National Center for Health Statistics. Current Estimates from the National Health Interview Survey, United States, 1988. *Vital and Health Statistics.* Series 10, No. 173, DHHS Pub. No. (PHS) 89-1501. Hyattsville, MD: U.S. Department of Health and Human Services, 1989.

411 LaPlante, M.P. *Data on Disability from the National Health Interview Survey, 1983-85.* An InfoUse Report. Washington, D.C.: National Institute on Disability and Rehabilitation Research (NIDRR), 1988.

412 American Academy of Audiology. Position Statement on Early Identification of Hearing Loss in Infants and Children. December, 1988.

413 Bess, F.H. *Hearing Impairment in Children.* Parkton, MD: York Press, 1988.

414 Norton, S.J. and Widen J.E. Evoked auto acoustic emissions in normal hearing infants and children: Emerging data issues. *Ear and Hearing* 11(2):121-127, 1990.

415 Prager, D.A.; Stone, D.A.; and Rose, D.N. Hearing loss screening in the neonatal intensive care unit: Auditory brain stem response versus crib-o-gram; a cost-effectiveness analysis. *Ear and Hearing* 8:213-216, 1987.

416 Stewart, I.F. After early identification: A study of some aspects of deaf education from an otolaryngological viewpoint. *Laryngoscope* 94:784-99, 1984.

417 Lynch, C. and Dublinske, S. Rehabilitation services and personnel needs for the communicatively impaired. Unpublished paper for the American Speech-Language and Hearing Association, Rockville, MD., November 7, 1985.

418 American Speech-Language-Hearing Association. Audiologic screening of newborn infants who are at risk for hearing impairment. *American Speech-Language-Hearing Association* 31:89-92, 1989.

419 Parving, A. Hearing disorders in childhood: Some procedures for detection, identification and diagnostic evaluation. *International Journal of Pediatric Otorhinolaryngology* 9:31-57, 1985.

420 Riko, K; Hyde, M.L.; and Alberti, P.W. Hearing loss in early infancy: Incidence, detection and assessment. *Larngoscope* 95:137-45, 1985.

421 Calogero, B; Giannini, P.; and Marciano, E. Recent advances in hearing screening. *Advances in Otorhinolaryngology* 37:60-78, 1987.

422 Duara, S.; Suter, C.M.; Bessard, K.K.; et al. Neonatal screening with auditory brainstem responses: Results of follow-up audiometry and risk factor evaluation. *Journal of Pediatrics* 108:276-281, 1986.

423 Cross, A.W. Health screening in schools. Part I. *Journal of Pediatrics* 107:487-494, 1985.

424 Zinkus, P.W.; and Gottlieb, M. Pattern of perceptual and academic deficits related to early chronic otitis media. *Pediatrics* 66(2):246-253, 1980a.

425 Zinkus, P.W.; Gottlieb, M.; and Shapiro, M. Developmental and physchoeducational sequelae of chronic otitis media. *American Journal of Disease of Children* 132:1100-1104, 1980.

[426] Occupational Safety and Health Administration. Occupational noise exposure: Hearing conservation amendment. *Federal Register* 46:4078-180. Washington, DC: U.S. Government Printing Office, 1981.

[427] Olson, R.A.; and Kittredge, D. Teaching anticipatory guidance: Pediatric residents' attitudes, knowledge, and behavior. Paper presented at the annual convention of the American Psychological Association, Washington, DC, August, 1986.

[428] Axelsson and Jesson. Noisy toys - A possible source of sensorineural hearing loss. *Pediatrics* 76:574-577, 1985.

[429] Corliss, L.M. et al. High frequency and regular audiometry among selected groups of high school students. *The Journal of School Health* XL, No. 8 400-405, 1970.

[430] Gallup. Research to Prevent Blindness, New York, 1988.

[431] Daubs, J.G., and Crick, P.P. The effect of refractive error on the risk of ocular hypertension and primary open angle glaucoma. *Trans Ophthalmol Soc UK* 101:121-126, 1981.

[432] Leske, M.C. The epidemiology of open-angle glaucoma: A review. *American Journal of Epidemiology* 118:166-91, 1983.

[433] American Academy of Ophthalmology. *Infants and children's eye care. Statement by the American Academy of Ophthalmology to the Select Panel for the Promotion of Child Health, U.S. Department of Health and Human Services.* San Francisco, CA: the Academy, 1980.

[434] Ehrlich, M.I.; Reinecke, R.D.; and Simons, K. Preschool vision screening for amblyopia and strabismus: Programs, methods, guidelines. *Survey of Ophthalmology* 28:145-163, 1983.

[435] Sanke, R.F. Amblyopia. *American Family Physician* 37:275-8, 1988.

[436] American Academy of Pediatrics. Vision screening and eye examination in children. Committee on Practice and Ambulatory Medicine. *Pediatrics* 77:918-919, 1986.

[437] Streissguth, A.P.; Barr, H.M.; and Sampson, P.D. Moderate prenatal alcohol exposure: Effects on child IQ and learning problems at age 7 1/2 years. *Clinical and Experimental Research*, in press.

[438] Kraus, J.F.; Rock, A.; and Hemyari, P. Causes, impact, and preventability of childhood injuries in the United States: Brain injuries among infants, children, adolescents, and young adults in the United States. *American Journal of Diseases of Children* 144:684-691, 1990.

[439] Belman, A.L.; Diamond, G.; Dickson, D.; et al. Pediatric acquired immunodeficiency syndrom: Neurological syndromes. *American Journal of Diseases of Children* 142(1):29-35, 1988.

[440] Epstein, L.G.; Sharer, L.R.; Oleske, J.M.; et al. Neurologic manifestations of human immunodeficiency virus infection in children. *Pediatrics* 78(4):678-687, 1986.

[441] Ullman, M.H.; Belman, A.L.; Ruff, H.A.; et al. Developmental abnormalities in infants and children with acquired immune deficiency syndrome (AIDS) and AIDS-related complex. *Developmental Medicine and Child Neurology* 27(5):563-571, 1985.

[442] Vinicor, F.; Cohen, S.J.; Mazzucca S.A.; et al. DIABEDS: A randomized trial of the affects of physician and/or patient education on diabetes patient outcomes. *Journal of Chronic Diseases* 40:345-356, 1987.

[443] Centers for Disease Control. Diabetes in pregnancy project—Maine, 1986-1987. *Morbidity and Mortality Weekly Report* 36(45):741-744, 1987.

[444] Centers for Disease Control. Impact of diabetes outpatient education program—Maine. *Morbidity and Mortality Weekly Report* 31(23):307-314, 1982.

[445] American Lung Association. *The Efficacy of Asthma Education—Selected Abstracts.* New York: the Association, 1989.

[446] Halpern, M. The impact of diabetes education in Michigan. *Diabetes* 38(2):151A, 1989.

[447] Guralnick, M. J., and Bennett, F. C. A framework for early intervention. In: Guralnick, M.J., and Bennett, F.C. (Eds.). *The Effectiveness of Early Intervention for At-Risk and Handicapped Children.* Orlando, FL: Academic Press, 1987. pp. 3-29.

[448] Bryant, D.M., and Ramey, C.T. An analysis of the effectiveness of early prevention programs for environmentally at-risk children. In: Guralnick, M.J., and Bennett, F.C. (Eds.) *The Effectiveness of Early Intervention for At-Risk and Handicapped Children.* Orlando, FL: Academic Press, 1987. p. 33-78.

[449] American Academy of Pediatrics. Data derived from the American Academy of Pediatrics' Periodic Survey #3, 1988.

[450] Northern, J.L.; Walker, D.; Downs, M.P.; and Guggenheim, S. Office screening for communicative disorders in young children. In Gottleib, M.I. and Williams, J.E. Eds. *Developmental Behavioral Disorders.* New York: Plenum, 1989.

[451] American Academy of Pediatrics. *Medicaid's EPSDT program: A pediatrician's handbook for action.* Evanston, IL: the Academy, 1987.

[452] Meisels, S.J. Prediction, prevention, and developmental screening in the EPSDT program. In Stevenson, S.W. and Siegel, A.E. eds. *Child development research and social policy* 1:267-317. Chicago: University of Chicago Press, 1984.

[453] American Public Health Association. APHA resolution number 8203: Children's vision screening. *American Journal of Public Health* 73:329, 1983.

[454] National Institutes of Health. *When Words Get in the Way. The Search for Health*. Bethesda, MD: U.S. Department of Health and Human Services, 1989.

[455] Coplan, J., et al. Validation of an early milestone scale in a high-risk population. *Pediatrics* 70:77-83, 1982.

[456] Walker, D.D. et.al. Early language milestone scale and language screening of young children. *Pediatrics* 70:77-83, 1989.

[457] Lass, N.J.; McReynolds, L.V.; Northern, J.; and Yoder, D.E. *Handbook of Speech-Language Pathology and Audiology*. Philadelphia, PA: B.C. Decker, Inc., 1988.

[458] Lubker, B. *Children with Communicative Disorders*. : Kirk and Gallagher, 1989.

[459] Shames, G., and Wiig, E. *Human Communication Disorders*. New York: Charles Merrill Inc., 1990.

[460] Coscarelli-Buchanan, J.E. Finding ears that do not hear. *Health and Environment Report* 39, 1986.

[461] Riko, K.; Hyde, M.L.; Corgin, H.; and Fitzhardinge, P.M. Issues in early identification of hearing loss. *Laryngoscope* 95:373-381, 1985.

[462] Clark, T.C. *Language development through home intervention for infant hearing impaired children*. Chapel Hill, NC: University of North Carolina, 1979,1 (University Microfilms International, 8013924).

[463] Northern, J.L.; and Downs, M.P. *Hearing in children* (3rd ed.). Baltimore, MD: Williams & Wilkins, 1984.

[464] Commission on Education of the Deaf. *Toward Equality: Education of the Deaf*. Washington, DC: the Commission, 1988.

[465] Coplan, J. Deafness: Ever heard of it? Recognition of permanent hearing loss. *Pediatrics* 79:206-213, 1987.

[466] Elssman, S. F.; Matkin, N. D.; and Sabo, M. P. Early identification of congenital sensorineural hearing impairment. *The Hearing Journal*. September:13-17, 1987.

[467] Freeman, R.; Malkin, S.; and Hastings, J. Psychosocial problems of deaf children and their families: A comparative study. *American Annals of the Deaf* 120:291-305, 1975.

[468] Luterman, D., and Chasin, J. The pediatrician and the parent of the deaf child. *Pediatrics* 45:115-116, 1970.

[469] Meadow-Orlans, K.P. An analysis of the effectiveness of early intervention programs for hearing-impaired children. In M. J. Guralnick & F. C. Bennett (Eds.), *The Effectiveness of Early Intervention for At-Risk and Handicapped Children*. Orlando, FL: Academic Press, 1987.

[470] Williams, D.; Darbyshire, J.; and Brown, B. Families of young hearing impaired children: The impact of diagnosis. *Journal of Otolaryngology* 7:500-506, 1978.

[471] Mahoney, T. M. Large-scale high-risk neonatal hearing screening. In Swigart, E. T. (Ed.) *Neonatal Hearing Screening*. San Diego, CA: College-Hill Press, 1984.

[472] Mahoney, T.M.; and Eichwald, J. G. The ups and "downs" of high-risk hearing screening: The Utah statewide program. *Seminars in Hearing* 8:155-163, 1987.

[473] Kisker, C.T.; Strayer, F.; Wong, K.; et al. Health outcomes of a community-based therapy program for children with cancer—a shared management approach. *Pediatrics* 66:900-906, 1980.

[474] Smith, P., and Levine, P.H. The benefits of comprehensive care of hemophilia: A five-year study of outcomes. *American Journal of Public Health* 74:616-617, 1984.

[475] Shelton, T. L.; Jeppson, E. S.; and Johnson, B. H. *Family-Centered Care for Children with Special Health Care Needs*. Washington, DC: Association for the Care of Children's Health, 1987.

[476] National Maternal and Child Health Resource Center. *A National Goal, Building Service Delivery Systems for Children with Special Health Care Needs and Their Families*. Iowa City, IA: the Center, 1990.

[477] Public Health Service. *Surgeon General's Report, Children with Special Health Care Needs, Campaign '87*. Pub. No. DHHS (HRS/D/MC)87-2. Rockville, MD: U.S. Department of Health and Human Services, 1987.

[478] Sirrocco, A. Characteristics of facilities for mentally retarded, 1986. *Vital and Health Statistics*. Series 14, No. 34. Hyattsville, MD: U.S. Department of Health and Human Services, 1989.

[479] Handsfield, H.H., Kreheler, B and Nicola, R.M. Trends in gonorrhea in homosexually active men: King County, Washington, 1989. *Morbidity and Mortality Weekly Report* 38(44):762-764, 1989.

[480] Dondero, T.J., Jr.; Pappaioanou, M.; and Curran, J.W. Monitoring the levels and trends of HIV infection: The Public Health Services's HIV surveillance program. *Public Health Reports* 103(3):213-220, 1988.

[481] Des Jarlais, D.C.; Freidman, S.R.; and Novack, D.M. HIV-1 Infection among intravenous drug users in Manhattan, New York City, from 1977 through 1987. *Journal of the American Medical Association* 261:1008-1012, 1989.

[482] Centers for Disease Control. Relationship of syphilis to drug use and prostitution: Connecticut and Philadelphia, PA. *Morbidity and Mortality Weekly Report* 37(49):755-764, 1988.

[483] Ginzburg, H.M.; Trainor, J.; and Reis, E. A review of epidemiologic Trends in HIV infection of women and children. *Pediatric AIDS and HIV Infection: Fetus to Adolescent* 1(1):11-15, 1990.

[484] American College Health Association. Task Force on AIDS, general statement on institutional response to AIDS. Rockville, MD: the Association, revised November 1988.

[485] Centers for Disease Control. Condoms for prevention of sexually transmitted diseases. *Morbidity and Mortality Weekly Report* 37(9):133-137, 1988.

[486] Food and Drug Administration. *Condoms and Sexually Transmitted Diseases . . . Especially AIDS* DHHS Pub.No. (FDA) 90-4239. Rockville, MD: U.S. Department of Health and Human Services, 1990.

[487] Centers for Disease Control. *HIV/AIDS Surveillance Report*. Atlanta, GA: U.S. Department of Health and Human Services, May 1990.

[488] Freidman, S.R.; Des Jarlais, D.C.; and Sotheran, J.L. AIDS and self-organization among intravenous drug users. *International Journal of Addiction* 22:201-220, 1987.

[489] National Center for Health Statistics. National Health Interview Survey. Centers for Disease Control, Public Health Service. Hyattsville, MD: U.S. Department of Health and Human Services, March, 1990.

[490] Centers for Disease Control. Guidelines for effective school health education to prevent the spread of AIDS. *Morbidity and Mortality Weekly Report* 37(Suppl. S-2): 1988.

[491] Centers for Disease Control. *Division of STD/HIV Prevention Annual Report, 1989*. Atlanta, GA: U.S. Department of Health and Human Services, 1990.

[492] Whittington, W.L., and Knapp, J.S. Trends in resistance of *Neisseria gonorrhoea* to antimicrobial agents in the United States. *Sexually Transmitted Diseases* 15:202-210, 1988.

[493] Washington, A.E.; Johnson, R.E.; Sanders, L.L.; Barnes, R.C.; and Alexander, E.R. Incidence of chlamydia trachomatis infections in the United States: Using reported neisseria gonorrhoea as a surrogate. In: Oriel, D.; Ridgway, G.; Schachter, J.; Taylor-Robinson, D.; and Ward, M. eds. *Chlamydial Infections* Cambridge, England: Cambridge University Press, 1986. p. 487.

[494] Centers for Disease Control. *Chlamydia Trachomatis Infections: Policy Guidelines for Prevention and Control*. Atlanta, GA: U.S. Department of Health and Human Services, 1985.

[495] Judson, F.N. Fear of AIDS and gonorrhea rates in homosexual men. *Lancet* ii:159, 1983.

[496] Pepin, J.; Plummer, F.A.; Brunham, R.C.; Piot, P.; Cameron, D.W.; and Ronald, A.R. The interaction of HIV infection and other sexually transmitted diseases: An opportunity for intervention. *AIDS* 3:3-9, 1989.

[497] Zenker, P.N., and Berman, S.M. Congenital syphilis: Reporting and reality. *American Journal of Public Health* 80:271-272, 1990.

[498] Cohen, D.A.; Boyd, D.; Prabhudas; I., Mascola, L. The effects of case definition, maternal screening, and reporting criteria on rates of congenital syphilis. *American Journal of Public Health* 80:316-317, 1990.

[499] Centers for Disease Control. Guidelines for the prevention and control of congenital syphilis. *Morbidity and Mortality Weekly Report* 37(S-1):1-13, 1988.

[500] Johnson, R.E.; Nahmias, A.J.; Magder, L.S.; Lee, F.K.; Brooks, C.A.; and Snowden, C.B. Distribution of genital herpes (HSV-2) in the United States: A seroepidemiological national survey using a new type-specific antibody assay. *New England Journal of Medicine* 321:7-12, 1989.

[501] Mertz, G.J.; Coombs, R.W.; Ashley, R.; Jourden, J.; Remington, M.; Winter, C.; Fahnlander, A.; Guinan, M.; Ducey, H.; and Corey, L. Transmission of genital herpes in couples with one symptomatic and one asymptomatic partner: A prospective study. *Journal of Infectious Diseases* 157:1169-1175, 1988.

[502] Koutsky, L.A.; Galloway, D.A.; and Holmes, K.K. Epidemiology of genital human papillomavirus infection. *Epidemiological Review* 10:122-163, 1988.

[503] Washington, A.E.; Arno, P.S.; and Brooks, M.A. The economic costs of pelvic inflammatory disease. *JAMA* 255:1735-1738, 1986.

[504] Wolner-Hanssen, P.W.; Kiviat, N.B.; and Holmes, K.K. Atypical pelvic inflammatory disease: Subacute, chronic, or subclinical upper genital tract infection in women. In: Holmes, K.K.; Mardh, P.A.; Sparling, P.F.; Wiesner, P.J.; Cates, W., Jr.; Lemon, S.M.; and Stamm, W.E., eds. *Sexually Transmitted Diseases* 2d ed. New York: McGraw-Hill, 1990. pp. 615-620.

[505] Centers for Disease Control. Changing patterns of groups at high risk for hepatitis B in the United States. *Morbidity and Mortality Weekly Report* 37(28):429-437, 1988.

[506] McEvoy, B.F., and Le Furgy, W.G. A 13-year longitudinal analysis of risk factors and clinic visitation patterns of patients with repeated gonorrhea. *Sexually Transmitted Diseases* 15:40-44, 1988.

[507] Darrow, W.W. Condom use and use-effectiveness in high-risk populations. *Sexually Transmitted Diseases* 16:157-160, 1989.

[508] Lewis, C., and Freeman, H. The sexual history taking and counseling practices of primary care physicians. *Western Journal of Medicine* 147:165-167, 1987.

[509] Grimes D.A.; Blount J.H.; Patrick J.; and Washington, A.E. Antibiotic treatment of pelvic inflammatory disease. Trends among private physicians in the United States, 1966-1982. *JAMA* 256:3223-3226, 1986.

[510] Centers for Disease Control. *Sexually Transmitted Diseases Treatment Guidelines, September 1989*. Atlanta, GA: U.S. Department of Health and Human Services, 1989.

[511] Rothenberg, R.B., and Potterat, J.J. Strategies for management of sex partners. In: Holmes, K.K.; Mardh P.A.; Sparling, P.F.; Wiesner, P.J.; Cates, W., Jr.; Lemon, S.M.; and Stamm, W.E., eds. *Sexually Transmitted Diseases* 2d ed. New York: McGraw-Hill, 1990. pp. 1081-1086.

[512] Centers for Disease Control. Partner notification for preventing human immunodeficiency virus (HIV) infection—Colorado, Idaho, South Carolina, Virginia. *Morbidity and Mortality Weekly Report* 37(25):393-402, 1988.

[513] Sutter, R.W.; et al. A new epidemiologic and laboratory classification system for paralytic poliomyelitis cases. *American Journal of Public Health* 79(4):495-498, Apr. 1989.

[514] Markowitz, L.E.; et al. Patterns of transmission in measles outbreaks in the United States, 1985-1986. *New England Journal of Medicine* 320(2):75-81, Jan. 12, 1989.

[515] Centers for Disease Control. Measles prevention: Recommendations of the immunization practices advisory committee (ACIP). *Morbidity and Mortality Weekly Report, Recommendations and Reports* 38(Suppl. 9), 1989.

[516] Sosin, D.M.; et al. Changing epidemiology of mumps and its impact on university campuses. *Pediatrics* 84(5):779-784, Nov. 1989.

[517] Centers for Disease Control. Pertussis surveillance: United States, 1986-1988. *Morbidity and Mortality Weekly Report* 39(4):57-66, 1990.

[518] Ad Hoc Group for the Study of Pertussis Vaccines. Placebo-controlled trial of two acellular pertussis vaccines in Sweden: Protective efficacy and adverse events. *The Lancet* 8592:955-960, Apr. 30, 1988.

[519] Ho, M.S.; et al. Diarrheal deaths in American children: Are they preventable? *Journal of the American Medical Association* 260:3281-3285, 1988.

[520] Williams, W.W.; et al. Immunization policies and vaccine coverage among adults. *Annals of Internal Medicine* 108(4):616-625, Apr. 1988.

[521] Centers for Disease Control. Recommendations for protection against viral hepatitis. Recommendations of the ACIP. *Morbidity and Mortality Weekly Report*, 39(Suppl. RR-2), 1990.

[522] Centers for Disease Control. Rabies surveillance, United States, 1988. In: CDC surveillance summaries, August 1989. *Morbidity and Mortality Weekly Report* 38(Suppl.1), 1989.

[523] Lurie, N.; et al. Preventive care: Do we practice what we preach? *American Journal of Public Health* 77(7):801-804, 1987.

[524] Ornstein, S.M.; et al. Compliance with Five Health Promotion Recommendations in a University-Based Family Practice. *Journal of Family Practice* 29(2):163-168, 1989.

[525] Palmer, R.H.; Strain, R.; Mauer, J.V.M.; and Thompson, M.S. A method for evaluating performance of ambulatory pediatric tasks. *Pediatrics* 73:269-277, 1984.

[526] Dawson, D.A.; Hendershot, G.E.; and Bloom, B. Trends in routine screening examinations. *American Journal of Public Health* 77(8):1004-1005, 1987.

[527] Gemson, D.H.; Elinson, J.; and Messeri, P. Differences in physician prevention practice patterns for white and minority patients. *Journal of Community Health* 13:53-64, 1988.

[528] The Robert Wood Johnson Foundation. *Access to Health Care in the United States: Results of a 1986 Survey*. Special Report Number Two/1987. Princeton, NJ: the Foundation, 1987.

[529] Alpert, J.J., and Charney, E. *The Education of Physicians for Primary Care*. DHEW Pub. No. (HRA)74-3113. Washington, DC: U.S. Department of Health, Education and Welfare, PHS Health Resources Administration, Bureau of Health Services Research, 1973.

[530] Hicks, W.H. *Community-Oriented Primary Care: The Health Center Experience*. Washington, DC: National Association of Community Health Centers, 1985.

[531] National Center for Health Services Research and Health Care Technology Assessment. *Program Note*. Washington, DC: U.S. Department of Health and Human Services, May, 1985.

[532] Nutting, P.; ed. *Community-Oriented Primary Care: From Principle to Practice*. DHHS Pub. No. (HRSA-PE)86-1. Washington, DC: U.S. Department of Health and Human Services, 1987.

[533] World Health Organization. *Primary Health Care. Report of the International Conference on Primary Health Care. Alma-Ata, USSR, 1978*. Geneva, Switzerland: WHO, 1978.

[534] Begley, C.; Aday, L.; and McCandless, R. Evaluation of a primary health care program for the poor. *Journal of Community Health* 14(2):107-120, 1989.

[535] Hubbell, A.; Waitzkink, H.; Mishra, S.; and Dombrink, J. Evaluating health care needs of the poor: A community-oriented approach. *American Journal of Medicine* 87:127-128, 1989.

[536] Mayster, V.; Waitzkin, H.; Hubbell, A.; and Rucher, L. Local advocacy for the medically indigent: Strategies and accomplishments in one county. *JAMA* 263(2):262-268, 1990.

[537] Thorpe, K.E., and Siegal, J.E. Covering the uninsured: Interactions among public and private sector strategies. *JAMA* 262(15):2114-2118, 1989.

[538] Hurley, R.: Freund, D.A.; and Taylor, D. Emergency room use and primary care case management: Evidence from four Medicaid demonstration programs. *American Journal of Public Health* 79(7):843-846, 1989.

[539] Gemson, D.H., and Elinson, J. Do doctors know cancer screening deadlines? *New York State Journal of Medicine* 12:643-645, 1987.

[540] Johns, M.B.; Hovell, M.F.; Ganiats, T.; Peddecord, K.M.; and Agras, W.S. Primary care and health promotion: A model for preventive medicine. *American Journal of Preventive Medicine* 3(6):346-357, 1987.

[541] McDonald, C.J.; Hui, S.L.; Smith, D.M.; Tierney, W.M.; Cohen, S.J.; Winberger, M.; and McCabe, G.P. Reminders to physicians from an introspective computer medical record. *Annals of Internal Medicine* 100:130-138, 1984.

[542] McPhee, S.S.; Bird, J.A.; Jenkins, C.N.H.; and Fordham, D. Promoting cancer screening: A randomized controlled trial of three interventions. *Archives of Internal Medicine* 149:1866-1872, 1989.

[543] Belcher, D.; Berg, A.; and Inui, T. Practical approaches to providing better care: Are physicians a problem or a solution? *American Journal of Preventive Medicine* 4(suppl.):27-48, 1988.

[544] American Public Health Association. *Model Standards*: A Guide for Community Preventive Health Services. Washington, DC: the Association, 1979.

[545] Health Resources and Services Administration, Bureau of Health Professions. *Sixth Report to the President and Congress on the Status of Health Personnel in the United States*. DHHS Pub. No. (HRS-P-OD)88-1. Rockville, MD: U.S. Department of Health and Human Services, 1988.

[546] Health Resources and Services Administration, Bureau of Health Professions. *Location Patterns of Minority and Other Health Professionals*. DHHS Pub. No. (HRS-P-OD)85-2. Rockville, MD: U.S. Department of Health and Human Services, 1985.

[547] Health Resources and Services Administration, Bureau of Health Professions. *Minorities and Women in the Health Fields*. 1987 Edition. DHHS Pub. No. (HRS-P-DV)87-1. Rockville, MD: U.S. Department of Health and Human Services, 1988.

[548] Health Resources and Services Administration, Bureau of Health Professions. *Revitalizing Health Professions Education for Minorities and the Disadvantaged: A Health Professions Deans' Forum on Issues and Strategies*. Contract N. 240-84-0119. Rockville, MD: U.S. Department of Health and Human Services, 1986.

[549] Health Resources and Services Administration, Bureau of Health Professions. *Seventh Report to the President and Congress on the Status of Health Personnel in the United States*. Rockville, MD: U.S. Department of Health and Human Services, 1990.

[550] American Association of Colleges of Osteopathic Medicine, personal communication, September 1990.

[551] National Restaurant Association. *Survey of Chain Operators*. Washington, DC: the Association, 1989.

[552] Smith, K; Crawford, S. Suicidal behavior among "normal" high school students. *Suicide and Lifethreatening Behavior* 16:313-325, 1986.

[553] Schwartz, M.D. Gender and injury in spousal assault. *Social Focus* 20(1):61-75, 1987.

[554] Pollock, D.A. and McClain, P.W. Trauma registries: Current status and future prospects. *Journal of the American Medical Association* 226:2280-2283, 1989.

[555] Day, N.E. Screening for cancer of the cervix. *Journal of Epidemiology and Community Health* 43:103-106, 1989.